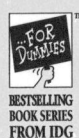

For Dummies

BESTSELLING
BOOK SERIES
FROM IDG

Alternative Medicine
For Dumm...

D0189045

Signs of Dangerous or Bogus Claims

If the alternative therapy you're considering involves any of the following features, you may be headed for trouble (see Chapter 2 for more information about using alternative medicine safely).

- Herbs or other substances your conventional doctor can't identify

- Secret ingredients

- Injections of any kind — unless they are investigated and approved by your conventional doctor

- Words such as "miraculous," "amazing," or "rejuvenating"

- Practitioners who won't tell you how long treatments will take, how much they will cost, and when you should expect improvement

- Alternative healers who are extremely hostile toward mainstream medicine

- People who claim that there are *no* questions about the safety or efficacy of their approach or product — or *no* limitations to what their approach or product can do

Steps Your Regular M.D. Should Take before You Try Alternatives

If you're suffering from a long-term or serious condition, don't try any alternative approach before asking your regular M.D. to take the following precautions (which we describe in more detail in Chapter 5).

- Rule out the possibility of serious illness.

- Make sure that the alternative doesn't interfere with any other medication or therapy you may be using.

- Make sure that the alternative you want to try is safe for you — based on your personal medical history.

- Evaluate the evidence on the safety and efficacy of the alternative you have in mind (if any evidence is available!).

...For Dummies: Bestselling Book Series for Beginners

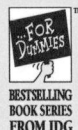

Alternative Medicine For Dummies®

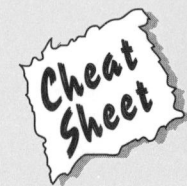

Cheat Sheet

Questions to Ask before You Agree to Treatment

Before you agree to let any alternative practitioner examine (or treat!) you, do a little examination yourself to make sure that this is the right person to provide the type of care you want. Ideally, try to set up a short office (or at least a telephone) consultation with the practitioner so that you can ask the following questions (see Chapter 6 for more information on finding the right caregiver).

- What will treatment involve? How will it affect my life — incapacitate me, alter my schedule, keep me home from work, and so on?

- How do results compare with results from conventional approaches — or just watchful waiting? What are the advantages and disadvantages of this therapy as opposed to other alternatives?

- Can I use this method together with conventional therapy?

- Does any scientific evidence show that this approach works — and is safe? Was the evidence published — and where?

- Have you (personally) used this therapy for other people with a health history or ailment similar to mine? If yes, what happened? Can I talk to some of these people?

- How often will I have to go to your office or clinic?

- How much will each session cost — and will anybody pay for it besides me? How much of this cost is for supplies and how much is for your time?

- How many sessions should I expect before seeing results? How long before we can decide whether the treatment is working?

- What are the potential side effects? (If the answer is "none," ask again. And then consider going elsewhere — because any effective treatment poses at least a slight risk to some people.)

- Are there any activities that I shouldn't engage in, or other drugs — prescription or over-the-counter, conventional or alternative — that I shouldn't take while using this therapy?

- Are you willing to talk to my regular doctor about the diagnosis and treatment plan? Will you place any limitations on what you are willing to talk about — and how often you are willing to talk?

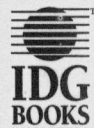

...For Dummies: Bestselling Book Series for Beginners

Praise For Alternative Medicine For Dummies

"Misunderstanding about alternative medicine abounds. *Alternative Medicine For Dummies* cuts through the confusion and presents a balanced, thoughtful viewpoint and a great deal of relevant information that will help patients and practitioners alike."
>— Brian Berman, M.D., Associate Professor/
> Director of the Center of Contemporary
> Medicine at the University of Maryland
> School of Medicine

"Out of almost 700,000 doctors in the United States, Jim Dillard is one of the three or four with the knowledge and experience to introduce this important topic. Anyone considering an alternative approach for themselves or a loved one need look no further than this excellent book."
>— David Edelberg, M.D., Northwestern University

"This book helps all 'dummies' to become knowledgeable about the basics of alternative medicine. It condenses a vast amount of material into a simple-to-use framework with concise definitions and directions for health and healing. The American Holistic Medical Association defines 'Holistic Medicine' as a new specialty that addresses the whole person — body, mind, and spirit. A 'Holistic Physician' combines conventional and alternative therapies to prevent and treat disease and to create optimal health. After reading this book, give it to your health practitioners to help them understand what we 'dummies' already know."
>— E.J. Linkner, M.D., Board of Trustees and
> Secretary of the American Holistic Medical
> Association; Clinical Instructor, University of
> Michigan Medical School

"This is a clear, crisp, tough-minded, and readable guide to alternative medicine — what it is, when to use it, and, perhaps most important of all, how to integrate it with conventional medicine."
>— James S. Gordon, M.D., Author, *Manifesto for a
> New Medicine: Your Guide to Healing Partner-
> ships and the Wise Use of Alternative Medicine*

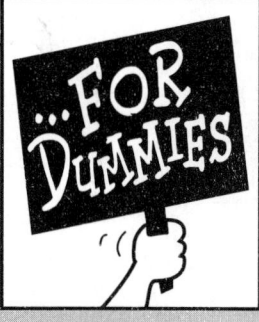

TM

References for the Rest of Us!™

BESTSELLING BOOK SERIES FROM IDG

Do you find that traditional reference books are overloaded with technical details and advice you'll never use? Do you postpone important life decisions because you just don't want to deal with them? Then our *…For Dummies*® business and general reference book series is for you.

…For Dummies business and general reference books are written for those frustrated and hard-working souls who know they aren't dumb, but find that the myriad of personal and business issues and the accompanying horror stories make them feel helpless. *…For Dummies* books use a lighthearted approach, a down-to-earth style, and even cartoons and humorous icons to diffuse fears and build confidence. Lighthearted but not lightweight, these books are perfect survival guides to solve your everyday personal and business problems.

> *"More than a publishing phenomenon, 'Dummies' is a sign of the times."*
> — The New York Times

> *"A world of detailed and authoritative information is packed into them…"*
> — U.S. News and World Report

> *"…you won't go wrong buying them."*
> — Walter Mossberg, Wall Street Journal, on IDG Books' …For Dummies books

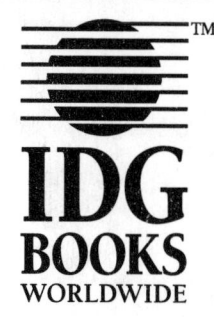

IDG BOOKS WORLDWIDE

TM

Already, millions of satisfied readers agree. They have made *…For Dummies* the #1 introductory level computer book series and a best-selling business book series. They have written asking for more. So, if you're looking for the best and easiest way to learn about business and other general reference topics, look to *…For Dummies* to give you a helping hand.

ALTERNATIVE MEDICINE

FOR

DUMMIES®

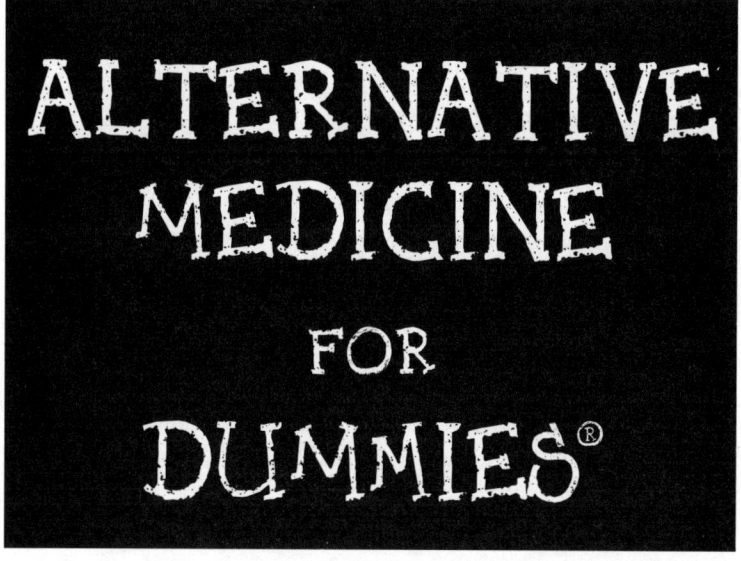

by James Dillard, M.D., D.C., C.Ac., and Terra Ziporyn, Ph.D.

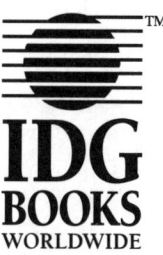

IDG Books Worldwide, Inc.
An International Data Group Company

Foster City, CA ♦ Chicago, IL ♦ Indianapolis, IN ♦ New York, NY

Alternative Medicine For Dummies®

Published by
IDG Books Worldwide, Inc.
An International Data Group Company
919 E. Hillsdale Blvd.
Suite 400
Foster City, CA 94404
www.idgbooks.com (IDG Books Worldwide Web site)
www.dummies.com (Dummies Press Web site)

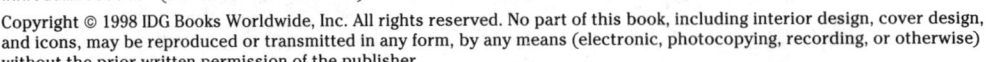
Library of Congress Catalog Card No.: 98-88391

ISBN: 0-7645-5109-4

Printed in the United States of America

10 9 8 7 6 5 4 3 2 1

1B/RX/RR/ZY/IN

Distributed in the United States by IDG Books Worldwide, Inc.

Distributed by Macmillan Canada for Canada; by Transworld Publishers Limited in the United Kingdom; by IDG Norge Books for Norway; by IDG Sweden Books for Sweden; by Woodslane Pty. Ltd. for Australia; by Woodslane (NZ) Ltd. for New Zealand; by Addison Wesley Longman Singapore Pte Ltd. for Singapore, Malaysia, Thailand, and Indonesia; by Norma Comunicaciones S.A. for Colombia; by Intersoft for South Africa; by International Thomson Publishing for Germany, Austria and Switzerland; by Distribuidora Cuspide for Argentina; by Livraria Cultura for Brazil; by Ediciencia S.A. for Ecuador; by Ediciones ZETA S.C.R. Ltda. for Peru; by WS Computer Publishing Corporation, Inc., for the Philippines; by Contemporanea de Ediciones for Venezuela; by Express Computer Distributors for the Caribbean and West Indies; by Micronesia Media Distributor, Inc. for Micronesia; by Grupo Editorial Norma S.A. for Guatemala; by Chips Computadoras S.A. de C.V. for Mexico; by Editorial Norma de Panama S.A. for Panama; by Wouters Import for Belgium; by American Bookshops for Finland. Authorized Sales Agent: Anthony Rudkin Associates for the Middle East and North Africa.

For general information on IDG Books Worldwide's books in the U.S., please call our Consumer Customer Service department at 800-762-2974. For reseller information, including discounts and premium sales, please call our Reseller Customer Service department at 800-434-3422.

For information on where to purchase IDG Books Worldwide's books outside the U.S., please contact our International Sales department at 317-596-5530 or fax 317-596-5692.

For information on foreign language translations, please contact our Foreign & Subsidiary Rights department at 650-655-3021 or fax 650-655-3281.

For sales inquiries and special prices for bulk quantities, please contact our Sales department at 650-655-3200 or write to the address above.

For information on using IDG Books Worldwide's books in the classroom or for ordering examination copies, please contact our Educational Sales department at 800-434-2086 or fax 317-596-5499.

For press review copies, author interviews, or other publicity information, please contact our Public Relations department at 650-655-3000 or fax 650-655-3299.

For authorization to photocopy items for corporate, personal, or educational use, please contact Copyright Clearance Center, 222 Rosewood Drive, Danvers, MA 01923, or fax 978-750-4470.

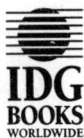

About the Authors

James Dillard, M.D., D.C., C.Ac., is the medical director for Oxford Health Plan's Alternative Medicine program and the chairman of the Oxford Chiropractic Advisory Board. A board certified medical doctor, doctor of chiropractic, and a medical acupuncturist, he's also a faculty member at Columbia University College of Physicians and Surgeons and a member of the medical staff at Columbia-Presbyterian Medical Center.

James conducted research in spinal biomechanics at Rush Presbyterian-St. Luke's Medical Center in Chicago while earning his medical degree at Rush Medical College, where he was elected to the medical honor society Alpha Omega Alpha. He also did cancer and transplantation immunology research at the University of California, Los Angeles while earning degrees from Cleveland Chiropractic College and California Acupuncture College.

When he's not windsurfing, surf kayaking, mountain biking, or scuba diving, James spends a lot of time talking up alternative medicine. He's been featured in such publications as *Newsweek, Town & Country, Mademoiselle, Shape, McCall's, Elle, Women's Sports & Fitness,* and *Parenting* and has appeared on *The Oprah Winfrey Show, Good Morning America,* National Public Radio, CBS News, *Good Day New York,* and many other broadcasts. He lives in Manhattan and Sag Harbor, New York, an old whaling town on the far East End of Long Island, enjoying consistent support and admiration from his six-month-old yellow Labrador, Hanna.

Terra Ziporyn, Ph.D., is a writer and historian who specializes in making science and medicine accessible to the public. She is the coauthor of the *The Harvard Guide to Women's Health, The Women's Concise Guide to a Healthier Heart, The Women's Concise Guide to Emotional Well-Being,* and *Future Shop,* as well as the author of *Nameless Diseases* and *Disease in the Popular American Press.* A former associate editor at *The Journal of the American Medical Association (JAMA),* she has written extensively on a wide range of health and medical issues in both professional and popular publications.

Terra is a summa cum laude graduate of Yale University with degrees in both history and biology. She was a Searle Fellow at the University of Chicago, where she earned a doctorate in the history of science and medicine. She's been awarded science writing fellowships from the American Association for the Advancement of Science, the American Chemical Society, and the Marine Biological Laboratory at Woods Hole.

Terra lives in the Chicago area with her political scientist husband, three children, Lhasa Apso, cello, and hundreds of cartons of papers and books that get carted around the country every time she and her family move.

ABOUT IDG BOOKS WORLDWIDE

Welcome to the world of IDG Books Worldwide.

IDG Books Worldwide, Inc., is a subsidiary of International Data Group, the world's largest publisher of computer-related information and the leading global provider of information services on information technology. IDG was founded more than 30 years ago by Patrick J. McGovern and now employs more than 9,000 people worldwide. IDG publishes more than 290 computer publications in over 75 countries. More than 90 million people read one or more IDG publications each month.

Launched in 1990, IDG Books Worldwide is today the #1 publisher of best-selling computer books in the United States. We are proud to have received eight awards from the Computer Press Association in recognition of editorial excellence and three from Computer Currents' First Annual Readers' Choice Awards. Our best-selling ...For Dummies® series has more than 50 million copies in print with translations in 31 languages. IDG Books Worldwide, through a joint venture with IDG's Hi-Tech Beijing, became the first U.S. publisher to publish a computer book in the People's Republic of China. In record time, IDG Books Worldwide has become the first choice for millions of readers around the world who want to learn how to better manage their businesses.

Our mission is simple: Every one of our books is designed to bring extra value and skill-building instructions to the reader. Our books are written by experts who understand and care about our readers. The knowledge base of our editorial staff comes from years of experience in publishing, education, and journalism — experience we use to produce books to carry us into the new millennium. In short, we care about books, so we attract the best people. We devote special attention to details such as audience, interior design, use of icons, and illustrations. And because we use an efficient process of authoring, editing, and desktop publishing our books electronically, we can spend more time ensuring superior content and less time on the technicalities of making books.

You can count on our commitment to deliver high-quality books at competitive prices on topics you want to read about. At IDG Books Worldwide, we continue in the IDG tradition of delivering quality for more than 30 years. You'll find no better book on a subject than one from IDG Books Worldwide.

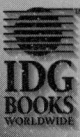

John Kilcullen
Chairman and CEO
IDG Books Worldwide, Inc.

Steven Berkowitz
President and Publisher
IDG Books Worldwide, Inc.

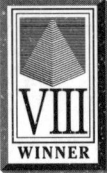

Eighth Annual Computer Press Awards ≥1992

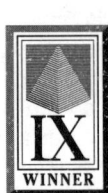

Ninth Annual Computer Press Awards ≥1993

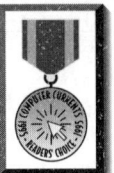

Tenth Annual Computer Press Awards ≥1994

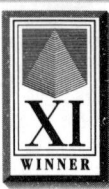

Eleventh Annual Computer Press Awards ≥1995

IDG is the world's leading IT media, research and exposition company. Founded, in 1964, IDG had 1997 revenues of $2.05 billion and has more than 9,000 employees worldwide. IDG offers the widest range of media options that reach IT buyers in 75 countries representing 95% of worldwide IT spending. IDG's diverse product and services portfolio spans six key areas including print publishing, online publishing, expositions and conferences, market research, education and training, and global marketing services. More than 90 million people read one or more of IDG's 290 magazines and newspapers, including IDG's leading global brands — Computerworld, PC World, Network World, Macworld and the Channel World family of publications. IDG Books Worldwide is one of the fastest-growing computer book publishers in the world, with more than 700 titles in 36 languages. The "...For Dummies®" series alone has more than 50 million copies in print. IDG offers online users the largest network of technology-specific Web sites around the world through IDG.net (http://www.idg.net), which comprises more than 225 targeted Web sites in 55 countries worldwide. International Data Corporation (IDC) is the world's largest provider of information technology data, analysis and consulting, with research centers in over 41 countries and more than 400 research analysts worldwide. IDG World Expo is a leading producer of more than 168 globally branded conferences and expositions in 35 countries including E3 (Electronic Entertainment Expo), Macworld Expo, ComNet, Windows World Expo, ICE (Internet Commerce Expo), Agenda, DEMO, and Spotlight. IDG's training subsidiary, ExecuTrain, is the world's largest computer training company, with more than 230 locations worldwide and 785 training courses. IDG Marketing Services helps industry-leading IT companies build international brand recognition by developing global integrated marketing programs via IDG's print, online and exposition products worldwide. Further information about the company can be found at www.idg.com.   10/8/98

Dedication

James Dillard, M.D., D.C., C.Ac.: To my father, who was an inspiration for many things in my life, including the virtue of "doing something worth a damn" in life, whatever that might be.

Terra Ziporyn, Ph.D.: To my aunt Cheryl, who taught me long ago that "alternative" was something worth considering.

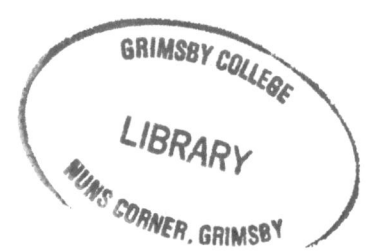
Authors' Acknowledgments

James Dillard, M.D., D.C., C.Ac.: First and foremost I want to offer belated thanks to my father, who died when I was 17 and to whom I have dedicated this book. Over the years I have fully debunked the myths that 17-year-olds have about "Dad," both good and bad, and have come to a reasonably balanced view of a flawed man with some distinct aspects of nobility. He has always inspired lawyer jokes, driving too fast, and a life outdoors.

As for more traditional acknowledgments, I want to thank Hassan Rifaat, M.D., my business and windsurfing partner, for his faith in my abilities and for pushing me to excel. I also want to thank Dr. David Eisenberg, my past and future research partner, for his inspiration and graciousness; Fredi Kronenberg, Ph.D., for consistent support, sound advice, and a strong, steady pace on kayak or bicycle; William Prensky, O.M.D., my advisor and friend, for his wisdom and humor; Asibi Abudu, M.D., for stimulating my desire to be a lifelong student; Terry Yokum, D.C., who taught me to look deeper; my terrific cowriter, Terra Ziporyn, Ph.D., who kept her sense of humor in the face of grueling deadlines; Thomas D. Selz, for his wise counsel; and our executive editor, Tami Booth, who is the best den mother a cub writer could want.

Last but not least, I want to thank my "kid sister" Kerri for keeping my life on the rails.

Terra Ziporyn, Ph.D.: I am eternally grateful to my husband, James Snider, for all the tension, screaming, and neglect he tolerated (even encouraged!) while I cranked out the manuscript for this book. I'm also grateful to my three children, Pallas, Sage, and Solon, for understanding that Mom had to get the book done (fortunately, this time they could appreciate my efforts, since ...*For Dummies* is famous even in elementary school circles!).

Thanks also to my agent, Carolyn Krupp, for introducing me to the ...*For Dummies* world and to my mother-cum-attorney, Charlotte Ziporyn, for her pro bono legal advice. Kelly Ewing and Diane Smith of IDG Books deserve credit for their devoted and diplomatic editing. Enduring thanks also go to Michael Fisher and Susan Wallace Boehmer for being so patient with me while I finished up this project. My brother, Brook Ziporyn, Ph.D., of Northwestern University, was immensely helpful in guiding me through the esoteric world of Chinese language and philosophy. And though there are way too many to mention, I'm also indebted to all the other supportive friends and family who helped pick up the slack in my life during the past year — chief amongst them are my father, Marvin Ziporyn, M.D., and my in-laws, Mary Ann and Stanley Snider.

Finally, many thanks to my coauthor, James Dillard, M.D., for being prompt, helpful, supportive, and — most of all — for thinking like me (most of the time!).

Publisher's Acknowledgments

We're proud of this book; please register your comments through our IDG Books Worldwide
Online Registration Form located at http://my2cents.dummies.com.

Some of the people who helped bring this book to market include the following:

Acquisitions and Editorial

Senior Project Editor: Kelly Ewing

Executive Editor: Tammerly Booth

Senior Copy Editor: Susan Diane Smith

Technical Editor: Ira D. Zunin, M.D., M.P.H.

Associate Permissions Editor:
Carmen Krikorian

Editorial Manager: Colleen Rainsberger

Media Development Manager:
Heather Heath Dismore

Editorial Assistant: Paul E. Kuzmic

Production

Project Coordinator: Karen York

Layout and Graphics: Lou Boudreau,
Maridee V. Ennis, Angela F. Hunckler,
Brent Savage, Jacque Schneider,
Janet Seib, Kate Snell

Special Art: Kathryn Born, Kathy Hanley

Proofreaders: Christine Berman, Kelli Botta,
Michelle Croninger, Rachel Garvey,
Nancy Price, Rebecca Senninger,
Ethel M. Winslow, Janet M. Withers

Indexer: Anne Leach

Special Help

Gwenette Gaddis, Copy Editor;
Maureen F. Kelly, Editorial Coordinator; and
Karen S. Young, Acquisitions Coordinator

General and Administrative

IDG Books Worldwide, Inc.: John Kilcullen, CEO; Steven Berkowitz, President and Publisher

IDG Books Technology Publishing: Brenda McLaughlin, Senior Vice President and
Group Publisher

Dummies Technology Press and Dummies Editorial: Diane Graves Steele, Vice President and
Associate Publisher; Mary Bednarek, Director of Acquisitions and Product Development;
Kristin A. Cocks, Editorial Director

Dummies Trade Press: Kathleen A. Welton, Vice President and Publisher; Kevin Thornton,
Acquisitions Manager

IDG Books Production for Dummies Press: Michael R. Britton, Vice President of Production
and Creative Services; Cindy L. Phipps, Manager of Project Coordination, Production
Proofreading, and Indexing; Kathie S. Schutte, Supervisor of Page Layout; Shelley Lea,
Supervisor of Graphics and Design; Debbie J. Gates, Production Systems Specialist;
Robert Springer, Supervisor of Proofreading; Debbie Stailey, Special Projects Coordinator;
Tony Augsburger, Supervisor of Reprints and Bluelines

Dummies Packaging and Book Design: Robin Seaman, Creative Director; Kavish + Kavish,
Cover Design

◆

The publisher would like to give special thanks to Patrick J. McGovern,
without whom this book would not have been possible.

◆

Contents at a Glance

Cartoons at a Glance

By Rich Tennant

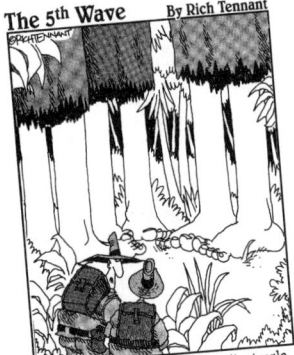

"Legend has it there's an herb in the jungle that, when eaten, imparts great size and strength. Let's ask these natives. Perhaps they've heard something."

page 219

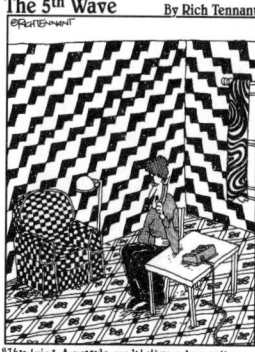

"I've tried Ayurveda, meditation, and aromatherapy, but nothing seems to work. I'm still feeling nauseous and disoriented all day."

page D-1

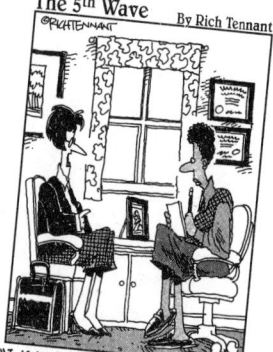

"I think my body's energy centers ARE well balanced. I keep my pager on my belt, my cell phone in my right pocket, and my palmtop computer in my inside left breast pocket."

page 281

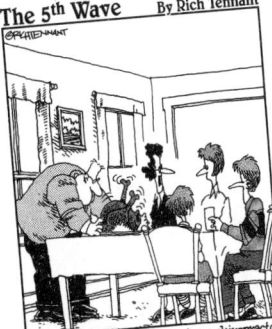

"This is what I get for marrying a chiropractor. Every Thanksgiving he's got to align the turkey's spine before he'll carve it."

page 137

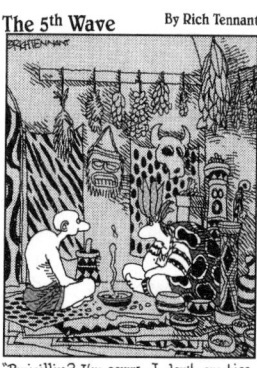

"Penicillin? I'm sorry—I don't practice alternative medicine."

page 55

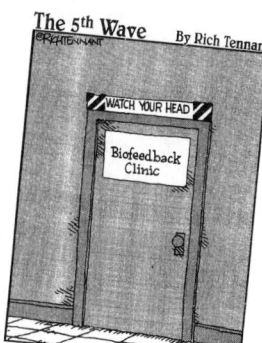

page 181

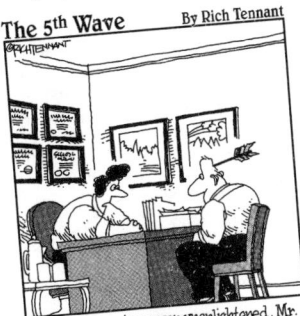

"I don't mean to appear unenlightened, Mr. Grave, but I don't think this is the time to explore alternative forms of treatment."

page 7

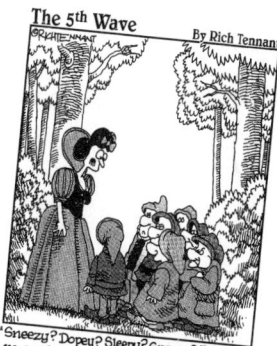

"Sneezy? Dopey? Sleepy? Grumpy? I take it no one here's ever heard of homeopathy?"

page 93

Fax: 978-546-7747 • **E-mail:** the5wave@tiac.net

Table of Contents

Part V: Mind-Body Medicine *181*

Chapter 17: Finding Ways to Relax 183

Chapter 18: Focusing on Hypnosis, Guided Imagery, and Biofeedback 197

Introduction

· ·

*I*f you feel bombarded by information about alternative medicine, you're not alone. No self-respecting magazine or newspaper can avoid the topic. No self-respecting bookstore can avoid it, either. You may have seen countless bookstore shelves sagging under the weight of alternative medicine books. You may have seen whole sections of bookstores devoted to them. If you live in a big (or hip) enough city, you may have even seen whole bookstores devoted to them.

You may also have noticed that every single one of these books is trying to sell you something, such as

- ✔ An esoteric system of healing that the author happens to practice
- ✔ An esoteric vitamin, herb, exercise, or philosophy that — on the faintest of evidence — is heralded as a universal cure
- ✔ A political philosophy
- ✔ A religion
- ✔ An axe to grind
- ✔ False hope

Guess what? We're not trying to sell you anything (except this book!). All *legitimate* healers and book authors share a common goal — and it doesn't involve knocking other healing systems or promoting one single system (a classic mark of the medical quack). The goal is to do whatever works to make patients well — and keep them that way. This openness to whatever works (and works without harm) makes this book different from the rest.

If you get nothing else out of *Alternative Medicine For Dummies,* get this: Books, doctors, or anyone else promising a single panacea are bad news. The same goes for anyone — conventional or alternative healer alike — who won't acknowledge that there's still a lot of uncertainty in the world of medicine.

Life would certainly be amazing if everyone alive today existed at the one time and place in human history when humankind knew everything there was to know about how to heal the body and keep it healthy. Too bad — like other amazing concepts, this one is also too good to be true. Although a lot of self-proclaimed experts would have you think otherwise, the medical world spans a vast wilderness of unknown territory. When you make decisions about your health care, you have to do the best you can with this muddle.

This book helps you do just that. It's full of straight answers about what works, what's safe, and what's worth trying, even in the face of all this uncertainty.

About This Book

One definition of alternative medicine is any health care practice that's not usually emphasized in conventional medical schools or practiced in mainstream hospitals. Think about this definition for more than two seconds, and you realize that the list of healing techniques that may be considered alternative is virtually infinite — including prayer, friendship, a good night's sleep, and anything else that may make you feel fitter.

Clearly, we can't mention every single one of these alternatives. Not only would we create the world's longest and most boring book, but we'd also create a book that would be obsolete the nanosecond it hit the presses. Hope springs eternal — and until disease and death are wiped from the face of the earth, new and creative theories about health care will abound.

Our approach to alternative medicine is more approachable, in our humble opinion. It's also more useful. Sure, we offer study guides for all the biggies — acupuncture, chiropractic, homeopathy, herbal medicine, touch therapy, and just about any method you may consider. But we also give you the jump on how to tell the good stuff from the bad, the hoax from the legitimate, the hype from the proven, and the innocuous from the dangerous. Whether you're thinking about an alternative approach right now or preparing for the future, you can find what you need to make an informed and safe decision.

Specifically, we focus on

- How to determine when alternatives are worth a try — and when they may be dangerous
- How to evaluate various alternative approaches
- How to use alternatives safely
- How to find a conventional doctor who is open to alternatives
- How to find an alternative practitioner

Foolish Assumptions

Pardon our assumption (and presumption), but we assume that you need this book if any of the following apply:

- ✔ Conventional medicine just isn't working for your problem.

- ✔ You feel uncomfortable dosing yourself up with potent drugs for every little ache and pain.

- ✔ You suspect that this alternative stuff is a bunch of bunk, but you have this back pain/headache/dry cough/whatever that just won't quit.

- ✔ You want to short-circuit your sister-in-law's constant prattling about some weird cure-all.

- ✔ Friends have suggested alternatives to you, but you're skeptical.

- ✔ You're sick of seeing mysterious signs for treatments such as "energy balancing," "naprapathy," and "reflexology" in professional buildings and feeling like you come from an alternate universe.

- ✔ Some of your friends are going to yoga teachers, massage therapists, or chiropractors, and you want to know what all the fuss is about.

- ✔ You've tried alternatives but want to know about any other options.

- ✔ You're interested in alternatives but feel overwhelmed by the number of choices.

- ✔ You're afraid you may be ripped-off — or even harmed — by trying certain (otherwise appealing) alternatives.

- ✔ You've read a book or two about alternatives but found them to be too flowery, commercial, or religious — and you're *still* confused.

On the other hand, we assume that you *don't* need this book if any of the following apply:

- ✔ You're looking for laundry lists of every remedy known to humankind alongside every single ache or pain that those remedies *may* help — even if the only "proof" comes from the writer's Great Auntie Griselda.

- ✔ You're looking for eternal life or the fountain of youth.

- ✔ You're Dr. Deepak Chopra, Dr. Andrew Weil, or Dr. Bernie Siegel.

- ✔ You've read (and understood) everything ever written by Dr. Deepak Chopra, Dr. Andrew Weil, or Dr. Bernie Siegel.

- ✔ You already own a copy.

How This Book Is Organized

Following is a summary of the information you can find in each part of the book.

Part I: What Everyone Needs to Know

This part brings you up to speed on the alternative phenomenon — what alternative means, who's doing it, and why. We offer everything you need to know about using alternatives safely and keeping clear of charlatans and hucksters. Then we tackle the million-dollar question — does this stuff work, and how can you figure out whether it does? We also describe all the basic alternative choices and where to get good information about them.

Part II: Complementing Your Medicine

In this part, we explain how to get the best out of alternative medicine — how to find (and pay for) good alternative care and use it together with conventional medicine. We show you how to broach the often-touchy subject of alternative options with your regular M.D. — and skeptical friends and family. We also guide you through the health food store, helping you shop for alternative products safely — and with your wallet intact.

Part III: The Big Picture: The Systematic Approach

This part introduces you to the big "systems" of alternative medicine — philosophies of healing that differ from conventional Western medicine.

Part IV: Hands-On Approaches

Part IV includes alternative approaches that involve the "laying on of hands" — or, in some cases, noninvasive tools. We demystify chiropractic, osteopathy, and acupuncture. We also let you in on the many healthful benefits of massage and bodywork. We also show you how to find a good therapist, healer, or teacher.

Part V: Mind-Body Medicine

This part describes the many effective (and often low-cost) approaches that rely on the mind's ability to affect the body. After discovering the amazing benefits of relaxation and finding out how stress can make you sick, you discover how to get these benefits from various relaxation techniques from around the world.

Part VI: Herbs and Other Natural Approaches

Part VI is all about the hidden healing powers that come from Mother Nature. You get a crash course in herbal medicine — including reasons to try herbs, facts explaining why herbs aren't necessarily harmless, and ways to make sure that you use herbal remedies safely. You discover what aromatherapy can — and can't — do for you and how to take advantage of simple and cheap lifestyle changes — such as better nutrition — without going overboard. You also get the bottom line on electricity, magnets, light, sound, and other natural forces that can supposedly affect your health.

Part VII: Specific Conditions

This part is the place to go if you're suffering from a specific ailment right now — and want to know whether any alternative approaches can give relief.

Part VIII: The Part of Tens

In ...*For Dummies* tradition, this part includes easy-to-use lists that can help you use alternative medicine more safely and effectively.

Icons Used in This Book

In the margins of this book, you can find little signposts (called icons) to highlight specific types of information.

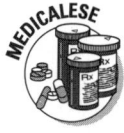

This icon warns you that a shot of "medicalese" is coming up. We inject jargon only when it helps you understand the ads, packaging, and promises in health care land.

This icon alerts you to myths, common mistakes, or just plain marketing hype that can waste your time and/or money.

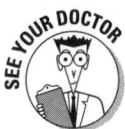

If you see this icon, conventional medicine is in order. See a medical doctor (an *M.D.*) as soon as possible.

We use this bullseye to earmark strategies for choosing the best health care provider, getting more for your time or money, or safeguarding your health.

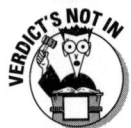

This symbol highlights practices that still have a lot of unknowns. They may turn out to be safe and effective (we tell you when we *know* they're not), but the final verdict awaits more scientifically valid experiments.

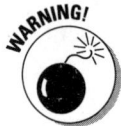

This icon introduces some product, action, or so-called advice that could be hazardous to your health. Steer clear.

Where to Go from Here

If you're considering a specific alternative practice or trying to find help for a specific health problem, you don't need to read this book cover-to-cover. Simply check out the table of contents or index and jump to the relevant section. If you have a particular health concern, you can also go directly to Part VII to see which alternative approaches may be helpful to you; then look them up in more detail in Parts III, IV, V, or VI.

If you want an overview of the state of alternative medicine right now — information that will come in handy for any future health concerns — this book is breezy enough to read straight through. For everyone, though, we highly recommend at least skimming through Part I for handy information to help you use any form of alternative medicine wisely and cost-effectively.

One more thing: The information in this reference is not intended to substitute for expert medical advice or treatment. If you're under a doctor or other qualified health care practitioner's care and receive advice contrary to information provided in this reference, the doctor or other qualified health care practitioner's advice should be followed, as it is based on your unique characteristics.

Part I

What Everyone Needs to Know

The 5th Wave · By Rich Tennant

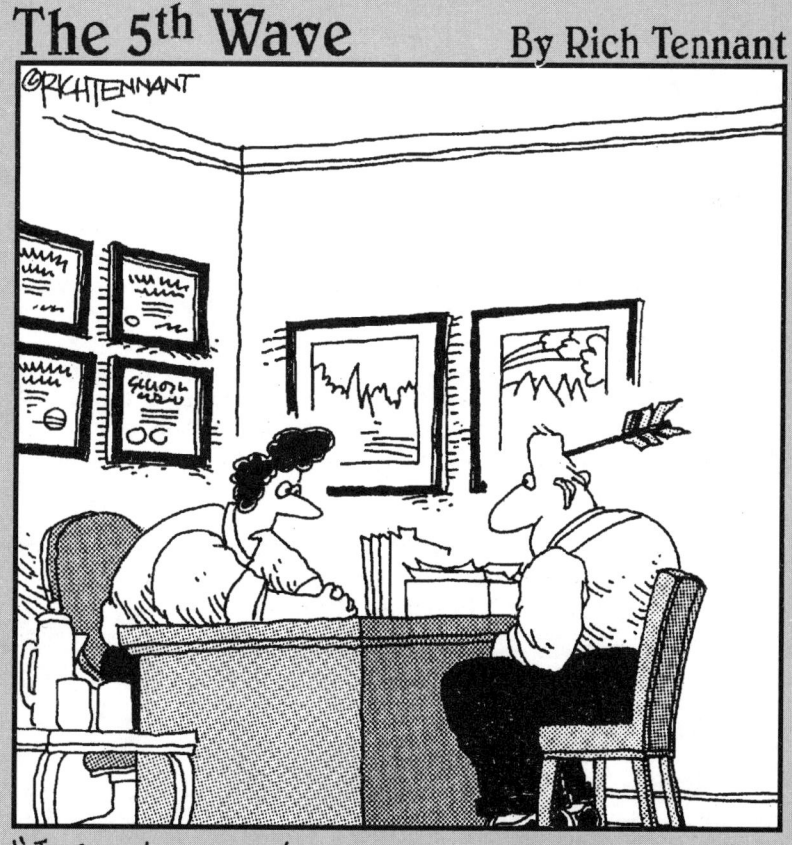

"I don't mean to appear unenlightened, Mr. Grove, but I don't think this is the time to explore alternative forms of treatment."

In this part . . .

Perhaps you have a long-standing health problem that conventional medicine hasn't helped much. Or perhaps you have a degenerative or noninfectious disease and aren't happy about the dangerous and painful side effects that often result from conventional options. In this part, you can find out whether alternative medicine may be worth a try — and which kinds of alternatives may be right for you. You get the scoop on choosing and using alternatives safely, plus tips for identifying which alternatives work and which ones don't. You also get a crash course in the basic alternative choices, together with quick and easy strategies for educating yourself about alternatives by using your telephone, library, or Internet service.

Chapter 1

The Appeal of Alternatives

At least one in three people in the United States has tried alternative medicine, most of them without ever mentioning that fact to their conventional physician. That ratio translates into approximately 85 million people. Huge as it is, that number is no big surprise. Throughout history, alternative medicine has been popular whenever people were frustrated with conventional treatments. Often they were frustrated because conventional treatments didn't work or were expensive, dangerous, and painful. (Think about leeches for a minute, and you'll see what we mean.)

Modern conventional medicine has worked wonders in certain areas — especially surgery, trauma, and (until recently) infectious disease control. It has a far worse track record, however, in the treatment and prevention of everyday woes — such as colds, flus, and ear infections — or chronic diseases — such as arthritis, autoimmune disorders, allergies, and depression. The same people who may once have succumbed to diphtheria or smallpox in childhood now grow to ripe old age, only to experience diseases that conventional medicine often can barely touch — such as heart disease, cancer, and diabetes.

This chapter looks at ways alternative medicine is stepping in to fill these gaps and brings you up to speed on what alternative medicine means in today's world.

Leave the Dictionary Behind — Defining Alternative

It's difficult to say what unites practices as different as acupuncture, yoga, macrobiotics, crystal healing, and chiropractic, but we'll say it anyway: The easiest way to know whether a method is alternative is to ask whether it's usually practiced by conventional M.D.s and taught in mainstream medical schools. In other words, the only thing all alternatives have in common is that, until recently, mainstream medicine has rejected them all.

The problem is, what's acceptable to the mainstream is changing all the time. Conventional medicine from time immemorial has swallowed up alternative approaches as they have proven themselves useful — and today's world is no exception. But today, more and more health care practitioners are picking and choosing from a variety of methods, making this the best of all possible worlds. The idea is to promote and restore health using whatever means is effective. Table 1-1 shows some of the most popular alternative treatments for common health problems.

Table 1-1   What the Joneses Are Doing (Popular Alternatives for Ten Common Complaints)

Complaints in Order of Frequency	Most Common Alternative Therapies
Back problems	Chiropractic, massage
Allergies	Spiritual healing, lifestyle, and diet changes
Arthritis	Chiropractic, relaxation techniques
Insomnia	Relaxation techniques, guided imagery
Sprains or strains	Massage (not for acute sprains or strains), relaxation techniques
Headache	Relaxation techniques, chiropractic
High blood pressure (hypertension)	Relaxation techniques, homeopathy
Digestive problems	Relaxation techniques, megavitamins
Anxiety	Relaxation techniques, guided imagery
Depression	Relaxation techniques, chiropractic, massage

Source: *The New England Journal of Medicine* 328 (January 28, 1993): 249.

The truth is, we're not all that wild about the term alternative. "Alternative" suggests a different approach from what's used conventionally. But lots of so-called "alternative" approaches *are* being used by conventional docs, and some are even being taught in the most conventional medical schools. On top of that, many M.D.s happily recommend that patients use these techniques to supplement more mainstream practices — an approach known as *complementary medicine*. But the term alternative has caught on, so we're using it.

We prefer to think of these health care practices as options to try together with more conventional approaches — not *instead* of them. The idea is to find the best approach — or combination of approaches — for the problem at hand, without emphasizing the labels all that much.

It's obvious that what's alternative and what's not is constantly changing. It's also obvious that alternative and conventional medicines are no longer at war — or don't have to be. This reconciliation really messes up definitions. But if it means that people have better health care choices — and it does — who cares?

You Already Use Alternatives

Plenty of approaches that were once alternative are now part (or almost part) of the mainstream — including biofeedback, stress reduction techniques such as meditation and yoga, and lifestyle approaches to health such as improving nutrition and exercising. Alternative no longer means exotic or countercultural — in fact, many everyday routines we all do for our health have roots in alternative practices. Here are ten "alternatives" you may have already tried:

- ✔ Massaging a sore muscle
- ✔ Icing a sprain
- ✔ Taking vitamins for tiredness
- ✔ Taking a "time out" after a heated argument
- ✔ Stretching to work out muscle stiffness
- ✔ Exercising to tone muscles or lose weight
- ✔ Soaking in a warm bath after a bad day
- ✔ Cracking your stiff or aching neck
- ✔ Buying your apartment (and yourself) some flowers
- ✔ Adding fish to your diet to reduce heart disease risk

Conventional Doctors Join the Club

There are still plenty of mainstream doctors out there who don't want to hear or talk about alternatives. And there are still plenty of people who think that they *can't* talk to their doctors about alternatives, or think that doctors are in a conspiracy to knock all alternatives — even those approaches that might help their patients — in order to protect their incomes. The good news is that all these attitudes are starting to change.

Top reasons for using alternatives

According to the *American Journal of Health Promotion,* the following are the top reasons that people in the United States give for using alternative medicine approaches:

- Frustration with what conventional medicine can do

- A sense that conventional (Western) medicine treats patients like machines and not like human beings with feelings and faith

- Increasing awareness of medical practices from different cultures

- Increasing scientific evidence linking diseases to nutritional, emotional, and lifestyle factors

- Desire — and expectation — of wellness, and not just absence of disease

- Desire to take fewer medications and experience fewer side effects

- Desire to cut personal health care costs

- Increasing support for alternative medicine by prominent M.D.s

Source: *American Journal of Health Promotion* 12 (November/December 1997): 112–122.

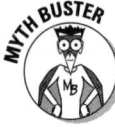

By the way, accepting this pervasive idea — that a conspiracy of M.D.s, government officials, and corporate fat-cats want to keep safe and effective alternative remedies from the public — can lead to an uncritical acceptance of any alternative method. Remember that accepting *every* alternative approach is just as misguided as rejecting *every* conventional approach.

More and more conventional doctors are incorporating the useful parts of alternative medicine. The very same medical centers and hospitals that were vilifying alternative medicine as quackery for most of this century have changed their tune. Now these esteemed institutions are opening their own alternative clinics and hiring their own alternative researchers and practitioners. Some are joining up because they recognize how narrow their treatment options have been. Others are just trying to capture the market share.

Bastions of the mainstream — including Harvard Medical School — now offer alternative, traditional, and in some cases even spiritually based alternatives to their patients. Highly esteemed M.D.s are writing books about the healing power of the mind, and some health plans even reimburse various types of alternative practitioners. The National Institutes of Health — for crying out loud — funds its own Office of Alternative Medicine (started in 1992), designed in part to fund studies that show just which alternatives really work. As we wrote this book, 75 of the 125 medical schools in the United States (64 percent) were offering courses in alternative medicine — elective courses, granted, but still courses. More and more centers for unconventional medicine were springing up at major universities.

The article that shook the world

The new openness of conventional medicine to alternatives can be traced — in large part — to an article that appeared in January 1993. This landmark article, in the esteemed publication *The New England Journal of Medicine*, was written by Harvard's Dr. David Eisenberg and colleagues.

Based on a telephone survey of 1,539 adults, this study showed that one in three respondents reported using an alternative therapy in the past year, and a third visited alternative health care providers. By extrapolating these results to the entire U.S. population, the researchers estimated that Americans made 425 million visits to alternative providers — in contrast to only 388 million to all U.S. primary care physicians. This amount translated into approximately $10 billion per year spent by Americans (not their insurance companies) — just $3 billion less than their out-of-pocket costs for all hospitalizations in the United States.

Money talks. It also erodes prejudices. Because although conventional medical schools and practitioners had scoffed at the "quacks" for decades, they couldn't argue with 10 *billion* bucks — bucks that were heading in the opposite direction of their pockets. The alternative options now sprouting up in many conventional medical settings around the country are the direct result!

Source: *The New England Journal of Medicine* (January 1993): 246–252.

Plenty of regular docs are sending patients off to chiropractors or acupuncturists for help with chronic pain, too. Many suggest herbal remedies for everyday complaints — such as cranberry juice to prevent urinary tract infections or chamomile tea to ward off insomnia.

Just because your M.D. claims to be alternative doesn't mean that he or she is competent — or appreciates the finer aspects of the alternative approach. After all, going through medical school doesn't automatically make you an expert at everything. Some M.D.s may prescribe an herbal remedy just because they read about it in a magazine — and may know less about it than you do. Some may think that they're trained herbalists because they listened to a lecture during a continuing medical education seminar in Palm Springs. Some may competently use certain therapies without "getting" what alternative medicine's all about.

The fact is, there's huge market and economic pressure for unscrupulous M.D.s to pretend to know something about these areas. At this point in time, *very* few true "crossover" docs with solid credentials are out there — and a lot of M.D.s with scant (or no) credentials would just like to make a bunch of money on alternatives. (One of us just met a brilliant doc, board certified in Internal Medicine and Infectious Disease and academic-based, who is also a fully trained acupuncturist, extensively trained herbalist, and who's finishing a long program in Chinese botanicals. But such people are *rare*.)

Your best bet (for complementary and alternative care) is to find a nonphysician practitioner who is very well schooled in one discipline, and just remember his or her limitations. This is just common sense: It's tough to find people who are real experts in more than one area, in any field.

Traits of All Alternatives — a Distinctive View of Health

Despite all the mixing, there *are* still some differences between alternative and conventional medicines, at least as they are practiced today. The following sections describe these differences.

Standards of proof

Alternative and conventional medicines often have different standards of proof. Conventional medicine prides itself on being "evidence-based," meaning that it values methods that have been proven to work in scientifically valid studies (more on this in Chapter 3). That doesn't mean that everything in conventional medicine has been proven — far from it — but new approaches in particular usually have to jump a lot of hurdles before they are accepted.

Alternative medicine, in contrast, is much more open to "what works" for the individual (*anecdotal evidence*) — even if the method hasn't been shown to work in a scientific clinical trial. Alternative medicine also relies on the kind of evidence that comes from experience — such as the approximately 5,000-year history of acupuncture.

Training

Alternative healers may have different training than conventional physicians. When you visit a conventional doctor (an M.D.), you pretty much know what credentials you're getting: someone who went to a four-year college, graduated from an accredited medical school, and then spent three to five more years in residency training. Some M.D.s have even more advanced training. All have passed standardized board examinations. This education is, at least in theory, based on a solid scientific foundation — that is, the knowledge that is learned is supposedly based on evidence.

When you see an alternative doctor, however, you're in murkier waters. Educational standards for alternative practitioners vary considerably, depending on where you live and what area of alternative medicine you're seeking. An "alternative" practitioner could be an M.D. with the usual training who has also been trained in some area of alternative medicine. That training could have been a weekend seminar (on a cruise ship) or three years of an advanced program in Chinese medicine. Just what the scientific foundation for these training programs may be varies considerably, too. A "trained" alternative practitioner could have completed many years of formal training in an accredited chiropractic, osteopathic, or acupuncture program and be licensed and/or certified by the state. Another practitioner could just be someone who took a mail-order course in crystal healing and put up a shingle.

Views of health and illness

Alternative medicine is based on a different (from conventional medicine) view of health and illness. Many conventional practitioners hold these views, but until recently they certainly weren't emphasized in mainstream medical schools:

- ✔ The whole person counts — not just the physical body.
- ✔ Therapy should exploit the healing power of nature.
- ✔ The individual patient is much more important than the disease.
- ✔ Preventing disease is as important as treating it.
- ✔ Patients should play an active role in their own health.
- ✔ Health care should be priced reasonably and be widely available.

A holistic approach: Emphasis on the "whole" person

For thousands of years, healers from all countries and backgrounds had recognized that health was a complex product of body, mind, and environment. As conventional doctors started "triumphing" over serious diseases with vaccines and drugs, though, they started overlooking this complexity and basing their medicine on what's known to philosophers as the *biomedical model* — that is, the view that disease is caused by a physical cause (such as a germ, a gene, or a knife in the back). This mechanistic view puts doctors in the role of expert technicians who can fix whatever is wrong by removing or altering that physical cause; the patient doesn't have to do anything but know how to choose the right doctor.

Alternative medicine, in contrast, takes a more "holistic" view of health — that is, it views health as a complex product of body, mind, spirit, even physical and social environment (to some people, "holistic" also means that the office smells like incense, but that's another story). The result is a much more patient-centered approach, and doctors and patients are partners in the journey toward better health.

Nature: A double-edged sword

Alternative medicine often emphasizes the body's natural power to heal itself. It tends to overlook the body's natural power to get sick and die. Deciding which of these two powers to emphasize for any given patient at any given time is what the art of medicine is all about — whether the healer is "alternative" or "mainstream."

The fact is, conventional medicine has long relied on the healing power of nature. True, now and then a fascination with new technology —

whether it was old-style bleeding and purging or today's computer-guided neurosurgery — have sometimes overshadowed letting nature do its thing. But it was actually the founder of Western medicine, good old Hippocrates, who is said to have coined the term *vis medicatrix naturae* (the healing power of nature — although how a guy who spoke Greek came up with a Latin phrase is another question).

Body, heal thyself

Many forms of alternative medicine play up the body's natural ability to heal itself. Instead of regarding medicine as a bunch of drugs, equipment, and procedures that work against or ignore the body's own natural defenses, it aims to boost the powers we have within us. For example, instead of viewing fever as something to "bring down" or a runny nose as something to "dry up," it tries to bolster the body's ability to heal itself by building up the immune system or even temporarily increasing these symptoms (which are only natural defenses).

Focus on the patient, not the disease

Statistics and studies are useful, but everyone has a unique set of circumstances, and the mathematical probabilities just don't apply in every case. Alternative healers emphasize that every patient is different, which often means that what works for one person won't necessarily work for another. The healer's job is to find the complex set of factors that bear on the individual patient's treatment.

Health promotion and disease prevention

Contrary to popular belief, conventional medicine has been talking about the importance of prevention for a long time. Talking and doing, of course, are rather different, and conventional M.D.s haven't been so great in the latter category. Alternative medicine frequently aims at taking steps to keep disease from ever happening in the first place — whether by encouraging the patient to adapt a less stressful lifestyle, change diet or exercise routines, or use various medicines that might bolster natural defenses (via the immune system). See Table 1-2 for some examples.

Table 1-2	Prevention: Conventional and Unconventional
Conventional Prevention	*Unconventional Prevention*
Immunization	Herbs, vitamins, "wellness" practices
Screening tests	Megavitamin therapy, diets
Physical examinations	Meditation, stress reduction
Standard hospital nutrition	Unusual "broader" nutrition
Exercise	Exercise, yoga
Health habit modification	Same, plus more extreme changes

Active role of the patient

One of the biggest appeals of alternative medicine is that it empowers people to be active participants in their own health care. Far too often, conventional doctors take on the role of gods (or are put there by patients) who issue orders to be followed unquestioningly. Alternative medicine takes the view that individuals are ultimately responsible for their own health.

Fun facts and figures

Who's using alternatives — and how often? A recent article in the *American Journal of Health Promotion* offers some eye-opening answers:

✔ In 1990, about one in three adults in the U.S. population said they used alternative medicine. And surveys since then estimate that alternatives have been tried by 30 to 73 percent of people suffering from conditions such as cancer, arthritis, AIDS, multiple sclerosis (MS), and acute back pain.

✔ The most commonly used practices are vitamins and health foods, herbal therapy, chiropractic, relaxation techniques, massage, and acupuncture.

✔ Most users are either between the ages of 25 and 49 or over age 65.

✔ Most alternatives are paid for "out-of-pocket" — that is, without insurance coverage.

✔ In 1990, people in the United States paid about $11.7 billion dollars to complementary and alternative medicine providers, and another $2 billion for commercial diet supplements and over-the-counter homeopathic remedies.

✔ In 1991, they paid $1.3 billion for herbal therapy. This market is supposed to be growing at a rate of about 20 percent per year.

Source: *American Journal of Health Promotion* 12 (November/December 1997): 112–122.

This can be a rather daunting view (because it also implies that each of us is responsible if we get sick). But all in all, it leaves people feeling empowered. They are not mere pawns of some drug or a godlike doctor; they can take positive steps to make themselves healthier. The doctor (alternative or otherwise) is best viewed as a partner in this process and not as some genie or dictator.

Affordability

The affordability issue isn't really a philosophy of alternative medicine so much as a fact. Alternative approaches are often real cost savers because they emphasize preventive, often simple and cheap, practices. Plus, they are performed by less costly non-M.D.s, outside of hospitals.

Because alternative medicines tend to be classified as "supplements" rather than "drugs," they don't have to go through the costly process of drug-testing required by the Food and Drug Adminstration (FDA) — and the consumer gets in on the savings. Of course, the downside to this lack of rigorous testing is not knowing if the stuff actually works — or is safe. But in terms of money, it can't be beat.

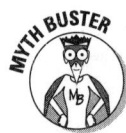

Whether alternative medicine as a whole is really more cost-effective than conventional medicine — an extremely common assertion — remains to be seen, however. Because so many people use alternatives without ever getting a good diagnosis of what was wrong with them in the first place, they may treat "nonconditions," psychic stress, or temporary symptoms, and mistakenly credit the treatment when the problem would have gone away by itself. This cost is unnecessary. Alternative medicine has many potential benefits, but until better studies are done on which ones actually help, the jury's still out on whether these practices can help contain healthcare costs.

Chapter 2

Do No Harm: The Number One Priority

In This Chapter

▶ How to use alternatives safely

▶ How even natural products can be harmful

▶ How to protect yourself from hoaxes, quacks, and frauds

Some of the pluses of alternative medicine can sometimes be minuses. In particular, the idea of empowered patients responsible for their own health care is great — but it can also be a burden. Separating the wheat (that is, safe and effective alternatives) from the chaff (that is, everything else) can be difficult. Regulations for alternative practitioners are often fairly lax. For many kinds of alternative care, just about anyone can hammer up a shingle, and there are far too many undertrained, uncredentialled healers around who may miss the signs of serious illness. This chapter and the next give you guidelines for navigating this jungle on your own — safely and effectively.

Telling Your Regular Doc about Alternatives

No question about it: The safest way to use alternative medicine is to let your regular doctor know what you're doing. Yes, you may get a strange response — such as "whatever," "they're all a bunch of quacks," or "you'd be better off buying a ticket to the Caribbean." Far too often, contempt or dismissal is a mask for ignorance. Don't take it personally, though. Remember that it's tough enough just to keep track of conventional medicine and practice it well, so knowing much about other disciplines is always a challenge.

But you may be surprised. More and more M.D.s are open to the idea of trying alternatives — particularly if they can't solve the problem alone.

By the way, if your conventional doctor can't handle the fact that you're trying alternatives — and you basically like your doctor — try to encourage (or challenge!) your doctor to get educated about the subject. You can be sure that you're not the only patient who is using alternatives. If your doctor ultimately stonewalls you, consider switching doctors or consulting with another doctor who is known to understand alternatives. Not all M.D.s will approve of what you're doing, of course, but if you're going to use the alternative method anyway, a reputable doctor will want to hear about it.

If you feel uncomfortable talking to your M.D. about alternatives, see Chapter 6.

Knowing When It's Safe to Try Alternatives on Your Own

If you're suffering from a health condition, a good basic rule for safety is to see a doctor first to make sure that you don't have anything seriously wrong with you. After you've ruled out anything serious, consider treatment options — alternative and otherwise. If you have a bone sticking out through your skin or crushing chest pain, you don't want to seek out an acupuncturist or herbalist.

This rule is good, but it has its problems — the biggest of which is that you have to decide whether your symptoms merit a trip to the doctor in the first place. In this book, your fate is ultimately in your own hands (as it should be). The ancient Chinese texts offer the axiom "the first doctor is always the patient himself." This truth will never change. Our goal here is to help better "train" that doctor.

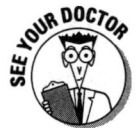

If there's any chance in the world that you may have a serious illness — that is, something that may threaten your life, incapacitate you, linger for years, cramp your style, and so on — don't even think about treating yourself. Go see a conventional practitioner and have that serious illness (such as heart disease, cancer, stroke, kidney failure, or diabetes) ruled out before you even consider alternatives.

A new or unusual injury or ailment — especially one that involves "vital signs" such as blood pressure, pulse, breathing rate, or temperature — needs a good professional diagnosis. For example, a new weakness in a leg accompanied by an up-and-down fever is not a good time to try an herbal remedy on your own.

The same rule is true if you're being treated for a serious illness — or using any kind of medication — and you suddenly develop what seems to be an unrelated symptom. Mixing and matching therapies on your own is a bad idea, even if one of the "mixes" is an over-the-counter "natural" therapy. In other words, if you're taking insulin for your diabetes or medication for your high blood pressure, don't assume that taking an herbal remedy for your cold is safe. It may be — but check with your primary doctor first. A doctor who doesn't know the answer (and bravo for admitting this!) should be asked to look it up and get back to you.

Those cautions aside, you can usually feel comfortable trying to treat yourself in the following situations:

- ✔ When you have an obviously common and nonlife-threatening problem — such as a cold, a simple bruise, occasional stress, a few extra pounds, and so on
- ✔ When you have a long-term, stable condition and you just want to augment your ability to heal

Identifying Ways Alternatives Can Be Harmful

Alternative medicine often bills itself as safer or more natural than conventional medicine, but don't let those claims fool you. The power to help (which some alternatives definitely have) goes hand-in-hand with the power to hurt. The following sections describe the potential dangers of alternative medicine.

Delay treatment for a serious problem

Sometimes, diagnosing and treating yourself — say, deciding your headaches are due to your mother-in-law and treating them with massage therapy or megavitamins — can be fine. Sometimes (though very rarely), self-diagnosis can be deadly — for example, if you really have a brain tumor.

Interfere with other treatments or medicines

Many natural substances that are usually safe alone can keep your other medicines from working right. For example, as difficult as it is to believe, even lowly grapefruit juice turns out to muck up potent heart medications called calcium channel blockers. And taking vitamin E and high doses of garlic can pose a risk of excessive bleeding if you're already taking the blood thinner Coumadin. There are undoubtedly many more herb and drug interactions that no one has discovered yet.

Cause direct damage

You're going to hear this from us a lot in this book, but we can't repeat it often enough: "Natural" and "safe" are not equivalent terms. Too many people assume that just because various herbs are "natural" that they cannot possibly cause harm, no matter how much or how often they are used. (It's interesting that these herbs are believed to have the power to make nearly miraculous positive change, but never any power to cause harm.)

Among "healing" herbs known to pose health risks are germander, sassafras, comfrey, chaparral, and even licorice root. Chapter 20 includes a table on potential health risks caused by many popular herbs. More to the point, we simply don't know the health risks of many alternatives — but that doesn't mean that those risks don't exist.

Ask anyone who tells you that a treatment is "perfectly safe" to show you the evidence (and see Chapter 3 to find out how to decide whether the evidence is valid). If that evidence is two clients who are still walking the earth or who happened to get well, consider the claim unproven. Individual cases of recovery can be intriguing and may stimulate more investigation — but they are not "proof."

Sometimes the problem comes from people using herbs and other alternative treatments incorrectly. People taking anticoagulant medications, for example, should avoid *ginkgo biloba,* (unless advised by a qualified practitioner), an herbal remedy gaining popularity as a memory enhancer. People with the muscle disease myasthenia gravis should avoid the so-called miracle pill GH3 (which is actually plain-old novocaine). And it could well be that dong quai doesn't work too well in treating the menstrual problems and menopausal symptoms of U.S. women because they don't use it the way Chinese herbal practitioners do — in combination with other herbs.

Sometimes danger comes from contamination. Because many alternative meds are not considered drugs, inspection procedures are often fairly lax. In the past, for example, many patent medicines coming in from Asia, especially from China, contained lead, steroids, benzodiazepines (anti-anxiety drugs), and other contaminants — but were regularly sold to unsuspecting consumers. Fortunately, in this particular case, a lot of publicity is inspiring the industry to clean itself up. But there's no guarantee that other nondrug alternatives are free and clear.

Recognizing False Claims

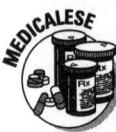

Just as there's no "safe sex," there's no 100-percent safe way to use alternative medicine. For that matter, there's no 100-percent safe way to use conventional medicine. There are plenty of stories of people who were harmed by prescription drugs, surgery, and even medical tests. The medical profession even has a name for these effects — *iatrogenic* — which simply means any problem caused by doctors or medicine.

Using alternatives safely

A few simple rules can minimize chances of trouble with alternative meds:

- **Use alternatives under the supervision of a qualified doctor if you have a serious medical illness.** That way, the effects can be monitored, and possible interactions between any conventional and alternative therapies can be weighed.

- **Avoid mixing and matching conventional and alternative therapies on your own.** Always let your conventional doctor know which alternatives you're trying. Too many people using conventional treatments try a little self-help on the side, without ever mentioning this to their physician. This self-treatment can lead to real interference trouble — because if problems arise, it's impossible to know whether the problem was from the conventional treatment, the alternative, or the combination of the two.

   This interaction can be a real problem for cancer patients undergoing chemotherapy. According to David Eisenberg, M.D., one of the world's leading authorities on alternative medicine, too many people decide to dose themselves with handfuls of herbs to prevent the nausea that often follows chemotherapy. If they still get nauseated and can't tolerate the chemotherapy while on all those herbs, he says, there's simply no way to know if they would have been able to tolerate it without the herbs.

- **Avoid the "more is better" fallacy.** Just as with conventional medicines, alternative meds have an optimal dose that allows them to get the job done with a minimum of damage. But there's always a balance between help and harm — and when you increase the dose, you could tip that balance in favor of harm. That's why it's risky to double or triple the recommended dose when you feel your headache is worse than usual, or worse than other people's. If the recommended dose doesn't seem to help, consult a qualified practitioner about trying a little more.

- **Mother was right.** Things that sound too good to be true generally are.

- **Above all, trust your instincts.** People who sound like they're trying to pull something over on you probably are. Try to find a practitioner who has some solid experience, a responsible attitude, and a good reputation to help guide your choices.

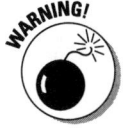

Even doctors should remember the old adage: "The physician who treats himself has a fool for a patient."

Read the box

Read package directions carefully before you use an alternative (or other) product. This is an obvious but too-often-ignored tip. Especially read the parts about who should use the stuff and who shouldn't. An even better approach is asking a doctor when you're not sure whether you fit into the "don't use" category.

Red flags — claims that should make you run in the other direction

Here are some tip-offs that often signal dangerous or bogus claims:

- Herbs or other substances your conventional doctor can't identify after a thorough literature search
- Secret ingredients
- Injections of any kind — unless they are investigated and approved by your conventional doctor
- Words such as "miraculous," "amazing," or "rejuvenating"
- Any alternative healer who won't tell you how long treatments will take, how much they will cost, and when you should expect improvement
- Alternative healers who are extremely hostile toward mainstream medicine
- Anyone who tells you that there are *no* questions about the safety or efficacy of his or her approach — or *no* limitations to what he or she can do

Spotting a charlatan

A charlatan or quack is usually defined as someone out to make a buck by trying to sell you a medical scheme or remedy that they *know* doesn't work. In reality, a lot of people out there truly believe that the junk they're selling *does* work. In both cases, they're worth avoiding because they're pushing bogus products.

What alternative medicine cannot do

We're not saying that it will never happen, but right now there's just little solid evidence that any alternative can

✔ Cure cancer, AIDS, diabetes, arthritis, or heart disease.

✔ Keep you from ever getting sick.

✔ Help you lose weight quickly, dramatically, effortlessly, or permanently.

✔ Test your body's overall "nutritional status" or make miraculous evaluations of your health status.

✔ Help you get well if you can't overcome a lousy attitude or bad emotional or spiritual state.

✔ Make you immortal or reverse aging.

Back in the good ol' days of patent medicine, quacks and charlatans were everywhere. They were notorious for hawking nostrums doctored with cocaine, soothing syrups full of heroin or opium, and medicinal "bitters" laced with alcohol — generally as cures for diseases untouchable by conventional medicine. Charlatans promoted their wares as cheaper, less invasive, and less painful than regular medicines, and portrayed M.D.s as purposely withholding cures to stay in business. They said that their cures were sure bets with no side effects either.

Sound familiar? The claims of the quacks and the claims of today's alternative medicine vendors have a lot in common — which is why they still make so many conventional doctors nervous. Worse, many of today's charlatans use sophisticated marketing tactics (including the Internet) — and many hold plenty of fancy degrees and credentials. You can get your pet hamster certain degrees and credentials, too, by filling out a form and sending off a check. So take that warning for what it's worth.

Even so, by screening out the following types of vendors, you can usually steer clear of these folks. Specifically, do everything you can to avoid people who do the following:

✔ **Rely completely on testimonials as evidence.** Hearing that a treatment or remedy worked for one or two people is encouraging. It's just not all that meaningful. First, you don't know whether the story is true. Second, even if it is true, you don't know whether the people really had the problem in the first place — maybe they *thought* they had heart disease, but they really had heartburn. Third, maybe the problem would have gone away by itself and did, in spite of — not because of — the alternative cure. Or perhaps the improvement in health was due to the power of suggestion (the *placebo effect*) and not the product.

Testimonials are fine, but without evidence from scientifically valid study, they don't mean very much. You have to figure that if good study results *were* actually available, it would be in this person's interest to tell you.

✔ **Advise you not to trust your doctor; or charge all drug companies, the government, or the mainstream medical profession with conspiracy; or refuse to talk to your regular doctor about the treatment.** This kind of advice comes from fear of exposure. Anyone who's selling you reputable treatment won't be threatened by another health care practitioner.

✔ **Refuse to tell you about what outcome you can expect, how long before you see results, and how much the treatment will cost.** These healers are a clear case of buyer beware.

✔ **Promise to cure your problem without a thorough examination and diagnosis.** If someone's giving out the same stuff to everyone — or assuming that you suffer from the same ailment as everyone else — steer clear. There's no such thing as a cure-all, and you want to make sure that you're not suffering from a serious condition before you try medicating yourself — or letting someone on the street tell you what's wrong with you.

✔ **Say that they can't give you evidence because they've been too busy treating patients.** Some questionable alternative healers claim that they've been treating patients with an unconventional treatment for years — leaving them no time to do quality, publishable research on what happens to these people. It seems to us that if a method really works, it's in that practitioner's interest to prove it to the world (including the skeptical mainstream world that likes research). If a procedure or remedy may not be working, though, this line is understandable.

✔ **Offer a long list of problems that a single device or pill can cure.** Again, cure-alls are phony.

Chapter 3

Does Alternative Medicine Really Work?

. . . .

In This Chapter

▶ How to know whether alternative medicine works

▶ How to tell which kinds of evidence are believable

▶ Why so many alternatives are difficult to prove

▶ When you need proof — and when you don't

. . . .

*E*vidence — scientific studies, trials, and data — sounds like a pretty heavy-duty topic. But once you fumigate the jargon, almost everything that matters can be reduced to simple common sense. Plus, knowing how to figure out whether a treatment or remedy does what it promises to do is key to using alternatives safely and wisely — and this issue is just where most guides to alternative medicine go wrong. How often have you seen those useless lists of 920 home remedies, 500 homeopathic cures, or 30 healing herbs or vitamins — without any guidance as to which of these have been proven to work, which may work, and which definitely won't work?

In this chapter, we give you all the information you need about evidence to make these decisions for yourself. We give you some tools to help you separate the sure-thing from the "who knows?" from the out-and-out hoax.

The Gold Standard of Evidence

Whatever old Doc Casey may tell you, the problem with alternatives isn't that they don't work. Plenty of them do (thousands of years of experience can't be *all* wrong!). The problem, though, is that identifying the ones that work from those that don't can be difficult. Plus, because anyone can get in on the alternative act, many people do — qualified and unqualified alike, honest and dishonest, and everyone in between. Along with the time-tested remedies prescribed to you by a trained practitioner of Chinese medicine, outlets are hawking aromatherapy bath soap or hand creams that may smell nice but probably won't cure your arthritis. All these products get indiscriminately lumped together in that sea of alternatives — hurting the legitimate ones.

A way to find out what works

Conventional doctors and researchers say that they distinguish effective from ineffective products and approaches by practicing "evidence-based" medicine. What they mean is that their practice rests on a solid scientific foundation — not wishful thinking, not armchair theorizing, but actual empirical studies that prove that their methods work and make sense according to accepted theories of nature.

At the same time, of course, everyone also knows that medicine is an art as well as a science. Healing is a matter of an individual physician's skill at assessing an individual patient's needs — in other words, sensing how and when to apply all the scientific knowledge, and when to call on other, perhaps less proven, forms of knowledge. One of the reasons conventional medicine has come under attack in recent years is that the science has overshadowed the art.

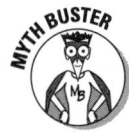

By the way, evidence, or lack thereof, is no way to distinguish the alternative from the mainstream. Conventional medicine tends to swallow up alternatives as they prove themselves useful. This assimilation has led some people to think that all nonevidence-based medicine is alternative, but that's a bunch of hooey. We like evidence as much as anyone, but plenty of methods already embraced by conventional medicine have never been proven. And plenty of alternatives *have* been proven.

The fact is, conventional medicine itself is based on the arts and traditions of practice as handed down from mentor to protégé. Most of it is not "evidence-based." This fact is also true of alternative systems of treatment. Of what is theoretically the sum total of all the knowledge about the workings of the human body and disease, the vast majority is still unknown. We are not on the Starship Enterprise in the year 2450 (too bad). Conventional and alternative proponents alike (and probably most humans) could stand to lose a bit of our arrogance about what we think we know.

The OAM to the rescue

Even though a lot of medical treatments have never been formally proven, scientific proof is nothing to scoff at. As a famous Chinese proverb puts it: "Real gold can withstand the heat of the hottest fire." For alternatives to receive full-scale acceptance by the mainstream medical community — and for you to feel most confident using them — they must be scientifically proven. Many alternatives have been scientifically accepted as safe and effective (see the sidebar "Trials and tribulations — scientific terms explained in plain English"). To help matters along, the United States Congress created The Office of Alternative Medicine (OAM) in 1992 as part of the National Institutes of Health. This office supervises the distribution of grants to researchers who want to evaluate the safety and effectiveness of alternative therapies.

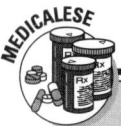

MEDICALESE

Trials and tribulations — scientific terms explained in plain English

Yes, the following list looks like a crib sheet for a biology test, but don't worry. You don't need to memorize these terms. We're just including this handy-dandy guide for those braving the waters of scientific literature on their own. Keep it nearby, and you'll soon be able to critique a scientific study with the best of them.

Anecdotal evidence: Data that comes from a single case. Most conventional scientists consider anecdotal evidence pretty meaningless, because there's no objective way to distinguish the effects that are due to the procedure being tested from the effects that are a result of chance, the power of suggestion, lunar rays, or whatever.

Case study: The kind of anecdotal evidence that conventional doctors like. The story of a single interesting "case" (that is, patient) can be printed in a distinguished medical journal, but it's really no more than food for thought. If many case studies — or anecdotal evidence — lead in the same direction, a more formal study may be called for.

Clinical trial: An experiment in which one group of human beings receives the treatment under investigation and is compared to an untreated, but otherwise similar, control group.

Clinically significant results: Results that make a noticeable difference in a person's disease — not just differences measurable in a test tube.

Control group: Subjects that have virtually everything in common with the group being treated in an experiment — except that they don't receive the treatment itself. Having a control group allows researchers to determine whether results were due to the treatment being tested or to some other factor affecting the study group.

Controlled study or trial: Any experiment with a control group and a treatment group (who gets to try the new method or pill).

Crossover trial: An experiment in which subjects switch from one approach (like Drug A) to another approach (like a placebo pill) in the middle of the study. Because certain alternative approaches are nearly impossible to study by conventional methods (with controls and "blind" subjects and researchers), crossing patients over from certain alternative treatments (such as acupuncture) to no treatment, and vice versa, is sometimes the best way to run a controlled experiment.

Double-blind study or trial: An experiment in which neither the researcher nor the subject knows whether they're using the treatment or the placebo (supposedly an ineffective sugar pill). This arrangement is supposed to help keep experiments bias-free — researchers who know their patients are getting the phony pill may unconsciously convey that information and, thus, dampen any response. In human trials, to continue this blinding is considered unethical if the effects of the drug become established.

Meta-analysis: A currently "in" type of study in which data from many small studies are pooled. Many researchers believe that this process allows them to draw conclusions that otherwise wouldn't be justified from smaller studies. Others argue that pooling a bunch of crummy studies — or studies with inconsistent methodologies — is meaningless. Garbage in, garbage out.

Placebo effect: Improvement due to the power of suggestion (placebo is Latin for "I will please"). This effect occurs, on average, in one-third of all subjects in clinical trials

(continued)

(continued)

(depending on the condition and responses being measured). So to prove that the positive result of a new cure is due to more than the placebo effect, researchers have to show improvement in more than a third of all subjects tested. The word placebo itself refers to the sugar pill or other supposedly powerless medicine or procedure.

Prospective study: A study that looks at the effects of a procedure over time — or just looks at what happens to a group of subjects over time without doing anything to them. For example, a study may take a group of women at age 30 and study them until age 65, seeing whether those who eat a calcium-rich diet over those years end up with a lower rate of osteoporosis later in life.

Randomized study or trial: A study in which researchers assign subjects to different treatment groups, as randomly as possible, so that each group will be as similar as possible. If the group getting a new drug were all women, for example, and the group getting the placebo were all men, findings that the pill "worked" would not necessarily be applicable to men.

Retrospective study: A study that looks back into the past to see whether people with a certain condition, such as lung cancer, have anything in common — say, smoking cigarettes. The more the subjects in retrospective studies have in common, the more valid the results.

Single-blind study or trial: An experiment in which only the researchers know who's getting the "real" treatment and who's getting the placebo. Although double-blind studies are considered preferable, they're not always possible — for example, if researchers are studying the effects of massage, it's impossible for the therapists not to know whether they're doing a real massage. If they do it wrong, or badly enough, however, it is possible for the subject not to know. (Good single-blind studies use "virgin" subjects and then ask them afterward if they got the sham treatment or the real thing.)

Statistically significant results: Effects unlikely to be due to chance alone. Statistically significant results mean that the treatment actually had a measurable effect in the test situation, but whether or not it will make a difference to a real-live patient is still unclear. Only clinically significant results have a (usually) noticeable effect on the patient's condition.

Subject: The person (or, in some cases, the animal) who is being tested in a study. If a study is to be statistically or clinically significant, it must include many different subjects suffering from the problem. (In technical language, the sample size must be big enough.)

One quick and dirty way to check whether a procedure or remedy is backed by solid evidence is to check out the literature from the OAM or its home page (see this book's appendix for relevant numbers). We wish we could say that you could also check the quality of the evidence with your personal M.D., but far too many conventional practitioners mask their ignorance of alternatives with contempt, although this response is changing — especially among younger doctors.

The evidence ideal

The alternative remedies that come up to snuff at the OAM have to satisfy scientific medicine's standards of evidence. The best of the bunch satisfies its gold standard — that is, these treatments undergo *controlled, randomized, double-blind clinical trials.*

If you want to know the nasty technical details of what each of these terms means, check out the sidebar "Trials and tribulations — scientific terms explained in plain English." Otherwise, just get this: The subjects in these studies are randomly assigned to one of two groups — the first gets the treatment, and the other *(the control group)* gets a placebo. Neither group knows who's getting the real thing, and neither do the investigators (thus, the term *double-blind*). Ideally, any sound study is approved by an impartial group of professionals in the field before it's published in a scientific journal. This process is called *peer review.*

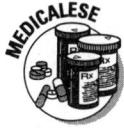

Actually, the best studies also include a no-treatment group in addition to the placebo group. These groups help distinguish the effects of both the treatment and the placebo from the effects of doing nothing ("the natural history of the disease") and other factors that are usually lumped together under the heading "placebo effect."

Too many alternative "studies" fall short of these standards, at least according to mainstream critics. We won't burden you with the details, but long lists of factors can go wrong with study design or execution and lead to invalid conclusions. The most common problems include

- ✔ Reliance on anecdotal evidence
- ✔ No way to rule out the placebo effect
- ✔ The expense — and slowness — of running valid tests
- ✔ Difficulty of running randomized controlled trials for many alternative techniques

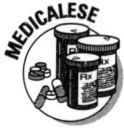

One solution to the latter problem is to follow large groups of people over a number of years who are using a certain treatment and see what happens to them (and preferably compare them to otherwise similar people who don't use the treatment). These studies (technically called sweeping *prospective clinical outcome studies*) are being increasingly advocated for alternative techniques that don't lend themselves to the gold standard (randomized clinical trials) and are likely to yield important (and valid) results.

Don't let "scientific studies" overwhelm you

Not all "scientific studies" are equal — and some are fake. Did you ever get one of those anonymous letters for a dietary supplement with a handwritten self-stick note attached reading "Try this — it works!" We have, several times. The people at *Consumer Reports on Health* debunked this scam years ago, and in February 1998, they revealed a new ploy. Now the company that sent out the notes, which uses the names Gero Vita Laboratories and Life Force Laboratories interchangeably, is sending out glossy, full-color booklets that supposedly contain scientific evidence for their claims.

These booklets cite actual studies but, according to *Consumer Reports on Health*, "twist the findings to support the company's own unsubstantiated claims. The deception only deepens when you purchase a product and receive a 'free' subscription to the *Journal of Longevity Research* — a grand-sounding publication that amounts to little more than a jargon-filled catalog for Gero Vita products."

Consumer Reports on Health regards many of the products hyped in this catalog to be overpriced at best and pure deception at worst. For example, they cite a vitamin and herb combo called G.H.3 that the company calls an "antiaging formula" and the Food and Drug Administration calls "an old health-fraud product." The company also describes a so-called remedy for "prostate problems" (including cancer and enlargement) called Prostata. "Along with many ineffective ingredients," says the article, "the formula includes an herb, saw palmetto, that has actually shown some promise against symptoms of an enlarged prostate in a few controlled trials. But if you want to give that herb a try, you could cut the monthly $29.95 price tag in half with single-ingredient saw palmetto pills from your local drugstore or health food store."

Anecdotes (The Alternative Bugaboo)

Books on alternative medicine are filled with amazing — and, on the surface, convincing — anecdotes about people miraculously healed by some alternative technique. But every time you read a story that ends "and after two weeks of [the alternative approach] my bronchitis was gone" or "just 24 hours after [the treatment] the fever was completely gone!", ask yourself how often could the explanation be that the illness would have gone away by itself anyway?

The antidote to anecdotes

One of our pet peeves is this type of really fun-to-read anecdotal story that is so often presented as some kind of proof. Almost always, they stand alone, without any confirmatory studies involving large numbers of people going through the same treatment. For that reason, these personal anecdotes mean nothing. They're good stories. And they may make us curious to look into the treatment more seriously (scientifically). That's all.

"It worked for me" doesn't cut it

"These natural alternatives are all a bunch of bunk, especially that St. John's wort stuff. I tried it for my depression — it didn't do a thing."

"I don't know why they say they can't cure the common cold. I take echinacea whenever I feel a cold coming on, and it's been working great. I'm almost never sick for more than a week after that, and the symptoms are just less severe than they used to be."

"Take one of these zinc lozenges for that cough! I just tried them for my last cold, and I was fit as a fiddle after three days!"

All these tales — overheard at recent cocktail parties and family gatherings — are worth about zero on the convincing scale. Just because a treatment or remedy did or didn't work for an individual tells you very little about which method will work for anybody else. When you hear these kinds of stories, always search for any other explanation besides the value (or lack thereof) of the treatment. (In these three cases, other factors may be responsible for the patient's experience, but you can't decide on the treatment's effectiveness from one person's statement.)

Don't forget the healing power of nature

People who rely on anecdotes often forget that most problems go away on their own no matter what you do. The human body has a built-in power to maintain and restore health, treatment or no treatment. Clean air and water, nutritious food, sufficient space, and relaxing thoughts can all enhance this most powerful of healing mechanisms.

Often when a fancy therapy seems to be doing the healing, it's your own body that should be getting the credit. For example, numerous studies show that all sorts of effective treatments are available for low-back pain. Among the methods that appear to work most of the time are chiropractic, patient education, pain medication, exercise, mini-injections, and bed rest. If you try any of these approaches, odds are in your favor it will work — and you'll swear by it. But it turns out that in 75 percent of cases, low-back pain goes away *by itself*.

So even though you may tell an anecdote about the time bed rest made your back pain disappear, you may actually have lowered the body's self-healing abilities with your new remedy. Your back may have healed *in spite of* this supposedly effective method! An experiment on one person — you — one time, doesn't prove anything.

It's great if you feel better, though. If you don't, however, don't blame the method. It just might not have been the right solution for this problem this time.

The Placebo Effect: A Bugaboo That's Not

Before you believe anybody's story about any health treatment, remember this: A lot of people get better because of the healing power of suggestion alone. Sometimes, just believing a pill will make a difference can lead to improvement — even if the pill is nothing more than a sugar or a "dummy" (we had nothing to do with this name) pill. Sometimes, just believing that a doctor can help you can make you better. Sometimes, just having anyone pay some attention to you is enough. This improvement caused by the mind is called the *placebo effect*.

One of the chief criticisms leveled at a lot of alternative medicine is that it "only" works because of the placebo effect. In some cases, there may be some truth to this accusation. The mistake is using the word "only." Healers of all stripes have known about this effect for millenia — and it's nothing to ridicule. If you get better because of a sugar pill (a *placebo*) or because a doctor pays extra attention to you — and not because of the $90 session with an electro-wand or whatever — who cares? You still got better.

We're not condoning blatant fraud, of course. More often than not, though, the healer's perfectly honest (if ignorant) belief that a treatment works — and a patient's trust in that healer — will make an otherwise useless treatment work. And that's nothing to scoff at.

Evidence-free advertisements

Beware the onslaught of ads and package labels going way beyond the actual evidence. A recent glossy magazine ad, for example, depicted a boy bundled up in coat and scarf, braving a blizzard by holding out a shiny metal shield in front of him. Next to the shield are the words: "This season your immune system will be under attack." Below the picture, we're told to defend ourselves with *New Halls Zinc Defense lozenges*. The ad then says that these lozenges "contain zinc acetate to support your natural immune system during this cold season and anytime during the year.*"

Just *how* do these peppermint- or cherry-flavored lozenges defend you? Well, if you follow the asterisk to the bottom of the ad page — and if your eyes are good enough to

read the tiny type — you get a more accurate explanation: "Halls Zinc Defense supports the natural immune system by defending against dietary zinc insufficiency." In other words, if you put zinc into your body, you're less likely to have a deficiency of zinc. (What a surprise!) The implication is that you're better able to fight off disease if you have all your vitamins and minerals. That's a pretty modest claim. In fact, if you keep reading the fine print, you also discover that "These statements have not been evaluated by the Food and Drug Administration. This product is not intended to diagnose, treat, cure, or prevent any disease."

So much for defending the immune system. You'd do just as well to stick to a balanced diet or perhaps take a multivitamin.

The placebo has gotten a bad rap from modern "scientific" medicine, resulting in a lot of cold "scientific" doctors. One person's placebo effect is another person's supportive, hopeful connection between patient and practitioner; or the sense of finally being cared for — some of the heart of the art of medicine.

Even so, if you're getting better because of the placebo effect, you'd probably prefer not to pay for the $90 session on top of everything else.

 If a treatment or remedy is working for you (and you don't feel ripped-off), don't get too concerned about whether the placebo effect is responsible. There's always the possibility that knowing about the placebo effect will destroy its power. And there's no reason on earth why we would want to do that.

Proof Isn't Always Necessary or Possible

Solid evidence can't be beat, but plenty of alternative approaches are worth trying even without it. Many potentially effective alternatives are inherently difficult — if not impossible — to prove by Western standards for a number of reasons:

- **The philosophy that illness is an individual experience makes testing difficult.** Scientific studies require a group of people who can be lumped together and called "the same" for the purposes of study. If you take the individualized view, though, it's clear that what works for one person won't necessarily work for another — whatever a "study" may say. A different genetic, physical, emotional, spiritual, or environmental make-up can make one person's reaction different from anyone else's.

- **Often, well-controlled experiments are impossible.** Finding a control (untreated) group for certain alternative practices is difficult. Without a good control group, determining whether the treatment itself made a difference is difficult — because many conditions get better on their own, and because of the power of the suggestion.

  Think of massage, for example. Suppose that you want to know whether a daily massage can help relieve allergy symptoms. Ideally, one group gets the massage and another one just *thinks* that they are getting a massage. That way researchers can know whether the massage itself helps, or just the random touching of the body.

  How do you make people believe that they are receiving a massage without really giving them one? What if you want to know whether just talking with cancer patients helps increase their chances of survival? How do you trick a control group into *believing* that they are being talked to every day without actually talking to them? Researchers have come up with some pretty clever solutions to these puzzles, but none are perfect.

✔ **Many alternatives depend on the skill of the healer as much (or more) than the treatment itself.** Alternatives such as homeopathy and acupuncture are notoriously difficult to prove for exactly this reason. If an alternative therapy doesn't work, the failure may be because the healer is untalented or inexperienced — and not because the treatment wouldn't have worked if done by the right person.

✔ **Some alternatives are based on unmeasurable, almost religious, assumptions.** Take *qi* (pronounced "chee"), for example, the concept of vital energy that Chinese medicine is built around. Supposedly, *qi* is coursing through the body, and its flow can be altered by inserting acupuncture needles at key spots. Alter the flow the right way, and you can block pain or maybe even treat certain symptoms. The problem, though, is that the *qi* itself is unmeasurable — and so it's impossible to show that stimulating a certain point has any specific effect on it. Ultimately, all you can do is ask: Do patients with problem X seem to get better when this happens? And does the method work without doing obvious harm? If yes, go with it. Even if the ultimate explanation is wrong, who cares? People get better.

Experience counts for something. Some of the approaches used by alternative practitioners have been used by so many people for so long that they are probably safe — and probably effective to some extent, too. Examples include many herbal remedies such as echinacea, valerian root, ginger, and *Ginkgo biloba*. (See Chapter 20 for more about these herbs.) The fact that these herbs may be effective doesn't mean that people are using them right, of course, but if used by someone trained in the ancient arts, they're probably a reasonable bet — formal studies or not.

Many conventional techniques are unproven, too. Certain routinely prescribed heart medications, for example, have never been shown to be safe or effective. Most of the drugs children receive have never been rigorously tested on anyone under the age of 12. After looking at inconsistencies in medical practices in different parts of the United States, researchers even estimate that 80 percent of conventional practice is based more on regional traditions and personal preferences than on scientific evidence.

Sometimes Proof Is Necessary

Again, just because a treatment or remedy hasn't been proven to work, or is difficult to prove, doesn't mean that it won't be effective. Before trying an alternative, though, find out whether some good evidence (and, remember, personal anecdotes don't count) is available that *may* prove that you're not throwing away good time and money. Also ask for evidence that the treatment is safe.

What the FDA can learn from the Ming Dynasty

We modern types like to think that we invented data collection. But the ancient Chinese were much better at it than today's federal regulators can hope to be in the next 50 years, at least according to Dr. William Prensky, one of the world's leading authorities on acupuncture and a speaker for the Oxford Health conference. During the Ming Dynasty in China about 1,500 years ago — the same time the number of herbal treatments there was skyrocketing — anyone who wanted to call himself a physician had to go through national tests to prove that he knew what he was doing and be ranked as a creditable doc by the emperor. And every one of these proven physicians also had to report all patient interactions to the imperial government.

According to Dr. Prensky, this government had "hundreds of millions of people who sat around and did nothing but tabulate these data" to see how many patients were being cured by any given doctor. Any doc who cured less than 68 percent of his patients was deemed a "physician of chance" — which was a nice way of saying useless. Interestingly, notes Dr. Prensky, we still use this 68 percent figure as a cut-off for the placebo effect — any treatment that works less than 68 percent of the time is thought to be working by chance and/or wishful thinking alone.

Anyway, this system gave the ancient Chinese a ton of data about how well their herbs were working — and who they were hurting — which should make people feel a little better about using the stuff. Of course, these ancient bean counters didn't check to see whether using a certain herb causes a tumor to form 35 years down the line. And, of course, these ancient records are no guarantee of the quality or content of the herbs people buy today down in Chinatown, health food stores, or mail-order— or that they're using them the way they were meant to be used!

Here are some kinds of proof you definitely should demand before trying a new treatment plan:

- ✔ **Proof that the treatment is safe for someone with your general background.** You should know what the possible risks and side effects are before trying anything, as well as how long you can use the treatment safely and what you can mix with it. Preferably, this proof should be in the form of controlled, scientific trials published in *peer-reviewed journals* (that is, journals impartially reviewed by other researchers before articles are accepted for publication).

- ✔ **Proof that the practitioner has acceptable training and credentials.** (See Chapter 6.)

- ✔ **Proof that the treatment won't cost you an arm and a leg.** Very expensive treatments start to smell fishy.

- ✔ **Proof that there's no known, reasonably well-proven conventional approach with an acceptable risk/benefit ratio for your problem.**

- ✔ **Proof that the practitioner will talk to your mainstream doctor, especially if you are not healing as expected.**

Bottom Line: Safety First, Efficacy Second

Scientific support is good and sometimes essential. But just because a treatment method isn't "proven" doesn't mean that it doesn't work or won't help you.

Just because a method is "proven" doesn't mean that it *will* work for you either. Some unfortunate people who are not responding as expected to appropriate treatment may just lack genetic strength, or they may suffer from poor nutrition, missing trace elements, unbalanced *qi,* subtle neural blockages (*subluxations* as they say in chiropractic land), the psychic and emotional drain of illness and life in general, the lack of human touch, and so on.

Getting someone like this to respond may call for fixing a lot of these factors with whatever treatments are available (proven or not) — improving "the healing milieu," so to speak. In other words, practitioners must integrate the best approaches from conventional and alternative worlds to work together synergistically. But the process of determining what integrations may help will continue to challenge even the best healers.

So stay tuned as far as efficacy goes. Researchers are learning more every day. In the meantime, staying safe is your first priority.

Chapter 4

Considering the Choices
Alternative Medicine Offers

· ·

In This Chapter

▶ Understanding the basics of hands-on therapies, mind-body medicines, and herbal/lifestyle approaches

▶ Using conventional treatments for unconventional purposes

▶ Getting good information on alternatives

· ·

*S*hould you try acupuncture for your aching back? What about chiropractic? Or that yoga program advertised at the coffee bar? The possibilities are mind-boggling. The first step to answering these questions — or finding the right approach for any condition — is to know your options. That's what this chapter helps you do.

The Three Basic Alternative Treatment Options

Alternative medicine comes in three basic flavors: hands-on therapies, mind-body approaches, and herbal healing and lifestyle approaches.

A lot of overlap occurs between these categories. Many practitioners use more than one approach, and some techniques fall into more than one category. Some big systems of healing — rivals of the conventional Western approach — use elements of all three approaches (see Part III).

Hands-on therapies

Hands-on approaches all involve touching or manipulating the body, either with hands or physical objects. Healers have been using manual or manipulative approaches — cracking bones, adjusting the spine, rubbing sore spots — since the beginning of recorded history, and probably before that, too. Many of the options today are safe, soothing, and cheap. If you want to know more after reading this brief introduction, check out the relevant chapters of Part IV.

- ✔ **Chiropractic.** Probably the best-known example — and certainly one of the most widely practiced alternatives in the United States — is chiropractic. Chiropractors believe that the spine is the center of human health and that a malfunctioning spinal column underlies many ailments (see Chapter 13).

- ✔ **Osteopathy.** Doctors of osteopathy *(osteopaths)* — who are trained much like conventional M.D.s and have all the same legal privileges — believe that the body's physical setup *(structure)* and the way it works *(function)* are intimately connected (see Chapter 14).

- ✔ **Acupuncture.** Used for between 2,000 and 5,000 years (history is not an exact science!) by practitioners of traditional Chinese medicine, acupuncture is used to relieve pain, improve general well-being, boost innate healing potential, and treat ailments of all sorts — particularly stress, headaches, whiplash, and sports injuries (see Chapter 15).

- ✔ **Massage therapy and bodywork.** Rubbing, stroking, tapping, kneading, rocking, or stretching applied to certain spots in specific ways (especially manipulations of the soft tissues) may help relieve a whole host of medical problems — including depression, labor pain, eating disorders, chronic fatigue, fibromyalgia, asthma, low-back pain, migraines, premenstrual syndrome, high blood pressure, attention deficit disorder, skin rashes — and more! It may even be part of treatment (though not a cure) for diabetes, cancer, and AIDS (see Chapter 16).

Mind-body medicine

The often inexpensive — and usually helpful — mind-body approaches are the "heart and soul" of alternative medicine. Based on the belief that mental and emotional states can affect the body, these practices may simply help relax you. But they may also challenge you to find a new and more healing way to think about and approach your life, leading you into releasing longstanding barriers and burdens. Do you have to go through this kind of spiritual and emotional make-over to benefit? Probably not, but it wouldn't hurt (check out Part V).

- ✔ **Relaxation techniques.** Many mind-body techniques are based on the premise that relaxation can help reduce the hazardous stress hormones in the body — and possibly undo some of their damage. So can feeling in control of your body and health. Scientists are just beginning to understand why; good evidence now suggests that thoughts and emotions can affect the nervous and immune systems (see Chapter 17).

✔ **Meditation.** One of the safest and simplest ways to relax is to keep your mind from wandering into what went wrong in the past or what may go wrong in the future — and keep it happily aware of the present. You can use various ways to achieve this "meditative" state, including yoga, Zen, and transcendental meditation (see Chapter 17).

✔ **Hypnotherapy.** People who are hypnotized go into a trance-like state in which they are more open to the power of suggestion — such as a suggestion to stop smoking, lay off glazed donuts, or get over a fear of heights (see Chapter 18).

✔ **Biofeedback.** People usually think of vital signs such as heart rate and blood pressure as automatic and uncontrollable, but it turns out that the mind can learn to change these physical processes — and many other so-called *involuntary* functions. During biofeedback, a person is hooked up to a machine that measures whatever function he or she wants to control. Using feedback from this machine, people can eventually learn how to control functions such as blood pressure, heart rate, body temperature, and muscle tension on their own (see Chapter 18).

✔ **Spiritual healing.** We can't explain how it happens, but believing in a higher power — or even believing that someone cares for you — can sometimes promote healing. So can a positive state of mind, a sense of control, a feeling of belonging, and even a good laugh (see Chapter 19).

Herbal healing and lifestyle approaches

Many alternative techniques use natural substances or forces (for example, herbs or electricity) to mend the body or bolster its natural healing abilities. Even more call for changes in diet or exercise habits. If you want to know more after reading this brief introduction, check out Part VI.

✔ **Herbs and botanicals.** Healers from time immemorial have used plants as medicine — and even many conventional drugs have vegetable roots, so to speak (see Chapter 20).

✔ **Aromatherapy.** Everyone knows that smells can affect mood — which in turn can sometimes affect health. Aromatherapy relies on this power — as well as the healing power of the concentrated essences of plants *(essential oils)* — even if they are absorbed into the skin rather than sniffed (see Chapter 21).

✔ **Nutrition and diet.** Although the science of nutrition is still primitive, to say the least, what we eat definitely affects our bodies. Aware of this fact, healers for thousands of years have tried different foods to build strength, cure disease, and even extend life (see Chapter 22).

✔ **Vitamins and supplements.** No one questions that the human body needs small amounts of certain vitamins and minerals to function. The question, however, is whether more is better — that is, more than the minimum requirements set by the government (see Chapter 23).

✔ **Electricity, magnets, light, and sound.** Many alternative practices assume that the human body is made up of *energy fields* — invisible waves of electromagnetic or some other form of energy. Illness occurs when these fields become blocked or unbalanced. Some alternative approaches use various natural substances — including crystals, magnets, electrical currents, light, and sound waves to detect and correct these blockages and imbalances (see Chapter 24).

Conventional Therapies "Alternative Style"

Somewhere down the line a health care practitioner may offer you one of the following therapies. Whether the doctor is conventional or alternative, the approaches are definitely "off-label." That is, each began as a conventional technique but is now being put to all sorts of unconventional (and generally unproven) uses.

Chelation therapy

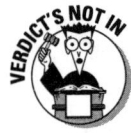

Chelation therapy began as a sophisticated technique developed during WWII to help clear the body of heavy metals. Basically, the patient gets injected with a chemical called *EDTA* (which stands for the mouthful *ethylenediamine tetraacetic acid* — chemists are so poetic!), which grabs onto lead and other bad-news minerals (the word *chelation* comes from the Greek word for "claw") hanging out in the bloodstream. The EDTA and whatever chemicals it grabbed get shuttled out of the body.

EDTA is a great way to get the lead out. But today, it's also a controversial "circulatory enhancer" hyped by some physicians and alternative practitioners. It's supposed to improve blood flow by clearing out calcium (a big part of artery-clogging plaque) from blood vessels — thus relieving leg cramps, lowering blood pressure, and helping prevent heart attack and stroke. Some people even think that it can relieve the pain and swelling of arthritis and many diseases of the joints, bones, and connective tissues. Others say that it may reduce the need for insulin in people with diabetes, prevent cancer, and slow the progression of Alzheimer's disease.

Does it work? To be honest, no one really knows. Right now, some studies of chelation therapy are going on at Stanford, but as of this writing no decent (controlled, double-blind) studies show that EDTA makes a difference in deaths or disability of any sort. And none show that it is safe. So, unless you have serious lead poisoning, avoid it for now!

Enzyme therapy

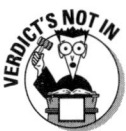

Enzymes are proteins that speed up *(catalyze)* chemical reactions in the body — such as the digestion of food, the build-up of tissue, and so on. If you don't have enough enzymes, vital processes can slow almost to a halt — and you can miss out on essential nutrients. So it's standard for a conventional doctor to prescribe enzyme supplements in these cases.

Conventional doctors also recommend enzyme supplements for certain intestinal problems. Probably the best-known is *lactase* (sold as Lactaid). This enzyme is necessary to break down lactose, a sugar in milk and dairy products. If you're lactase-deficient (lactose-intolerant), a glass of milk or a grilled cheese sandwich can lead to a bout of bloating, gas, cramping, and/or diarrhea. If you can't avoid dairy, taking lactase can help.

Another conventional enzyme supplement is *alpha galactosidase* — more popularly known as Beano. This enzyme helps break down sugars found in beans and peas — keeping the sugar out of the intestine where it can incite excessive gas and flatulence.

Some alternative healers, though, are prescribing enzymes for just about everyone and everything. Some of the enzymes used in enzyme therapy come from plants, others from the pancreases of animals. The plant stuff is supposed to promote general health and help you digest fiber. The pancreatic enzymes are supposed to cure a wide variety of otherwise incurable woes — including multiple sclerosis, cancer, arthritis, and viral infections. Even healthy people supposedly suffer all sorts of dire consequences from not taking these enzymes on a regular basis.

No good scientific evidence proves any of these claims. A couple of studies suggest that *bromelain,* an enzyme derived from pineapple plants, may help relieve swelling and inflammation. But basically, unless you are lactase-deficient or have a problem eating beans, skip this alternative.

IV vitamins

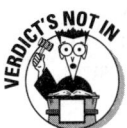

Some people with certain medical or inherited conditions can't absorb enough vitamins and minerals the natural way — through the gut after eating. So they need injections of these vital substances right into their veins, a process known as *intravenous* (or *IV) therapy.*

Alternative medicine has extended this idea to healthy people whose guts are perfectly fine absorbers, thank you very much. The idea is that by shooting megadoses of the stuff into the veins, you can get much more dramatic effects than by swallowing pills. To relieve your cold or asthma symptoms, for example, someone may suggest infusing a "cocktail" of 25 grams of vitamin C (over 400 times the recommended daily dose!) along with huge amounts of other vitamins and minerals. Other people suggest the same cocktail for treating heart disease and speeding recovery from surgery, fatigue, chronic infection, arthritis, or just plain inundation with the "toxins" of daily life. Even better, they'll tell you that this approach presents no proven negatives, other than possible reactions to preservatives or low blood pressure if the mineral magnesium is "pushed in" too quickly.

In reality, some evidence suggests that IV vitamin C *may* speed the healing of wounds after surgery — though probably at some cost to the kidneys and other organs. As for the other claims, stay tuned. Like any therapy that's supposed to work for just about every ailment on earth, and without any side effects, this approach should be viewed with extreme skepticism.

Environmental medicine

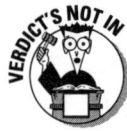

There's no question that what goes in and around our bodies — air, water, food, pesticides, synthetic dyes, and the like — affects our health. Public health officials who evaluate and try to control these effects work in the field of *environmental medicine*. They do research such as studying the health effects of pesticide-infested food or asbestos-laden buildings. Or they may try to explain why unusually high rates of cancer, lung disease, or birth defects show up in towns near landfills or toxic dumps.

There's a big leap between recognizing that modern life exposes people to many potentially toxic chemicals, and claims to *know* — no question about it — that someone's particular health problem is due to an environmental "allergy." Based on very little evidence, certain alternative practitioners insist that environmental toxins underlie a huge array of health problems, including migraine headaches, arthritis, eczema, depression, colitis, nerve disorders, hyperactivity and attention deficit disorder, chronic fatigue syndrome, memory loss, incapacitation, and even death.

It's an even bigger leap to say that you *know* how to cure all these problems (except death, of course) simply by changing a patient's environment. The alternative practitioners of environmental medicine believe that not just the *allergen* (the substance provoking allergic reactions) is at fault. Many other factors — such as genetics, poor nutrition, infections, chemical exposure, and stress — are also involved.

Using terms such as "multiple chemical sensitivities" or specific "food or nutrient sensitivities," doctors who practice the alternative form of environmental medicine say that blood tests can detect substances released into the body of people allergic to these toxins. Too much exposure to the allergen, they claim, wreaks havoc with the immune system.

Bloodwork of the alternate kind

Part of environmental medicine involves checking out your blood and tissues for residues of pesticides, hydrocarbons, or other toxic chemicals that supposedly explain weight problems, indigestion, fatigue, irritable bowel syndrome, bloating, chronic sinus infections, ear infections, and headaches. Practitioners say that they can check your blood for "signs" of a challenged immune system (such as high levels of white blood cells and natural antibodies) and "mediators" released by sensitive body cells when troublesome toxins (foods) are lurking. Some practitioners like to check your hair or urine for heavy metals, too. The result is a huge industry offering elaborate, expensive tests with little justification — and, of course, the tests are followed by expensive supplements that will supposedly fix all the bad readings. In our opinion, this whole field rests on shaky ground. Buyer beware!

The only answer, say practitioners (other than retreating to a rustic home in the mountains or desert), is to detoxify your system — that is, purge it of nasty poisons — and build up your immune system. This detoxification involves taking massive doses of vitamins or various herbs or oxygen therapy (see the upcoming section, "Oxygen therapies"). They may try to sell you various "ecomasks," air and water filters, hypoallergenic vitamins, "negative ion generators" (whatever they are), and chemical-free clothing. You may also be asked to cut the offending substances from your diet, or rotate possible culprits to try to figure out what's causing the problem.

This approach may be helpful if you're really reacting to environmental substances inappropriately, but check the practitioner's credentials carefully and watch your wallet. More often than not, the treatment will cost you a pretty penny — out of your own pocket — for questionable results.

Cell therapies

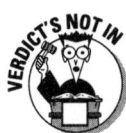

No matter what your problem is, someone trying to sell you cell therapy will claim to be able to treat it. Want your arthritis, heart disease, menstrual cramps, infertility, cancer, herpes, lung disease, epilepsy, Down's syndrome, Parkinson's disease, or hot flashes to go away? Want sexual prowess, youthful skin, a stronger heart, or even immortality? Nothing is too much to ask.

Whether you'll get it or not is highly doubtful. What isn't doubtful is that the treatment will cost you a bundle. If you live in the United States, include travel costs in your calculations, too. Cell therapy is unapproved in the United States, though it's popular in Europe and many other countries. Ever since it was first developed in Switzerland in 1931, it has attracted throngs of the world's rich and famous, many of whom assumed that they could buy themselves eternal youth and beauty.

Conventional doctors transfer cells from healthy to sick people all the time. Think of blood transfusions, for example, or bone marrow transplants. More recently, there have been some intriguing attempts to treat diseases such as diabetes, Alzheimer's disease, and Parkinson's disease with transplanted cells from human fetuses.

In the alternative form of cell therapy, however, the transferred cells (which are usually injected into the patient) come from an animal, usually glands from sheep or pigs. Ideally, these cells are freeze-dried, sterilized, and finely filtered to prevent rejection (and, yes, the freeze-drying idea came right out of the coffee business!). Cells from the animal's liver are said to go right to the liver of a person with hepatitis, cells from the pig's gonads go right to the man's testicles to cure impotence, and so on. Meanwhile, these cells are supposedly bolstering the entire immune system. That's why some alternative practitioners use it as a "helper therapy" alongside other treatments and why others think that it may be useful in treating AIDS.

The trouble is, there's just no convincing evidence that any of this stuff works. Anecdotes and testimonials abound, some of them even from prominent scientists. But until someone does some hard-core studies, we advise you to avoid cell therapy altogether.

Oxygen therapies

Lots of people take antioxidants such as vitamins C and E to *prevent* a chemical process called oxidation that may be involved in cell destruction. Oxidizing agents are chemicals that do this oxidizing. So why on earth would anyone use them to promote healing?

Good question. The thinking here is that oxygen — the main agent that does the oxidizing — is a good thing (even though it can be highly toxic!). We need it to breathe, right? Sick people often need extra oxygen, right? And *hyperbaric oxygen therapy* (which involves inhaling pure pressurized oxygen) can reduce air bubbles that can form in blood vessels during medical procedures, reverse carbon monoxide poisoning, spur regrowth of crushed or irradiated blood vessels, cure chronic wounds and bone infections, help heal burns, and offset "the bends" that can kill deep-sea divers.

However (and it's a big however), using this therapy to treat or relieve symptoms of AIDS, stroke, cancer, senility, and multiple sclerosis is much more speculative — and right now too uncertain to justify using this costly therapy. Claims that hyperbaric oxygen therapy can help with other problems — such as heart disease, ear infections, and recovery from drug addiction — have even less evidence. Plus, oxygen under high pressure can cause serious damage (including ruptured membranes, collapsed lungs, and cataracts), so this is not a technique to be undertaken lightly.

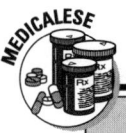

Superfluous stuff about oxidation and oxidizing therapy

Oxidation is a chemical reaction during which one molecule donates electrons to another. The molecule getting the electrons is said to be "*oxidized*" (and the one losing electrons is said to be "*reduced*"). Quite often the electrons come from an oxygen (O_2) molecule — hence the term "oxidation." A certain amount of oxidation has to happen for the body to function. Oxidation therapy is based on the theory that repeated environmental stress cuts down on the ideal amount of oxidation. Restoring it with extra doses of oxygen — in one of several forms — is supposed to rev up these reactions and, in the process, heal just about any ailment.

Even more speculative — and dangerous — is using oxygen in other forms to treat disease. The two most popular of these methods are *hydrogen peroxide therapy* and *ozone therapy.*

Hydrogen peroxide therapy

To some people, hydrogen peroxide sounds like the yucky stuff in the brown bottles that your dentist wants you to swish around in your mouth or that your mother used to dab on your cuts to prevent infection. And, in fact, it is. But it's also an abundant natural chemical (H_2O_2 to be precise — a water molecule with an extra oxygen atom attached).

It's one thing to rub a tiny bit of 3 percent hydrogen peroxide solution into a scrape, and quite another to drink, inject, snort, gargle, or soak yourself in higher concentrations of this stuff. No evidence we know of shows that hydrogen peroxide douches, footbaths, enemas, or injections can "detoxify" your system, boost your immunity, cure your arthritis, or anything else.

Worse, hydrogen peroxide can hurt — even kill — you if used incorrectly. Don't worry if you swallow or spill a bit of the 3 percent stuff (the amount in standard mouthwashes, toothpastes, skin cleansers, and the like), but don't even think of buying any higher concentrations, and throw out any that may be lurking in your medicine cabinet.

And if you're considering drinking 35 percent hydrogen peroxide to treat your arthritis or other ailments, think again. We can't say for sure what it will do for your symptoms, but chances are you won't be around to find out. Also stay away from anyone who wants to inject you with high concentrations of hydrogen peroxide to treat AIDS, cancer, yeast infections, depression, lupus, multiple sclerosis, fractures, and all manner of woes.

Oxygen-ozone therapy

Although banned in many countries including the United States, ozone therapy is used in Cuba, Brazil, Israel, Australia, and some parts of Europe to treat many serious health problems, including cancer, HIV-related disorders, arthritis, herpes, blocked arteries, and prostatitis.

The ozone used in "ozone therapy" is pretty much like oxygen, except that it's made up of molecules that have three oxygen atoms instead of the usual two. It's just as natural as oxygen — in fact, it's the same ozone that's being destroyed in our atmosphere. When the O_3 hits the bloodstream, it happily gives away its extra oxygen atom — boosting the body's oxygen.

Advocates say that this extra oxygen can destroy microorganisms; alleviate arthritis and prostatitis; clear blocked arteries; destroy cancer cells; and even cure AIDS, herpes, and hepatitis. Even if you're not sick, they add, you can probably use the immune boost of ozone therapy — especially because in today's polluted environment none of us gets enough oxygen.

The oxygen or ozone is put into the body through a variety of methods — some of them innocuous and others pretty petrifying (such as blowing the ozone into women's vaginas to treat yeast infections) or gruesome (such as a method called *rectal insufflation* — need we say more?). The most common method — called *autohemotherapy* — involves removing a pint of blood from the patient, bubbling ozone through it, and injecting it back through a vein.

There have been very few human studies proving the extravagant claims for ozone therapy — and even fewer with enough subjects or legitimate research techniques to be convincing. On the plus side, increasing evidence (though further study is needed) shows that ozone therapy can at least improve quality of life for AIDS patients and may even help clear blocked arteries. Also, except for the blow to your bank account, ozone therapy — if (and this is a big if) used correctly — doesn't have any known side effects.

Finding Good Information on Alternative Medicine

Even more choices are out there than we mention in this chapter — but don't despair! On the slight chance that we've overlooked some therapy you're anxious to check out, you can almost certainly find someone willing to tell you about it. Of course, the competence of that person doing the telling can be tough to gauge. That's where we can make your life a lot easier. Read on!

Decoding scientific information

Way too often, evidence comes tangled up with scientific jargon (researchers seem to think that the more obscure they are, the more profound). It's helpful to remember that every single one of these words can be translated into plain English with a good dictionary. An even better way of getting a quick translation is enlisting the services of a scientifically savvy friend — or a health care provider.

You don't have a friend like this? S.O.S. your local public or medical librarian. Or contact the U.S. National Library of Medicine (NLM) Web site at www.nlm.nih.gov; phone them at 888-FINDNLM (888-346-3656) or 301-594-5983; or send snail mail to The National Library of Medicine, 8600 Rockville Pike, Bethesda, MD 20894.

Here are some other helpful "information decoding hints" to remember:

- Don't believe everything you read.

- Never rely on a single source.

- Always ask, "How do they know that?" If the answer doesn't seem like real proof (see Chapter 3), consider the claims unproven.

- Be careful about any information that you get off the "Web." A lot of horse-hockey is out there, plus a lot of sites designed merely to sell you something.

- Remember that one or two scientific papers are not "proof."

Using your computer to get (good!) alternative information

One great way to keep on top of new or obscure therapies is the Internet — which can change its information from day-to-day in a way no published text can do. As you undoubtedly know (or have heard), however, the Internet really is the wild West — everyone's out there by (and for) themselves. Stick with the following sites, though, and the five basic "information decoding hints" (see the sidebar, "Decoding scientific information"), and you won't go far astray.

By the way, even Internet novices can easily access information with the help of *The Internet For Dummies,* 5th Edition, by John R. Levine, Carol Baroudi, and Margaret Levine Young (published by IDG Books Worldwide, Inc. — not that we're biased or anything). And not owning a computer is no excuse — most public libraries offer free access, and surfing lessons to boot!

Web sites of worth

Here are a few of the most helpful Web sites (at least the last time we checked!):

- ✔ **Health WWWeb: Integrative Medicine, Natural Health and Alternative Therapies** at `www.healthwwweb.com`. This easy-to-use site lets you call up information on a growing list of alternative therapies, plus find references to health organizations, discussion groups, training programs, upcoming events, and useful books. The site is maintained by an alternative-minded health care corporation.

- ✔ **NIH Office of Alternative Medicine (OAM)** at `altmed.od.nih.gov`. This official government site includes an Information Clearinghouse, text of quarterly newsletters, and links to other government sites.

- ✔ **World Health Organization (WHO)** at `www.who.org/pll/dsa/cat95/trad5.htm`. Check out what the World Health Organization (WHO) has to say about various types of traditional medicine at this site.

Advice from cyberspace

Web sites offering advice on medical alternatives:

- ✔ **Ask Dr. Weil** at `cgi.pathfinder.com/@@0uvdrwUAC803dy7b/drweil`. (Yes, it's a lot of letters.) Click on <u>Ask your Question</u> at the upper-right corner of this page, and the renowned Andrew Weil, M.D., will respond. Go back to the home page for access to bulletin boards, polls, home remedies, a Dr. Ruth sex clinic, and more fun stuff.

- ✔ **HealthWorld Online Alternative & Complementary Medicine Center** at `www.healthy.net/clinic/therapy/index.html`. Here you can ask selected experts about various aspects of alternative and complementary medicine, plus find other gems. The site also offers free access to the MEDLINE database (see the next section).

Databases of distinction

If you want to dive into the research papers themselves, here are some relatively easy ways to find them:

- ✔ **MEDLINE.** The National Library of Medicine (NLM) has crammed 20 million printed references into one computer-based retrieval system known as MEDLARS (Medical Literature Analysis and Retrieval System). This system includes over 40 online electronic databases, but the one to check out for alternative medicine data is MEDLINE at `www.nlm.nih.gov/databases/freemedl.html`. Because the NLM maintains rigorous standards for accepting journals into its databases, you can feel pretty good about the studies you pull up. Two Web-based products, PubMed and Internet Grateful Med, provide this access.

By searching this database for relevant terms (such as "color therapy," for example) you can get citations and often brief summaries ("abstracts") for relevant studies — and order the complete papers. The articles you pull up are written by and for professionals, but once you have them in hand, cracking the code is easy (see the sidebar "Decoding scientific information").

Navigating MEDLINE takes a little time and practice, but if you surf to the NLM's MEDLINE Web site listed in the preceding bullet, they'll walk you through the process. Or call 800-423-9255 to get Internet Grateful Med software (another way to access MEDLINE). You can also contact the Office of Alternative Medicine's Clearinghouse (altmed.od.nih.gov/oam/clearinghouse), which offers information to the public about alternative medicine, and ask for the fact sheet, *Alternative Medicine Research Using MEDLINE.*

✔ **NLM's other databases.** If you don't find what you're looking for in MEDLINE, you can also try the many other health-related databases maintained by the National Library of Medicine. Check out the NLM Home Page (www.nlm.nih.gov) for details, or call the NLM at 888-FINDNLM (888-346-3656) or 301-594-5983. While you're on the home page, by the way, don't forget to look over their many other publications, all of which are available online.

✔ **The CRISP System.** This huge database offers information about biomedical studies funded by certain U.S. government institutions. Access it at www-commons.dcrt.nih.gov; click on the CRISP button in the left column. If you need navigational help, go to NLM's Internet home page (www.nih.gov) or contact the Research Documentation Section of the Office of Extramural Research, National Institutes of Health at 6701 Rockledge Drive, MSC 7772, Bethesda, MD 20892-7772, phone 301-435-0650, or e-mail: DRT@CUOD.NIH.GOV.

Directories of alternative information

Fortunately for us, other folks have put together directories of links to alternative information on the Web. Here are a few worth checking (the Web offers many others, but too many indiscriminately include lots of junk):

✔ **Alternative Medicine — Health Care Information Resources** at www.hsl.mcmaster.ca/tomflem/altmed.html. Lists both general resources (such as Web pages) on alternative medicine, as well as links to information on specific practices. They tell you up front that "The inclusion of a site in this list of resources is not an endorsement of its claims."

✔ **SPAN IT Health & Medicine** at www.spanit.com/Health.html. This list includes some unusual links to both conventional and unconventional sites that offer advice on alternatives.

✔ **Yahoo! Home: Health: Alternative Medicine** at `www.yahoo.com/Health/Alternative_Medicine`. This site offers a simple-to-use list from the well-known search engine.

✔ **Internet Medical and Health Care Resources** at `www.healthwwweb.com/LinksIndex.html`. Brought to you by the same folks who bring you the Health WWWeb Website, this is another fairly comprehensive list of links to alternative topics.

Finding other sources of information

If you don't have/like/understand the Internet, plenty of other relatively accessible, reliable, and up-to-date resources are available. Here are the sources we think are best bets:

✔ **Your health care provider.** Yes, we know that we said that many conventional M.D.s don't know a whole lot about alternative medicine. And we stand by that — though, again, that situation is changing for the better. But that lack of physician knowledge doesn't mean that you shouldn't ask your conventional doc about alternative options (the next chapter explains how to interpret what your doctor says). Conventional doctors can help steer you away from out-and-out fraud, and — by doing what they do best — they can also help rule out serious conditions that may require more conventional treatment.

Talking to alternative health care providers can help, too, especially when it comes to therapies they don't offer themselves. A great way to get good information is to ask people about their competitors — some of the stuff you'll hear may be based on jealousy or ignorance, but you can also glean some real problems that you won't hear by asking practitioners directly about the potential dangers of their particular approaches.

✔ **The telephone or the mails.** Many of the resources listed under "computers" are also accessible via more traditional means. Probably the best, though, is the Office of Alternative Medicine's Clearinghouse in Silver Spring, MD. Their toll-free telephone number is 888-644-6226; this is also the TTY/TDY number for the hearing impaired.

The Clearinghouse's toll-free number is answered by trained information specialists from Monday through Friday, from 8:30 a.m. to 5:00 p.m. Eastern Time. Information specialists can answer inquiries in both English or Spanish. If you're put on hold too long, just leave your name and number, and someone will call you back.

You can also ask for fact sheets to be sent to you via fax by writing them at P.O. Box 8218, Silver Spring, MD 20907-8218.

✔ **The library.** With all the to-do about computers and the Internet, too many people overlook a time-tested resource: the public library. If you have access to a university or medical school library, all the better. Besides shuffling through the card catalog (or the computerized version), you can use various indexes of magazine articles to see what has been written on your topic (start with the *Reader's Guide to Periodical Literature*). If you can get to a medical or university library (and some public libraries), you can also check the *Index Medicus* for articles published in over 3,000 health-science journals.

Online versions of these guides can sometimes bring the actual articles to your fingertips — and can be a great introduction to the world of online information if you don't have a computer at home.

Even if you can only get yourself to a small library, the Interlibrary Loan system allows you to borrow books from virtually any library in the world. Just ask a reference librarian about it.

One of the best things you can do for yourself is to make friends with a reference librarian. These usually knowledgeable and helpful people are among the few "free" resources left in this world. Tell them what you want to know about, and they'll ladle out information until it hurts. They'll even teach you how to use the library's information resources.

✔ **Health information services.** If you don't like hunting for information yourself, you can hire someone to do the work for you — and tell you what it means! These information services can cost you real money (usually at least $80 to $200) — but if you don't want to wade through technical medical indexes yourself or translate medical jargon into English, they can be lifesavers. If you've been diagnosed with a serious or life-threatening condition, they can be a worthwhile investment.

For a fee, these services will do a database search on your condition and write an individualized (and understandable) "research report" that lets you know what treatment methods have been tried by other people. They'll also direct you to support groups, reference materials, and both conventional and alternative therapies.

Probably the most-established among these services is Health Resource in Conway, Arkansas at 800-949-0090. Another good bet is the Planetree Health Resource Center in San Francisco at 415-923-3681.

Remember, though, that the people writing these reports for these services have not examined you personally — and are not licensed to practice medicine. Check with your health care practitioner before taking action on any information you read — especially if you may have a serious condition.

✔ **Support groups.** Misery loves company. Support groups provide plenty of that, and they exist for just about any disease you can think of. Besides providing validation and possibly even health benefits (see Chapter 19), these groups can be great sources of ideas about how to live with your condition. After all, the other members aren't talking theoretically. They know what it's like to have chronic fatigue syndrome and desperately need to get out of the house each day. They know what it's like to have back pain so intense that life doesn't seem worth living. If some treatment method seems to work — however alternative it may be — chances are members will share it with the group.

Remember that testimonials aren't too meaningful for determining whether a treatment will work for *you* — or whether it's safe. But they can give you some ideas about what approach *may* work, especially if you can find any controlled scientific trials supporting claims.

✔ **Advocacy associations.** Some support groups are affiliated with (or sponsored by) advocacy associations. These groups usually try to influence legislation to help victims of particular diseases — especially by improving insurance benefits, disability payments, research funding, and so on. They also often provide educational materials to promote public awareness and to help victims of the disease and their families. Quite often newsletters published by these groups discuss alternative treatments as well. To find a support group or advocacy organization for your particular condition, just check local papers, bulletin boards, and hospitals. Or check out Chapter 6 for advice about how to contact various organizations that help link people and support/self-help groups.

Part II
Complementing Your Medicine

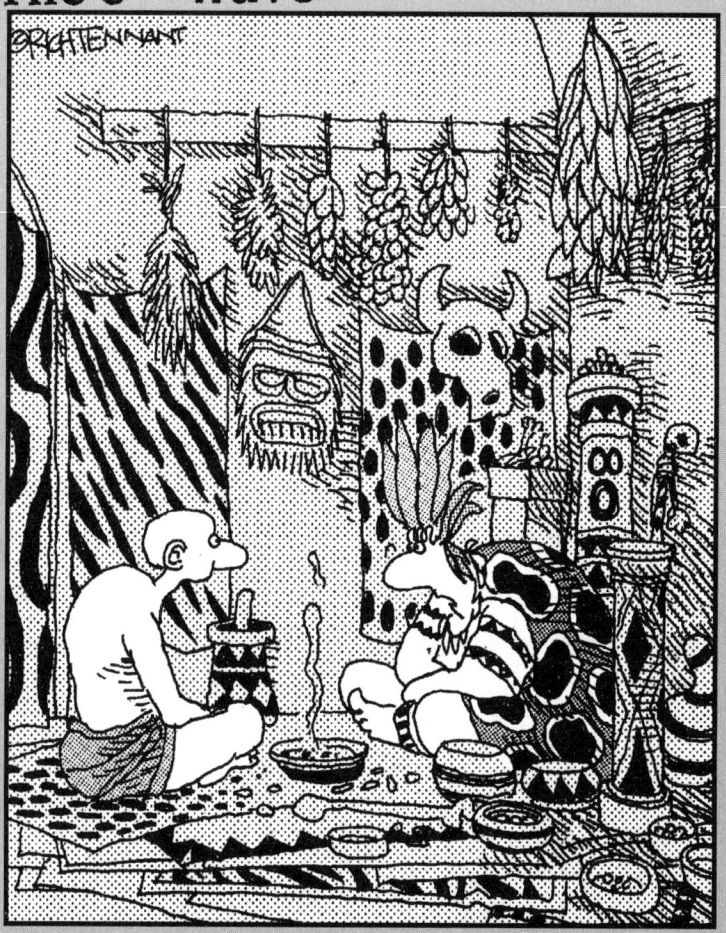

"Penicillin? I'm sorry— I don't practice alternative medicine."

In this part . . .

In this part, you find out how to use alternative medicine most effectively. We explain why using alternatives alongside conventional medicine is often the way to go, plus we show how you can reap the benefits of both approaches without losing your mind, your money, or the good will of your conventional doctor. Along the way, you discover how you can sometimes get your insurance company to help pay for alternatives — not a bad deal! For those of you who are shy or conflict-averse, we offer tips for broaching the often touchy subject of alternative medicine with skeptical friends, family, and physicians. And finally, we arm you with all the information you need to navigate a modern health food store or pharmacy — and to zero in on marketing hype.

Chapter 5

Mixing Conventional and Alternative Medicines

● ●

In This Chapter

▶ Why using alternatives together with conventional medicine is the way to go

▶ How to work alternatives into a conventional approach

▶ What to do if your conventional doctor hates alternative medicine

▶ What to do if you hate conventional medicine

▶ How to find out who pays for alternative treatments

● ●

*V*iewing alternative and conventional medicine as two battling armies is a thing of the past. If you're interested in getting healthy and staying that way — and who isn't? — the solution is to take what's best from any system of medicine, however it labels itself. The key is finding out how to do that effectively, which is what this chapter is all about.

How to Have Your Cake and Eat It, Too

It's obvious that alternative and conventional medicines are joining forces all around us. Lots of people have their M.D. prescribe an antibiotic for an infection but see a chiropractor or try botanicals to calm chronic indigestion. Other people who take prescription anti-anxiety drugs also try stress-relieving herbal remedies, yoga, or massage therapy on the side.

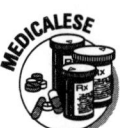

Boosting or "complementing" mainstream treatment with one or two alternatives is sometimes called *complementary medicine*. Sometimes it's also called *CAM* — which is simply a short version of the mouthful "complementary and alternative medicine."

What integration is all about

The ideal health care draws on whichever traditions, practices, and philosophies make sense for the individual patient. A lot of words for this approach are being kicked around right now by people who like to label things. We use these three terms:

- ✔ **Complementary medicine:** Using an alternative or two to boost conventional treatment (see the preceding section).

- ✔ **Integrative medicine:** Turning to any valid (and relevant) method of healing rather than sticking to one particular system.

- ✔ **Pluralistic health care**: People using a lot of different systems to heal themselves. Unlike integrative medicine, which describes two or more approaches used by a single practitioner, this term is used by policy wonks to describe two or more approaches used by a single *patient* (or a whole population of patients).

A lot of these labels are nothing more than hair splitting. The good news, though, is that they all mean that more and more people are forgetting about labels and just using whatever methods they can to get and stay healthy. That's what integrative medicine is really all about.

If you've ever gone to a "wellness clinic," you may have seen integrative medicine in action. More and more groups of various health care professionals — maybe a mainstream M.D., a chiropractor, a massage therapist, a nutritionist, and/or a physical therapist — are working together as equal players to offer a fairly holistic treatment plan. In the old-fashioned clinic (such as the famous Mayo Clinic), M.D.s may have worked with other health care professionals, but they were the top dogs. In integrative medicine, everyone's on an equal footing.

Why combining alternative and conventional medicines is smart

If you're lucky enough to have an M.D. who is treating you effectively (and that includes cost effectively), there's no reason to seek alternative care. If you're not satisfied with what conventional medicine is doing for you, though, don't throw out the baby with the bathwater—that is, don't forget that some parts of your conventional care are worth keeping. For safe and effective care, your provider needs a complete picture of your overall treatment plan — both the conventional and alternative aspects. That's why letting your conventional doctor know about your alternative treatments — and vice versa — is a smart move.

Unfortunately, most of the "complementing" and "integrating" that's happening right now is being done by the patients — with M.D.s left out of the loop.

Dr. David Eisenberg of the Harvard Medical School estimates that over 70 percent of patients using alternative medicine have never mentioned it to their physicians. This lack of disclosure is bad news. It leaves people open to all sorts of risks — risks from mixing together incompatible treatments, missing out on a serious diagnosis, or using herbs, botanicals, and supplements incorrectly. (See Chapter 2 for more on what can go wrong.) The widely reported deaths from overdoses of ma huang (a Chinese herbal medicine) in 1996 — as well as a recently reported death from the popular herb pennyroyal — are just some of the sad examples.

Unless you have a temporary, obviously minor problem, don't even think about trying an alternative (even a preventive approach) until you check with your regular doctor to:

- ✔ Rule out the possibility of serious illness.

- ✔ Make sure that the alternative doesn't interfere with anything else you're doing.

- ✔ Make sure that the alternative is safe for you — based on your personal medical history.

- ✔ Give you a built-in expert to help evaluate (and, if you're lucky, even supply) the often hard-to-find or inadequate evidence on the safety and efficacy of alternatives.

When you can use alternatives alone

Checking with an M.D. isn't always essential, of course. If you have a common, non-life threatening problem — or just want to help speed the healing of a long-term but stable condition — you can often start by trying one or more simple alternatives on your own, without too much risk. Almost all mind-body approaches fall into this category, as do many kinds of hydrotherapy (soaking sore muscles, icing sprains, and the like) and other home remedies. Make sure that you get professional care if the alternatives don't work — or if there's any chance that your symptoms may be due to a more serious condition.

A plan for complementary care

The following plan is based on a process proposed by Harvard's Dr. David Eisenberg, one of the gurus of the CAM (complementary and alternative medicine) world. The plan assumes a lot of stuff that probably isn't true in everyone's case — such as an M.D. who is completely sympathetic to alternative adventures, and an insurance plan that will pay for all the visits and phone calls to that M.D.. But the plan is a good guidepost anyway for the kind of give-and-take relationship between doctor and patient that you can work toward. Follow these steps:

1. **See your regular M.D.** If you don't have one, get one. Explain your main symptoms. After listening (politely, please) to conventional wisdom, ask whether any alternative approaches are applicable. If you know about a possible alternative that your M.D. isn't aware of, don't be afraid to mention it and at least get the doc's opinion (bringing in articles about the approach — or relevant chapters from this book — can help). Talk about starting a *symptom diary* — where you can record every instance of your problem and describe what else was happening when it hit (such as eating chocolate ice cream, screaming at your kids, being screamed at by your boss, and so on).

2. **Actually keep a symptom diary.** Down the line, a diary is a much better way than hindsight to see what *really* sets off your symptoms, how much the symptoms *really* bother you, and how often they *really* occur. You may be surprised. After they start a diary, many people who think that they have migraines "all the time" find that they only have them about once a week. Some people who think that taking the hormone melatonin makes their insomnia milder find that the frequency doesn't differ at all — they just thought that they used to have more trouble sleeping than they actually did. A symptom diary is also a great way to see for yourself whether a treatment — alternative or otherwise — makes any difference. Keeping this record is like doing your very own science experiment on the most important subject in the world (you!).

3. **Select an alternative therapy.** Make a choice based on what you find out from this book (and other sources — see Chapter 4 for suggestions) and what your M.D. has told you. Find an alternative provider (see the next chapter if you need help). Make an appointment — but don't start treatment yet.

4. **See your M.D. again before starting alternative treatment.** Review questions you plan to ask the alternative provider and ask for suggestions. The right questions can help you rule out dangerous, wasteful, or fraudulent practices — and incompetent providers.

5. **Visit the alternative provider.** Ask a lot of questions about what treatments will be like, how many you'll need, how long you can expect to wait before seeing some results, what the treatment is going to cost, and any conflicts with conventional treatments. Also ask about that particular provider's experience with your particular problem as well as training, certification, and licensing. (See Chapter 6 for more specific questions to ask.)

6. **Call or visit the conventional M.D. again.** Review the treatment plan you worked out with the alternative provider. The idea is that your doctor should assess the safety of the plan and be on call to monitor its effects. Meanwhile, you should continue your symptom diary.

7. **Try the alternative approach.** Visit your doctor as often as you've agreed to and follow the treatment as planned. Keep writing in your diary, and let your M.D. know what's happening.

8. **Follow up with your M.D.** After you've tried the alternative long enough to expect some results, see your M.D. another time. Together, you can review the experience and your diary. Decide together whether the alternative seemed to help.

When You and Your M.D. Disagree

We admit that bringing up the subject of alternatives with a conventional doctor can be daunting — and, more likely than not, you won't get the approval you want. (Check Chapter 7 for tips on how to discuss alternatives with your M.D.) But this discussion is key if you want to use alternatives safely.

If your conventional doctor just won't listen, try to change doctors. (Almost all health plans allow you to do this if you squawk loud enough.) If you basically like and trust your doctor, though, you can try educating him or her (see Chapter 7) about the virtues of alternative medicine. With the right ammunition (including a copy of this book!), you can expect a lot more open-mindedness.

You can also agree to disagree — especially about alternatives for which little scientific evidence of safety and efficacy is available. Many M.D.s feel uncomfortable sanctioning a therapy about which little is known — and rightly so — but that doesn't mean that you can't decide to take the risk on your own shoulders if you can persuade your doctor to monitor your health as you're trying the therapy.

This approach is easy if you just think of yourself as a partner in the health care process — capable of actively participating in decisions involving your own body. Just remember that with this power comes responsibility — and when you take some of the responsibility onto yourself, you take some away from your doctor.

When You Just Won't Take Conventional for an Answer

Even if you think that physicians are the root of all evil and doctors do more harm than good, do yourself a favor and have a thorough medical exam; then do what you want with what the doctor tells you. Sure, it's nicer to keep believing that your woes are due to a vitamin imbalance and not cancer. But no reputable physician — or author — is going to encourage you not to go after the truth. Of course, no one (least of all us) can force you to go to a doctor. Just remember, though, that if you make this choice, you can't blame anyone else when you don't get better.

Note that providing a basic medical history and undergoing an examination is not the same thing as agreeing to an invasive medical treatment. It's simply a way to give yourself peace of mind about not having a serious disease — especially the life-threatening kinds that conventional medicine is best at helping. Remember that acupuncturists, massage therapists, nutritionists, herbalists, and homeopaths are usually not licensed or trained to diagnose any medical illness and generally do not want that responsibility. You don't have to agree to uncomfortable or expensive tests (such as CAT scans) if you don't want to, but you should at least hear the M.D.s opinion as to why you might benefit from these.

After you hear your options, you can choose which, if any, treatments you want to use — conventional and/or alternative. This is *real* integrative (and holistic) medicine!

Who's Going to Pay for Alternative Care?

A lot of people have come to expect someone else to pay for their health care (that's one of the reasons costs have gotten out-of-hand — why shop cost if someone else is paying, at least in the short term?). But one of the biggest testaments to the appeal of alternative medicine is that so many people have been paying for it out of their own pockets — to the tune of $10 billion per year in the United States.

Until better research shows that alternative therapies work — and (probably even more important) save money — don't expect too much help from insurers. Even so, for certain types of alternative treatment, we suggest looking into your insurance policy. You may be surprised. In fact, many insurance plans offer at least some coverage for the following types of treatment: acupuncture, biofeedback, chiropractic, nutrition counseling, osteopathy, and preventive medicine.

According to a study in the *American Journal of Health Promotion* 12 (November/December 1997): 112–122, some insurers also cover herbal medicine, guided imagery, hypnotherapy, meditation, *Qi Gong*, support groups, yoga therapy, Ayurveda, homeopathy, naturopathy, Tibetan medicine, Chinese medicine, acupressure, Alexander technique, craniosacral therapy, massage therapy, naprapathy, reflexology, Reiki, Rolfing, shiatsu, and Tragerwork.

Many insurance companies have plans in the works to reimburse at least some forms of alternative care. Most states (41 at last count) already require private insurers to pick up costs of chiropractic care for low-back pain, and a handful of states require them to cover certain acupuncture and other alternative treatments. Some insurance companies also offer discounts on health food and vitamins, as well as health education books and tapes. And if you're lucky, you may even belong to (or be able to join) one of the growing number of insurance companies with specific policies covering alternative care — either through special alternative plans or as part of their regular plans. So before you pull out your wallet, ask some questions!

Even the best policies have limits, though. Don't expect reimbursement if:

- ✔ Treatment isn't "medically necessary" for your specific ailment.
- ✔ Treatment isn't a covered service in your particular policy.
- ✔ You're getting "wellness" treatment rather than care for a specific medical condition.
- ✔ Treatment exceeds a set number of visits or a dollar limit.
- ✔ No good scientific evidence shows that the treatment works.
- ✔ The provider is improperly trained and/or licensed or doesn't meet national quality assurance standards.
- ✔ The provider doesn't belong to the insurance company's network (unless the policy includes some "out of network" benefits).

Watch out for token coverage that's used mainly to bait consumers into buying policies. Insurance companies know that the public is showing a lot of interest in alternative medicine, so promoting plans that cover it is smart marketing. In the fine print though, a lot of this coverage is so limited that it can't really help you. Other companies are so anxious to beat the competition — or worse, to save themselves some dough — by offering alternative care that they pay for treatments not yet proven safe or effective.

Chapter 6

How to Find an Alternative Caregiver

- -

In This Chapter

▶ Discovering the qualities you want in a healer

▶ Getting names of alternative care providers

▶ Screening potential candidates — without paying a penny

▶ Identifying the pros and cons of licensing

▶ Deciding whether you've found the right practitioner

- -

*W*e hate books that tell you how to be a "good health care consumer" by listing a thousand questions you need to get answered — and then throwing you out to the wolves to find those answers. Most of the questions we discuss in this chapter are answered in this book. But you will have to answer a few questions about yourself and your provider before agreeing to pay anyone to help you get better. Fortunately, finding the answers doesn't involve a lot of legwork, and no library research (we promise!).

Finding "Dr. Right"

Too often, people think that they have to take whatever they get in health care — and, unfortunately, the policies of HMOs and insurance companies often encourage this thinking. One of the beauties of alternative care is that — although you often have to pay for it yourself — you also have the power to pick and choose your practitioner and your treatment method.

Knowing thyself

Before you can choose the right practitioner for you, you have to know what will make you happy. A lot of people get jumpy if they have to be so specific. But when you think about it, you'll realize that you definitely know what you *don't* like in a health care practitioner (such as doctors who phone their stockbrokers in the middle of your exam or offices with X-ray machines that date back to World War I). Flip your negatives over, and you'll know more about what kind of care you want.

You can also ask yourself what kind of doctor or healer makes you most comfortable. Think about what you care about — not what you *should* care about. If the gender, race, age, or religion of a practitioner matters to you, consider that issue. Do you like a "let nature heal you" approach — or all-out artillery attacks on disease? Do you want a practitioner who shares uncertainties with you — or someone who takes charge and makes you feel cared for? Knowing your likes and dislikes helps you eliminate healers who will only make you feel scared, uncomfortable, angry, or frustrated.

Finally, don't forget about the amount you're willing to pay (or what services your insurance company will pay for). You can eliminate a number of possibilities on this factor alone.

Finding the best places to get referrals

You can get the names of alternative health care practitioners from many sources. Remember, though, that no recommendation guarantees competence. At best, the referrals you get are only a starting point. After you have a list of names, you still have to make sure that the practitioner is the right one for *you* — and only you can make that determination. Even so, don't underestimate the time and agony you can save by getting a good list of possibilities. Try these sources:

- ✔ **Your regular M.D.** In most cases, asking your family doctor for a good massage therapist or chiropractor is an exercise in futility. It's always worth asking, though. More and more, conventional doctors are recognizing that they just can't do everything — and they are sending patients to alternative providers to perform the services they can't. If you do get a name from a conventional M.D., you can feel pretty comfortable about the person's competence (and willingness to work with conventional doctors).

- ✔ **Professional associations of alternative caregivers.** Most alternative specialties have national professional associations that will provide names of local practitioners (and sometimes estimated costs of treatment) for the asking. Their recommendations tend to come in the form of long and sterile lists (which are no guarantee that you and the practitioner will click), but the information should give you some peace of mind. You'll only be given names of caregivers who have acceptable training and credentials — and you can ask what these are if you don't feel like looking them up in this book. Check the Appendix to get the names of these associations.

✔ **Medical regulatory and licensing associations.** Many states license practitioners who provide certain alternative therapies, including acupuncture, chiropractic, massage therapy, herbal medicine, homeopathy, and naturopathy. You can contact these associations and ask for names of qualified practitioners close to home.

You can also use state and local regulatory agencies (including state consumer affairs departments) to check the credentials of a given practitioner or the going rate for a particular service. Ask if the practitioner is properly trained, licensed, and accredited to perform the offered services. While you're at it, ask whether any complaints or lawsuits have been reported. You can often get the names and numbers of regulatory agencies by asking the relevant professional association (see the preceding section).

✔ **Other alternative caregivers.** If you have a great chiropractor, by all means ask her if she knows a reputable massage therapist. Alternative healers often run in the same circles, and the professional opinion of someone you already know and trust is worth its weight in gold. Ask alternative healers whom you already trust which caregivers they use themselves. Just as you would with a regular doctor, ask if they would recommend the same healer (or approach) for their spouse or children. If you get a thumbs up, you can feel confident about the recommendation.

✔ **Schools of alternative care.** If you're gutsy enough to call the dean's office, you can often get a school of an alternative practice to refer you to its graduates who work near you (as well as to faculty members, if you live nearby). Assuming that the school is reputable, you're getting the name of someone with adequate training. Whether or not this person has kept up by getting proper credentials or, when relevant, licensing, is something you'll have to find out for yourself though.

✔ **Illness-related self-help groups.** Just as you can often find out about alternative therapies for a specific ailment through a self-help or support group (see Chapter 4), you can often pick up information on quality providers. People in these groups tend to be more like you than people on the street — you have the same ailment — and so it pays to listen to their stories about which method or healer helped them. Of course, the treatment or remedy that helps somebody else may not help you, but hearing that a healer is reputable — and helped other people suffering from the same problem — is a good beginning, especially when you hear this stuff several times over.

To find a national organization for people with your particular ailment, call the American Self-Help Clearinghouse in Denville, New Jersey at 973-625-7101 or The National Health Information Center at 800-336-4797. The American Self-Help Clearinghouse also lists relevant organizations in their *Self-Help Sourcebook*. Internet fans can also turn to HealthWorld Online (at `www.healthy.net/pan/cso/cioi/index.html`) — another U.S. government service, partly supported by the National Health

Information Center — for a list of national medical and health organizations (for specific ailments) that are reachable via cyberspace. For additional information, check out these Web sites:

- The National Health Information Center at nhic-nt.health.org
- The Self-Help Sourcebook at www.cmhc.com/selfhelp
- Healthfinder at www.healthfinder.gov/moretools

✔ **World Wide Web.** A huge number of Web sites offer referrals to alternative practitioners or places that will give you referrals. Some of them aren't too picky about who they're willing to include, though. So make sure that you check out the criteria for inclusion before you rely on Web sources too heavily.

✔ **Friends and family.** Just mention your ailment, and chances are high that someone you know will offer you a solution — often in the form of an alternative treatment. It's a simple step then to ask who (if anyone) provided the treatment. Voilà! Instant referral.

Of course, just because Aunt Matilda raves about the way Dr. Massage kneaded her back doesn't mean that Dr. Massage can help your chronic fatigue — or even *your* aching back. If you hear the same name several times from people you trust and respect, though, that person is probably a good bet.

Don't forget the power of "negative referrals" from friends and family. If you hear several people complaining about any given practitioner, that's good reason to stay away.

Recognizing the worst places to get referrals

No referral is useless — but some require more work on your part to make sure that the practitioner is reputable. That extra effort is necessary because the names you get may reflect practitioners' networking and marketing skills (and cash reserves) more than their abilities to heal.

✔ **Advertisements and telephone directories.** Sure, you can add to your list of possibilities by trying advertisements and telephone directories. But just because someone plunked down money for a fancy listing or radio spot — or made the effort to photocopy an ad and pin it up on a bulletin board — doesn't mean that they know what they're doing as a health care practitioner. Promises of free services and other marketing gimmicks should make you particularly suspicious.

Feel free to call these people and find out what they do and what their background is — especially if you're having trouble getting referrals any other way. But just remember that you'll have to screen even more rigorously if you get the names from these sources.

✔ **Paid referral services.** Some alternative practitioners pay money to have their names given out by referral services. These services often run ads on radio and TV claiming that they can help you find a qualified practitioner. The danger here is obvious — just because someone can pay to be included in a referral database doesn't mean that he or she is a good practitioner. Sure, many of these services require that their clients meet minimal standards, but the emphasis is on the word "minimal." Stick to referral services that work in the interest of the customer (you), not the interest of the person trying to sell you goods or services. Because plenty of these reputable services are around (see the previous section, "Finding the best places to get referrals"), you don't need to go to one of these paid referral services.

✔ **Salespeople in health food stores.** Because local health food stores are often centers of a town's alternative circle, salespeople can have firsthand knowledge of community caregivers. The problem is that they have knowledge of them as people (nice guy!) but often not as healers. The same is true for the many patients who pass through the stores and share their stories. All the reports the salespeople hear are second-hand. Plus, you never know who's paying who off.

So, sure, you can ask the clerk in the homeopathy store which herbalist she likes. But unless she's used her personally (and, better yet, can refer you to several other people who have, too — and will talk to you), don't take the recommendation too seriously. Use the name as a place to start — but have the practitioner's competence confirmed through better sources (see "Finding the best places to get referrals," earlier in this chapter).

Screening and interviewing tactics

Once you have a list of possibilities, you have to eliminate the duds. Some of this screening you'll have to do one-on-one, in the practitioner's office (anyone who won't give — or sell — you fifteen minutes to talk this way should be crossed off your list).

Five cheap and easy screening steps

Before you start running around town or paying for initial meetings with potential practitioners, take advantage of the free "screening" you can do over the phone. Follow these steps:

1. **Check with the state licensing agency (if one exists) for the practitioner's specialty to see if that person meets basic standards or if anyone has complained.**

   While you're on the phone, ask which credentials you should be inquiring about.

2. **Find out where the practitioner is located and decide whether you can live with the cost, time, and any inconvenience of getting there.**

   How long will commuting take? How will you travel — car, bus, subway, or taxi? Will you have to deal with rush-hour or city traffic? Will you have to pay $15 to park in a covered garage at each appointment?

3. **Call the office and say that you're thinking about becoming a new patient and you'd like to ask some questions.**

   Evaluate the way you're treated over the phone. Is the receptionist (or other staff member) friendly and helpful? If no receptionist is available, does the practitioner return your call promptly? Don't be put off by an answering machine or a busy receptionist — better that someone is paying attention to patients than chatting on the phone. But at the very least you should be able to talk briefly to someone within minutes. (What if you had an emergency, after all?)

4. **Ask whether this is a good time to ask a few questions about the office and the practitioner you're interested in.**

   If not, set up a phone interview at a mutually agreeable time.

5. **Get as much information as possible over the phone.**

   Inquire about the following issues:

   - How many patients the practitioner sees per day, how long most patients have to wait, how often the appointments run late, and how much time is spent with the average patient.

   - The hours patients can be seen, the best way to reach the provider after hours, and arrangements for emergencies.

   - The procedures usually performed during a first appointment.

   - Cost per treatment, the possibility of negotiating fees or making installment payments, and arrangements, if any, with insurance companies.

   - The practitioner's area of expertise and her training (both conventional and alternative), number of years in practice, credentials, and philosophy of care.

   - The practitioner's personality. Some doctors are all business, others like to tease their patients or engage in small talk, still others give everyone a hug before they leave the office. One woman we know asked a receptionist about a chiropractor for her kids and was told: "My kids love him — he makes them laugh. But I know other kids who are scared by his size and loud voice." If you know what kind of relationship you want to have, these kinds of answers can save you a lot of grief.

   - Whether you can set up a 15-minute interview (free or for a reasonable fee) with the practitioner before making a formal appointment.

If any of the answers don't feel right to you (or don't meet the standards listed in this book for the particular specialty), cross off the name.

Questions to ask before agreeing to treatment

After you've narrowed down your list to a few top prospects, set up a short consultation with your top choice. There should be no formal examination — and definitely no treatment — going on here. The goal is just a straightforward discussion to let this person know the type of care you're looking for and to find out if he or she is the right person to provide it. Before you agree to let anyone treat you, go over the following points:

- ✔ What will treatment involve? How will it affect your life — incapacitate you, alter your schedule, keep you home from work, and so on?

- ✔ How do results compare with results from conventional approaches — or just watchful waiting? What are the advantages and disadvantages of this therapy as opposed to other alternatives?

- ✔ Can you use this method together with conventional therapy?

- ✔ Does any scientific evidence show that this approach works — and is safe? Was the evidence published — and where? (If the provider can give you a copy of relevant studies, decide whether they are valid — or get the opinion of your M.D.)

- ✔ Has the practitioner (personally) used this therapy for other people with a similar health history or ailment? If yes, what happened? Can you talk to some of them?

- ✔ How often will you have to go to the caregiver's office or clinic?

- ✔ How much will each session cost — and will anybody pay for it besides you? How much of this cost is for supplies and how much for the practitioner's time?

- ✔ How many sessions does this healer expect that you'll need?

- ✔ How many sessions should you expect before seeing results? How long before you and the practitioner can decide if the treatment is working?

- ✔ What are the potential side effects? (If the answer is "none," ask again. And then consider going elsewhere — because any effective treatment poses at least a slight risk to some people.)

- ✔ Are there any activities you shouldn't engage in, or other drugs — prescription or over-the-counter, conventional or alternative — that you shouldn't take while undergoing this therapy? Is there anything you shouldn't be using or doing while undergoing this therapy?

- ✔ Is the alternative practitioner willing to talk to your regular doctor about the diagnosis and treatment plan? Will the alternative caregiver place any limitations on what he or she is willing to talk about — and how often is the caregiver willing to talk? You should also ask your M.D. to give the alternative caregiver information about your health status, use of prescription drugs, and so on to avoid conflicting recommendations. (Physicians aren't permitted to release private information about you without express written permission to do so.)

Disclosing personal information

Your healer shouldn't be the only one giving answers if you expect to have a full partnership. Before embarking on any long-term treatment plan, your healer needs to know some information about you, too. Because many healers aren't trained to ask these questions, you often have to volunteer them yourself. Speaking up about your expectations, values, and concerns before any treatments or services is a good way to prevent future misunderstandings, frustrations, and even lawsuits.

Here's what a potential healer needs to know about you:

- ✔ Your basic health (and family health) history
- ✔ Past problems you may have had with a related treatment
- ✔ Drugs or other treatments you're currently using
- ✔ The amount of information you want from your healer and the value you place on open communication (if you do)
- ✔ Any aspect you don't understand about the treatment or anything else that doesn't make sense to you
- ✔ Any procedure in the proposed treatment that you don't want to be part of — and why
- ✔ Fears or concerns about the treatment, the office, or the type of medicine in general
- ✔ A statement that you expect to be an active decision-maker in any treatment choice

Remember — no question or concern is too trivial, too confrontational, or too dumb when it comes to your own health. If the healer thinks that it is, say good-bye.

Ten ways to be a partner with your practitioner

If you want to take charge of your own health, you have to act like a partner with your practitioner — and not a passive recipient of advice from "on high." Here are some top ways to start your relationship on the right foot — and keep it that way:

- Make clear from the beginning that mutual respect and open communication are important to you.

- Find out as much as you can about your illness and how it can be treated.

- Speak up if a remedy, treatment, or procedure hurts, scares, angers, or confuses you.

- Bring along a friend or relative to act as your advocate if you find speaking up for yourself difficult.

- Remind the healer about the factors that make your situation unique — and why a treatment that works for someone else may not apply to you.

- Arm yourself with a list of questions so you don't forget anything.

- Respect the healer's time by staying focused on your questions.

- Consider asking the staff members to explain details the healer may not have time to tell you. Receptionists often know a lot more about a healer's philosophy and personality than you may think, and they certainly can tell you about average waiting times, billing obstacles, and so on. And nurses often have the time, training, and people skills to explain details about diseases and medical procedures even better than their employers.

- Ask whether other options exist for treating your problem — and the pros and cons of each.

- Be prepared to get a second opinion — or go elsewhere — if you're at all uneasy about the healer or the approach.

Knowing What to Expect and What to Reject

If you want a "good" doctor-patient relationship, expect your practitioner to

- Act as your "partner" (see the sidebar, "Ten ways to be a partner with your practitioner").

- Respect and listen to you (and vice versa).

- Offer clear information about the cost, length, and nature of the treatment — and the results you should expect from it.

- Give you freedom to ask questions.

- ✔ Be willing to talk to your regular M.D. about your condition and the effectiveness of the treatment plan.

- ✔ Offer a clean, safe setting that meets regulated standards for medical care.

- ✔ Charge a reasonable price for the service provided.

You should reject potential health care providers on the spot (or at least spark a good deal of skepticism about anything they tell you) who:

- ✔ Make extremely hostile or gratuitous nasty remarks about mainstream medicine as a whole (not just certain aspects of it) or other philosophies of health care.

- ✔ Claim to be able to cure everything, or claim that the treatment has no possible side effects.

- ✔ Refuse to estimate the cost or time required for treatment.

- ✔ Won't communicate with your regular M.D.

- ✔ Advise you not to consult your regular M.D. or any other health care provider.

- ✔ Don't listen to you.

- ✔ Ask you to commit to long-term and costly care.

Recognizing the Pros and Cons of Licensing

Do you need to have a licensed healer? If you live in a state that requires practitioners of your chosen alternative approach to be licensed, the answer is an obvious yes. And if you live in a state that doesn't license these practitioners, the answer is obviously no. Most of the time, though, you'll need to rely on other measures of competence — such as training, experience, and other credentials — to evaluate a healer's (potential) competence.

Which alternatives are licensed

If you're seeing a chiropractor or osteopath and live in the United States, you're in luck. All fifty states require these practitioners to be licensed.

All other forms of alternative medicine vary widely from place to place. Because more and more states are licensing alternative practitioners, we suggest checking with the Federation of State Medical Boards of the United States, Inc. for updated information (Federation Place, 400 Fuller Wiser Road, Suite 300, Euless, TX 76039-3855, phone 817-868-4000 or e-mail webmaster@fsmb.org).

You can also contact the national organization of practitioners of the alternative practice you're interested in (see Appendix) for up-to-date information about legislation, certification, or registration laws. If you want all the gory details about the current (and ever-changing) legislation for most alternative practices, check out the overview of alternative care legislation on the HealthWorld Web site at www.healthy.net/public/legal-lg/regulations/fetzer.htm. Unless you're an aficionado of legalese, though, go there at your own risk.

What are the pros of licensing?

Because standards for training are generally loose for alternative healers, a license is a good way to start separating out competent healers. It's essentially a short-hand way of letting you know a healer meets minimum educational standards, has jumped through the right testing hoops, and hasn't been indicted on too many counts of gross incompetence or malpractice. Licensing also means that insurers may have to pay for these treatments — if treatment is deemed "medically necessary" (and if the HMO or insurer includes that particular provider).

If no license is available, other similar standards of minimal competence may apply. Many national associations of alternative practices certify healers who meet set standards of training and testing. Some states have similar voluntary certification or registration procedures. A certified or registered practitioner often meets standards just as rigorous as those for a licensed practitioner, but certification or registration aren't *required*.

What are the cons of licensing?

Even if licensing requirements apply, having a license by no means guarantees competence. As the logicians like to say, a license is necessary in these cases, but not sufficient. And just because a certain alternative approach is licensed is no guarantee that the approach is valid to treat all conditions — or, more to the point, to treat your particular condition.

Critics also object to medical licensing in general (even of M.D.s) because licenses are by definition exclusionary — they keep the "in" group "in" and the "out" group "out." During the age of populism in the mid-19th century United States, certain alternatives flourished for this very reason — people objected to the high-and-mighty doctors who thought they were the only ones entitled to heal people. Old licensing laws were overturned as a result.

A lot has been written on how licensing laws have been set up more to protect the economic interests of service providers rather than the rights of consumers. To this day, many people complain that licensing laws keep health care costs high, squelch competition, stifle new ideas, mask incompetence, and keep people from learning how to care for themselves. These claims are somewhat valid. Still, on the whole, we think that licensing requirements for healers set some standards for quality care and help to keep the unscrupulous and incompetent out of business.

Knowing Whether You've Found "Dr. Right"

You can gather information until you're blue in the face. But after you've used this information to rule out the charlatans, the rip-offs, the inconvenients, and the plain old jerks, you're ultimately left with an emotional decision. After all, in choosing an alternative healer (or any healer, for that matter), you're looking for someone who's going to be your partner in health care. In that sense, finding the right caregiver isn't all that different than finding the right mate.

The choice ultimately comes down to intangibles — do you two "click?" Do you feel that you're on the same wavelength when it comes to a basic approach to health? Are you comfortable together? Is this practitioner someone you respect — and who respects you? If the answer to all of these questions is yes — and you've eliminated the unqualified or overpriced — you have a match.

Above all, trust your gut. If what you're hearing seems too good to be true, it probably is.

Chapter 7

Talking to Other People about Alternatives

In This Chapter
▶ How to ask your regular M.D. about alternatives — what to do if you're afraid to ask
▶ How to convince skeptical M.D.s
▶ How to get friends and family to take you seriously
▶ How to convince skeptics to consider alternatives

*F*or all the enthusiasm out there about alternative medicine, the public also maintains plenty of skepticism. Some of this skepticism is understandable, but a good deal of it is based on pure and simple prejudice. This chapter helps you rout out unwarranted skepticism — whether it's from your otherwise reasonable M.D. or your bedridden grandfather who has given up on conventional solutions but refuses to consider alternatives.

Talking to Conventional Doctors

As we say in Chapter 2, part of using alternative medicine safely is filling your M.D. in on what you're doing — especially if you have a serious condition or any kind of new problem.

Why you should tell your M.D.

Mainstream docs still have the most extensive training and experience in diagnosing life-threatening conditions, and you want to have these ruled out before trying alternatives. Plus, to make sure that your alternative treatment isn't interfering with some underlying health problem or ongoing conventional treatment, you want all your care providers to know the treatment methods and remedies you are using — and, preferably, to communicate with each other.

Unfortunately, most M.D.s probably won't give you an immediate A-okay. After all, assuming that all of alternative medicine is a bunch of bunk is a lot easier than getting educated about it. So you shouldn't be surprised if you diligently inform your doctor that you're considering an alternative approach — or you ask whether any alternatives are available — and all you get is a roll of the eyes, or worse, a lecture on the foolishness or dangers of alternatives. This response is especially true of doctors who weren't trained in the past few years — when more and more medical schools started including aspects of alternative medicine in their curricula.

What if your doc laughs?

Remember that all too often ridicule and dismissal are simply masks for ignorance. So don't get flustered if your doctor won't take you seriously. Instead, take a deep breath. And while you're taking it, listen to what the doctor has to say. There's a chance that the advice may be somewhat valid. It is always possible, after all, that you're proposing a truly dangerous or risky practice (but if you've read this book that's less likely!). It's also possible that the doctor really does know some new and important information about this practice that should make you think twice.

If, after listening, you're convinced that your doctor's response comes more from ignorance or prejudice than real information, you're going to have to steel up the courage to do some mind-opening. Fortunately, we're going to help you do that.

If you think that your doctor is ridiculing you or that your relationship lacks mutual respect, it may be time to consider switching doctors. Ignorance is one thing; personal ridicule is another.

What if you're a scaredy-cat?

If you're one of those people who worries a lot about what other people think of you, you may not even be able to imagine getting yourself into a situation where you question your doctor about alternative treatment. Maybe you're afraid that your conservative family doctor would think less of you for mentioning alternatives. Maybe you're afraid to "challenge" authority.

If this sounds like you, don't just sneak off to an alternative practitioner (even though this approach can be tempting). Instead, try consulting a different M.D. whom you know is more open to alternative medicine (for example, one who is also licensed in acupuncture, or who works with alternative practitioners at a wellness clinic).

Which information to give your doctor

If you basically like and trust your doctor, you need to arm yourself with certain paper weapons to come off as a well-informed, reasonable patient (and partner in health care). The best weapons for winning over M.D.s are research papers. If you can, bring in copies of Dr. David Eisenberg's two landmark papers from *The New England Journal of Medicine* and the *Annals of Internal Medicine*. The first of these papers documents the enormous popularity of alternatives — and makes it clear that no M.D. can afford to ignore them. The second gives lots of concrete advice about how even the stodgiest of M.D.s can get up to speed about alternative medicine issues — and why doing so is vital.

If you can't get a hold of these papers through a medical library or computerized database (see Chapter 4), just write the following citations on a notecard and present them to your doctor, who will know what to do with them: *The New England Journal of Medicine* 328 (January 28, 1993): 246–283 and *Annals of Internal Medicine* 127 (July 1997): 61–69.

What to do if your M.D. won't listen

If, after your best attempts at education, you still can't convince your doctor that an alternative is worth trying, don't despair. If you can get your doctor to agree to monitor your health — even if he or she doesn't approve of the alternative treatment you have chosen — the two of you can still work together. If, along the way, you find that your doctor may have been right, there's no shame in changing your mind. If, along the way, it appears that *you* were right, we can only hope your doctor will see the light.

On the other hand, if your best efforts to show off your reasonable attitude and killer evidence don't make a dent in your doctor's skepticism — and your doctor refuses to hear anything at all about your alternative adventures — politely ask to be referred to an M.D. more open to alternatives. If you get no suggestions, you may have to find one on your own.

How to get your M.D. to talk to other healers

Suppose that you do have an M.D. who's willing to let you try alternatives — and to keep an eye on your health while you do so. Or suppose that you manage to convince your M.D. to take on this attitude. Your next step is to get your M.D. to communicate with the alternative healer you choose.

Many doctors, however open-minded, don't have a clue about how to interact with an alternative practitioner. They think that calling a massage therapist is akin to calling a Martian. So help them out. A copy of Dr. David Eisenberg's article — from the *Annals of Internal Medicine* 127 (July 1997): 61–69 — on advising patients should do the trick for most of them. It's kind of a *Talking to Alternative Practitioners For Dummies;* it handholds M.D.s through the whole process.

Another option is to have your alternative practitioner do the work for you by calling the M.D. — or sending a note — about your proposed treatment.

Talking to Skeptical Friends and Family

If you're sold on an alternative approach, you may want to spread the word to people you care about — but, then again, maybe not. Not everyone will share your enthusiasm, and some will be downright suspicious, shocked, or sarcastic. This section tells you how to deal with these inevitable encounters.

The downside of spreading the word

No matter how excited you are about the way echinacea helped your cold or the way acupuncture treatments are controlling your son's asthma, you're going to meet someone who acts like you're a kook. Not so long ago, anything alternative was generally considered downright radical — the stuff of mystic gurus, wacko hippies, ignorant illiterates, and spaced-out cultists. Right or wrong, this was the common perception. And a good number of people still think this way.

When you run into these people, some may say nothing and just leave you with a sense of disapproval. There isn't much you can do about these people because they haven't actually made any criticisms. Others may try to "help" you — by reminding you of the importance of evidence and scientific medicine or telling you horror stories they've heard about the stuff you're using (conveniently forgetting that a lot of conventional medicine is also based more on habit and hunch than on solid evidence).

Your best defense is to make clear that you know as much as you can about why this approach may work, why it makes sense for *you,* and why you feel reasonably confident that it's safe. Because you're reading this book, this explanation won't be a problem.

The choice to say nothing

One other possibility is to say nothing to critical or skeptical people. You have a treatment method that works for you. You're a good citizen for trying to spread the good news, but if all you get is grief, why bother? Besides, continuing to live a happy, healthy existence is the best response. You don't have to say anything else to make your point.

How to get reluctant relatives to try alternatives

Sometimes you want to speak up about alternative methods. Maybe you've had to listen to your grandmother complain about her arthritic knee one too many times. Maybe you're sick of your dearest friend saying that she can't jog with you because her sciatica is acting up. Maybe you're convinced that your husband's headaches would stop if he'd just try yoga or some other relaxation technique.

But whatever you do, these people just roll their eyes — or look at you like you're nuts. You know you're supposed to mind your own business, but you care about these people. You know they've tried all sorts of conventional therapies to no avail — and, in some cases, are living with serious side effects from all the drugs they're taking. And you think that they're closing their minds to treatment methods that could really help them.

Probably the most convincing approach you can take in these situations — after presenting your views as clearly as possible — is to put your money where your mouth is. If you think that Grandma would benefit from a massage, take her along when you're getting one and let her see for herself. Remember that nobody gets better because somebody else wants them to — but good examples can inspire people to *want* to get better.

Surefire facts to make your case

Here are some killer convincers to win over the most die-hard mainstreamer:

- ✔ As of this writing, nearly two-thirds (75 of 125) of the accredited medical schools in the United States are offering courses in alternative medicine. Not good enough? Reel off some of the esteemed institutions we're talking about: Columbia University College of Physicians and Surgeons, Harvard Medical School, Johns Hopkins School of Medicine, and Mount Sinai School of Medicine.

- ✔ Not only has the United States Congress looked into unconventional cancer treatments, but in 1992 it established an Office of Alternative Medicine at the National Institutes of Health to facilitate scientific research and evaluation of these practices and spread the word to the public.

- ✔ Other hotshot (and widely respected) health organizations — including the World Health Organization, the World Bank, and the United Nations — are working to raise international awareness and formulate policies about traditional medicine.

✔ Several well-publicized studies have concluded that chiropractic is the treatment of choice for low-back pain. And in nearly every country outside the United States, chiropractic schools are part of the university system and financed by the government.

✔ Approximately two-thirds of a group of 700 heart doctors (cardiologists) said that they took antioxidants (dietary supplements that may lower risk of heart disease) — according to B. Jancin, *Family Practice News* (March 1, 1994): 10. And about half of family practice physicians have tried or recommended alternatives — according to N. Elder, A. Gillcrist, and R. Minz, *Archives of Family Medicine* 6 (March 19, 1997): 181–184.

✔ Big-name cancer centers are including alternative practices to boost conventional approaches. The big names include Columbia-Presbyterian Medical Center and Memorial Sloan-Kettering Cancer Center in New York City and the Duke Comprehensive Cancer Center in Durham, North Carolina. Among the most popular complementary approaches are stress reduction techniques such as biofeedback, meditation, prayer therapy, therapeutic massage, and touch therapy, as well as certain forms of herbal medicine.

✔ Herbs have been used in almost every culture for thousands of years to treat almost any ailment imaginable. In fact, about one-fourth of modern pharmaceutical drugs are derived from herbs.

✔ Since 1979, the World Health Organization (WHO) has recommended acupuncture as an effective treatment for over 100 physical illnesses. And many hospitals throughout the United States offer acupuncture as a standard treatment to help people overcome substance abuse and other addictive behaviors.

If nothing else works, try talking turkey. Remind skeptics that health care currently makes up 16 percent of the Gross National Product in the United States and that the high cost is in part due to Americans' over-reliance on expensive, high-tech, "scientific medicine" solutions. By picking and choosing from the best of both conventional and alternative medicine, people all over the world can open up the door to appropriate, low-tech, generally inexpensive, user-friendly approaches to common and chronic conditions.

Yes, a lot of unnecessary and even dangerous stuff is out there in alternative land. But instead of always going immediately for a "million-dollar work-up" to test for every conceivable problem and the often unnecessary medications with wicked side effects, why not start with the affordable work-up and then get on a better diet, find ways to de-stress, get more sleep and exercise, maybe try a gentle botanical or two to relieve symptoms, fluff your *qi* (or whatever you want to call it), or get some human touch and massage? You can always call in conventional medicine's big guns later if your condition proves to be more serious or resists alternative approaches.

Even the most conservative of critics should find this approach worth considering — both for their own personal health and the state of the world's pocketbook.

Chapter 8

How Not to Lose Your Mind or Money in the Health Food Store

· ·

In This Chapter

▶ How to shop in health food stores without feeling intimidated or confused

▶ How to know which products are safe to buy — and where to buy them

▶ Who to trust for product information

▶ When to order products by mail

▶ How to avoid being ripped-off

· ·

The north side of Evanston, Illinois is often considered one of the more conservative areas of the United States, home to descendants of the Women's Christian Temperance Union and prospective debutantes. But today in a two-block stretch of shops, which still hosts a Christian Science Reading Room and a family-owned stationery shop, you can find a chiropractic clinic, an herb store, a homeopathic medicine shop, and a locally-owned coffeehouse with a bulletin board advertising massage therapists, Tibetan healers, and yoga classes.

This neighborhood is hardly unique. No major mall in the United States is complete without a General Nutrition Center or a Garden Botanika (often where the Hickory Farms used to be), and every even half-hip town has some nonchain health food or medicine shop. You can't even go into a mainstream grocery or drugstore without seeing aisles of herbal and homeopathic remedies, vitamins promising quick cures, natural remedies for arthritis pain or motion sickness, and even goodies such as ginseng gum and soy protein bars at the check-out counter.

Walking into a drugstore may leave you feeling like you've gone back a century or two in a time capsule — or maybe off into the future (one store we know bills itself as "Medicine for the 21st century"). For those of us who grew up thinking of pharmacies as places with neat rows of slickly labeled boxes, it can feel odd to face rows of mysterious brown bottles, exotic teas, preserved stems and leaves in jars, giant vats of egg protein, and weird homey-looking labels, much like you see in the re-creations of the town pharmacy in living history museums.

If you're intimidated by these products and places — you don't know what to buy or what to make of the advice you're given — this is the chapter for you.

How to Navigate the Health Food Store

Health food stores can give the impression that someone out there — the whole medical and pharmaceutical profession included — has been hiding something from you. Why didn't anyone ever tell you that there *is* a cure for arthritis, a natural way to cure yeast infections, simple tablets to prevent colds, and cancer-cures in a bottle? Why didn't anyone ever tell you that regular people should take enzymes to improve the absorption of food? Boy, were you ever dumb, you believe, for not knowing about this stuff.

If you're not totally intimidated (and you don't head right back to Walgreens — where, surprise, you'll also face a row of homeopathic remedies and nutritional supplements), you may feel relieved. Often the people in these stores are more than willing to help you. They may listen to you describe your situation and suggest remedies for it. They may offer an "information bar" of books and other reference materials. They may invite you to free lectures or even provide a list of healers who practice alternative medicine.

This attention all sounds neighborly-like. And in the responsible health food stores, it can be a great service. The problem, though, is that far too many irresponsible health food stores are out there trying to make a buck by exploiting people's vulnerabilities and fears.

That's why we generally recommend that you go into these places with your guard up. If you're going in to get a remedy that a reputable practitioner has prescribed — particularly a specific brand, size, and formulation — that's great. Go in, get what you were planning to get, and get out.

Impulse purchases of stuff that sounds interesting — or of stuff that the clerk suggests is right for you — is a risky business.

Understanding "Natural Products"

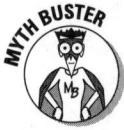

Many health food stores pride themselves on selling only "natural products." This phrase sounds like a good thing — "natural" sounds as noncontroversial as motherhood and apple pie. Unfortunately, though, the term "natural products" is pretty open-ended — and certainly no guarantee that the product is good for you, or even safe.

The fact is, buying an unknown product at a health food store can be risky just because of the nature of "natural products." Because so-called natural products are very loosely regulated (especially in the United States), what the label seems to say and what the product actually is (and does) can often differ significantly. We get into this subject more in Part VI.

Meanwhile, remember that just because a product is natural doesn't mean that it's harmless (is this beginning to sound familiar?). In fact, if you're buying it because it may do something *good* to your body, you must realize that it also has the potential to do something *bad*.

Of course, some natural products are truly harmless. And if you want to buy them because they make you feel better about yourself (and, as Chapter 19 explains, feeling better about yourself can be as good for your health as any drug), go ahead. In general, these are the kinds of products you can buy on your own without worrying too much about ill effects (except, of course, possibly wasting your money):

- Vitamins and minerals (but avoid high-dose, fat-soluble vitamins, such as vitamins A and E — greater than 5,000 I.U. of vitamin A and greater than 400 I.U. of vitamin E per day are considered high doses)
- Common cosmetic products such as "homeopathic" toothpaste, herbal hair rinse, natural bristle brushes, or carrot facial scrubs

For any product that is at all unusual, though, start with expert advice from providers or from medical databases.

Do They Know What They're Talking about at Health Food Stores?

Even the most reputable health food store has its limitations. No matter how well-meaning — or even well-informed — the salespeople are (and it doesn't hurt to ask them if they have any formal training), they are not qualified to prescribe a specific treatment or lifestyle plan for you. That's because they haven't conducted a thorough physical examination and medical history. Even if they have an M.D. and have studied Ayurvedic healing with Dr. Deepak Chopra himself, plus earned a Ph.D. in human physiology on the side, they can't responsibly tell you what to do merely by listening to your tales of woe in the antioxidant aisle.

Many clerks speak with total authority and assurance about anything that happens to be on the shelves. But you do have to wonder if this enthusiasm is because they really believe the product works or because they sense that they can make some money. In the responsible stores, both can be true, and that's fine. But in far too many stores, a healthy dose of suspicion is in order. This need for caution is particularly true of stores that change their product lines every time the media hypes a new trend, or those that emphasize expensive devices and overpriced and relabeled versions of the same stuff you can get at Wal-Mart.

What's the bottom line? Even if your salesclerk *isn't* a teenager recently laid off from Burger Barn, don't expect him or her to be able to say what remedy or method is right for *you*. Only your practitioner can tell you

- Whether the new product will interfere with anything else you're doing or taking

- Whether the new product is right for someone with your underlying health condition

- Whether you have a medical or family history that makes this product dangerous for you

- Whether an approach that is simpler, cheaper, and more fundamental to your problem — such as changing your diet or stress level — may work better for you

Who Can You Trust?

So who should you be getting information about alternative products from? Well, as we said before, your alternative care provider or regular M.D. is the ideal source. If you can find a registered nurse with experience in this area, all the better — many nurses have made it part of their life's work to find out about alternative methods. Research you've done outside the store — particularly if it comes in the form of credible scientific studies — is also good.

Try the pharmacist — but don't hold your breath

Another person to trust is your local pharmacist, who, at least in theory, is one of the last expert consultants on earth who can give you free advice on all aspects of substance-taking. A good pharmacist should be able to fill you in on which products are known to work, which may work, which are harmful, which can be mixed together, and which you shouldn't use.

In reality, though, you probably don't talk much to your pharmacist, especially if you buy your supplies at impersonal chain pharmacies, supermarkets, warehouse clubs, or discount superstores. Plus, we believe that most pharmacists in conventional drugstores today know almost nothing about alternative medicine. In our opinion, no longer do we have very many independent pharmacists who have a personal interest in attracting customers; rather we have hired hands whose work comes second to the grocery or lawn chair department. And in any kind of pharmacy, too often the emphasis is on business — making it all too tempting to push products with the best profit margin.

Still, if pharmacies were smart, they'd be able to use their pharmacists as advisors and still turn a profit. How? If the chains would send their pharmacists back to school to be trained in the old science of *pharmacognosy* — the pharmacology of plants and botanicals that all drug dispensers *used to* know (and they still do in many countries) — everyone could win. Not only would pharmacists have the training and background to be natural advisors to customers, but the chains could advertise this service to their customers.

On the off chance that the chains won't listen to our advice, we suggest that you use every opportunity you have to push your pharmacist to get up to speed on supplements, vitamins, and botanicals. Remember, it's okay to put a bit of pressure on your local pharmacist to check some remedy out for you, respectfully of course. It's part of their job.

Information sheets — proceed with caution

Some stores try to make shopping easier for you by providing studies — or summaries of studies — right there for you on the shelves. You may well find some of these professional-looking papers lying beside specific products. Or you may see large laminated signs summarizing a study's conclusions for you and depicting impressive-looking charts and graphs.

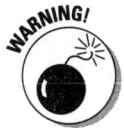

On the surface, these explanations look bona fide — they claim to give solid scientific explanations about what the product does. Some even include intimidating references to obscure professional journals. The problem is, these information sheets and pamphlets are generally written by the same people trying to sell you the product. Did someone say conflict of interest? Needless to say, they more often than not rely on anecdotal evidence (see Chapter 3 for an explanation about why that evidence isn't so convincing) and speak in the voice of God — as if there's no question that this, and only this, product is the final word in cure.

Even when the pamphlet or sheet comes from the store management, it usually doesn't contain enough information for you to know whether the study was valid or not.

A good way to eliminate at least some of the doubtful stuff is to ignore any health information that plugs a specific radio show, clinic, Web site, or company.

When to Buy from the Practitioner

An often safe and convenient place to buy alternative products (especially when you're using them for the first time) is from your alternative practitioner — assuming that yours is trustworthy and properly credentialed. You may not be getting the stuff at the cheapest price possible, but at least you can have more confidence in the product you're getting — and someone to take responsibility for its effects, too.

Make sure that those credentials are related to the products being sold, though. Just like fantastic hairdressers who try to sell designer dresses on the side, your great chiropractor may not know all that much about the herbal remedy he's trying to push on you.

Here are a couple of other issues to consider:

✔ **Know what you're getting.** A gracious "no thanks" is in order if the practitioner can't explain why you need this product or tell you much about its potential adverse effects or track record — or if the cost seems exorbitant. You should also be told how long the remedy will take to work — but keep in mind that many botanicals and supplements act gently and gradually, so they may take longer to kick in than conventional medicines.

✔ **Don't forget your M.D.** No matter how much you trust your alternative provider, prudence requires that you seek the advice of a knowledgeable M.D. if you intend to use a product for a long time — particularly in high doses.

What about Mail Order?

One way to avoid the intimidation factor in health food stores — not to mention the problem of pushy salespeople — is to order by mail. The number of natural and other alternative products available this way is mind-boggling.

Many books on alternative health care offer toll-free numbers and coupons through which you can order highly specialized teas, herbs, guidelines, and devices. Then there's the classified sections in the back of natural health and healing magazines. By calling toll-free numbers or writing to obscure post office boxes you can get all sorts of esoteric products such as magnetic wrist supports, vitamins, tapes on oral chelation, juicers, colloidal silver, Chinese herbs and teas, and a whole assortment of "miracle" products for pain. Plus you can find scores of quick, easy, and "free" ways to become "accredited" and "certified," or even earn a Ph.D, in metaphysics, hypnotherapy, parapsychology, tarot, naturopathy, herbology, nutrition, energy healing, *Feng Shui*, aromatherapy, and so on — all without leaving your home.

Ordering this way presents some basic problems (some of which we suspect that you've guessed by now):

✔ **Ordering by mail means that you're less likely to get checked out by a reputable healer first.** As we've said countless times already, neglecting to see a reputable healer before beginning any treatment is a bad move, especially if there's any chance that you have a serious or new condition. Remember the famous saying: The doctor who treats himself has a fool for a patient.

✔ **Ordering by mail also gives you less chance to check out what you're buying before you buy it — and less chance to check out the company.** Sure, you can always return a product if it doesn't turn out to be what you thought it was. But as you probably know from other areas of life, this process is often more of a headache than it's worth. Sometimes you have to pay hefty postage. Sometimes you've violated some obscure rule that prohibits returning the item. Sometimes the company doesn't exist any longer by the time you return the product — or they just won't send a refund.

Mail order can be a good idea, however, if you've used a product before and have trouble finding it in local stores. In other words, if you know *exactly* what you're buying and you have reason to believe that the company is trustworthy, the convenience (and often cost) factor can make mail order worthwhile.

How to Escape without Spending a Bundle

If you get nothing else out of this chapter, you can still feel comfortable shopping for natural remedies and products by keeping a few simple principles in mind. As the following sections explain, they're really not all that different from the guidelines you should remember when you shop for anything! But somehow when people start thinking about the possibility of a health answer that they haven't heard of, they throw all caution to the wind. So don't do that, okay?

The basics of smart shopping

The following principles will go a long way toward making you a savvy shopper:

✔ **Avoid impulse purchases.** Stick to products that your practitioner has recommended and/or you've used before. Know what you want when you go into a store — and get out with it as soon as possible.

✔ **Read labels — including lists of ingredients.** Often the new "cure for colds" is plain old vitamin C with a new label. You may be able to get the same thing for less by shopping around.

✔ **Avoid products that sound too good to be true.** Nothing new here.

✔ **Try one remedy at a time.** If you start using three products at once, you'll never know which one made a difference or which produced side effects.

✔ **Watch for slick marketing tactics that make products sound like they do more than they do.** In other words, watch for rip-offs (see Figure 8-1)!

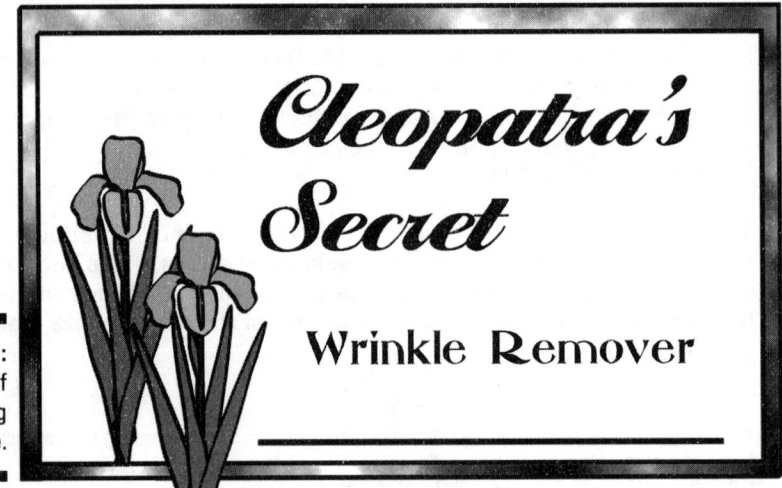

Figure 8-1:
Beware of marketing hype.

Rip-off warning signs

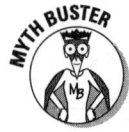

We don't mean to sound paranoid, but there really are a lot of companies that are "out to get you" by using promotional tricks — or at least "out to get you" to buy stuff you don't need. When we look at the marketing of natural remedies, it sometimes seems like we're back in the days of snake oil and elixir hawkers and patent medicine vendors. The following sections describe a few common tactics to watch for.

Promises to cure diseases generally considered incurable

Theoretically, manufacturers of nondrug supplements in the United States are not allowed to promise to cure diseases. If they do claim to cure a disease, then the product they're selling is considered a drug — and they have to prove safety and efficacy to the FDA.

But marketers will go to incredible lengths to get around these official requirements. Without actually naming a disease, a label may quote a health care provider who *does* name the disease or claim to "nutritionally support" people who have that disease — all suggesting a cure without stating the claim directly. Instead of directly claiming to cure depression, a product may claim to "support feelings of well-being" or "help maintain a healthy emotional outlook." Instead of directly claiming to cure Alzheimer's disease, a product may claim to "improve mental sharpness." Other products imply that they can cure; they make vague promises such as claiming to protect membranes, improve circulation, boost immune systems, or remove toxins.

Probably the most clever tactic of all showed up on an unproven arthritis cure. The label contained the words "as seen in *THE ARTHRITIS CURE*" — but the last three words were much larger than the first three so "The Arthritis Cure" popped out. *The Arthritis Cure* is just a book that mentioned the product, but a casual buyer would think that this substance is a "cure" for arthritis — a claim that the manufacturer cannot legally make, and, in fact, has not made.

Fine print that undoes all the promises

All packages and ads for natural "remedies" are required by law to contain the following disclaimer: "These statements have not been evaluated by the Food and Drug Administration. This product is not intended to diagnose, treat, cure, or prevent any disease." In other words, no matter what the manufacturer says about the ability of its product to "help your heart" or "boost your immune system," this disclaimer basically says that there's no promise to do *anything*.

This disclaimer makes distinguishing legitimate products from snake oil impossible. So think twice whenever you see it. Until some legislation gets passed to guarantee minimum safeguards and standardization requirements, make your purchasing decisions based only on the advice of a practitioner — or the results of your own research.

Vitamins or other supplements repackaged as "special formulas"

Some vitamins and other supplements are just repackaged as "special formulas." We recently saw a box for a product that claimed to be "an exclusive patented formula" and "recommended formulation" to promote cartilage regeneration and healthy joints. The package promised that when taken regularly, the product would promote healthy cartilage by supplying dietary ingredients that stimulate the production and repair of cartilage. What did the wording on the package really mean? Just that the stuff contained *glucosamine sulfate* (a chemical that *may* be helpful in treating osteoarthritis) together with *chondrotoin sulfate* (another chemical that probably makes no difference at all). But one thing is for sure: No evidence proves that this *particular* formulation is better than any other product containing glucosamine sulfate.

Watch out, too, for fancy products that are really nothing but plain old vitamins, repackaged and repriced (usually upward). Recently, for example, we saw an ad for a heart formula implying that it could lower levels of *homocysteine* (an amino acid linked to a higher risk of heart disease). Really this stuff is nothing but folic acid, B6, and B12 — a bunch of vitamins. Yes, like the ad copy says, these vitamins can (or, more accurately, *may*) help lower levels of homocysteine. But what the ad doesn't tell you is that you're probably not getting any more "defense" against heart disease by using this particular product than from taking the vitamins.

If you really want to be a guinea pig in a completely haphazard and unregulated experiment — which we don't recommend — at least save yourself some money by avoiding the fancy packaging and get the same ingredients in a cheaper formulation. Better yet, go see a licensed health care provider and find out which product is right for *you*.

Products that claim to be cure-alls

Some packages and promotional materials promise quick and easy relief for a whole range of symptoms — and don't first suggest that you get a diagnosis. We recently saw an ad for a "dietary supplement" — basically blended herbs and fiber — that is supposed to help "flush out wastes" without being a "laxative." Endorsed by "a nutripath," this product is supposed to help anyone suffering from poor digestion and elimination, fatigue, stiff joints, mood swings, or poor skin. The ad contained all sorts of blather from the nutripath, who assumed that anyone with *any* of these problems had a "sick colon" and could be helped with his herbal product within seven days. He didn't even mention the possibility that mood swings may be due to a serious psychological disorder or that stiff joints, poor skin, and fatigue may be signs of an underlying systemic disease.

Promises to solve problems you didn't know you had

Remember when advertising whizzes created "diseases" such as halitosis in order to sell mouthwash? Well, a lot of similar stuff is going on in the world of alternative products as well. Ads may tell you that you need to "cleanse your liver" to boost your energy. They may tell you that "intestinal toxins" are the cause of your fatigue, dry skin, stiff joints, and moodiness. They may tell you that you need to "neutralize the acids in your system" to reverse the aging process.

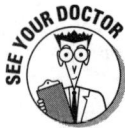

You can believe this stuff if you choose to. But we suggest that you get some convincing evidence for these kinds of claims before you take out your wallet. And if you really have troublesome ailments, get them checked by an M.D. before you let people selling products diagnose you.

Part III

The Big Picture: The Systematic Approach

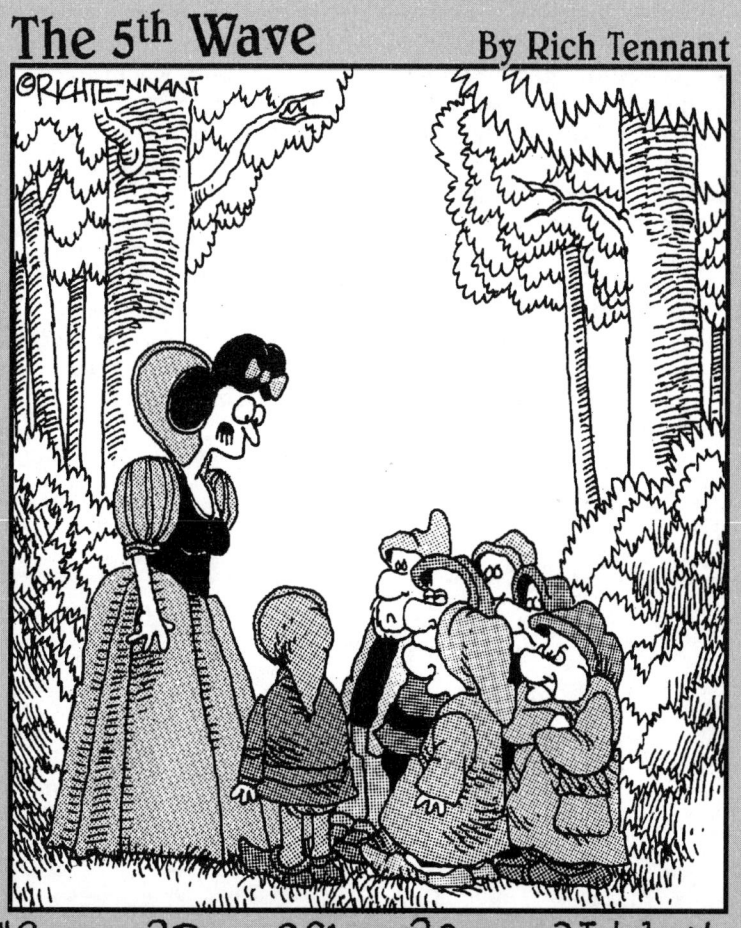

The 5th Wave
By Rich Tennant

@RICHTENNANT

"Sneezy? Dopey? Sleepy? Grumpy? I take it
no one here's ever heard of homeopathy?"

In this part . . .

Thinking about Chinese medicine, Ayurveda, naturopathy, or homeopathy? In this part, we introduce these big "systems" of alternative medicine one by one, describing — in plain English — how each system views health and disease and how these views differ from those in conventional Western medicine. Even more to the point, we show you how these different ways of thinking about health play out when it comes to the care you get. You find out when (and when not) to consider each system, the strengths and weaknesses of each, and what experiencing various techniques is like. You can also find tips on how to locate a reputable practitioner and, in some cases, how to increase the odds of getting your insurance company to help pay.

Chapter 9

Exploring Chinese Medicine

● ●

In This Chapter

▶ Recognizing the roots of Chinese medicine — diverse Asian traditions

▶ Understanding the basics of Tao, yin-yang, and *qi*

▶ Discovering what goes on in the healer's office

▶ Considering the evidence for the effectiveness of traditional Chinese medicine

▶ Knowing when to try Chinese medicine — and when not to

▶ Finding a reputable healer

● ●

*C*hinese medicine has been around for nearly 5,000 years and is still used by more than a quarter of the world's population — and yet this field still mystifies Westerners. That confusion is partly because instead of emphasizing that people get ill, it emphasizes that they stay well. Plus, it uses a whole different language (and we're not talking about Chinese) to describe the body and how it works.

Multiple Asian Traditions

Actually, Chinese medicine is more than Chinese. What's called Chinese medicine today can trace its origins to several related traditions of healing that developed over the past 5,000 years in China, Japan, Korea, and parts of Southeast Asia. That's why some authorities prefer to call these practices "Oriental medicine" (even though the term "Oriental" has fallen out of favor in the Asian community). The national organization of healers in this tradition, for example, calls itself The American Association of Oriental Medicine.

Among the practices included in "Chinese medicine" are

✓ **Traditional Chinese medicine (TCM).** Don't let the name "traditional" fool you. TCM was given full "modern" status in 1958 during the Chinese communist government's attempt to handle the health needs of a huge population. After determining that TCM was often effective, they tried integrating rural TCM doctors into Western-type modern hospitals. Today, you can find M.D.s, TCM doctors, and dual-trained doctors in China. Because TCM involves the largest number of techniques (acupuncture, herbs, massage, and so on) — and is probably the most widely practiced version of Oriental medicine — we devote most of this chapter to it.

✔ **Ethnic Chinese traditional medicine.** This approach is the more old-fashioned kind of Chinese medicine — the kind you may find practiced in a big-city Chinatown. Many of the techniques resemble those used in TCM — acupuncture, herbs, and the like — but don't be surprised if you're sent home with a jar of raw ma huang and don't really understand how to use it. Many practitioners of ethnic Chinese traditional medicine cater to a Chinese-speaking clientele — so brush up on your Mandarin if you plan to visit one.

✔ **Classical acupuncture.** This approach, also known as "The Worsley School" and developed in England, uses acupuncture alone to do the healing. It's sometimes called "five element acupuncture" because it's based on the ancient Chinese theory that the universe is made up of five interrelated elements: earth, fire, water, metal, and wood. Human health is the direct product of the interactions and relationships between these elements, and every organ system of the body corresponds to one. The acupuncturist's job is to help get all the elements into perfect harmony.

✔ **Japanese acupuncture.** In this kinder, gentler version of acupuncture, the needles tend to be thinner and less intimidating. Plus, you're more likely to have the points stimulated with fingertips rather than needles. Unlike Chinese acupuncture, no herbal remedies are used.

✔ **Auricular acupuncture.** In this approach, the ear is a signpost and the road to better health. A healer may look at your ear, for example, and tell you that your spleen is out of whack! Not only can the ear give clues to what's wrong in many different places in the body, but these diseases can be treated by putting acupuncture needles or staples into (or taping them onto) strategic points of the ear. Auricular acupuncture is often used to relieve pain or ease withdrawal symptoms.

✔ **French/Helms-style acupuncture.** This school of acupuncture, also known as *medical acupuncture,* is used by M.D.s (and D.O.s, or osteopaths) who draw on any of the previous techniques to supplement more conventional treatments. If you live in the United States, chances are high that this is the kind of Chinese medicine you're going to get from a physician. That's because most physician acupuncturists in the United States were trained in this approach. Its leading proponent is Dr. Joseph Helms at UCLA, and his course in medical acupuncture trains more physician acupuncturists by far than any other program in the United States. Plus, in 23 states (as of this writing) medical acupuncture is the only *legal* form of acupuncture.

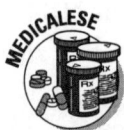

Many, if not most, practitioners of "Chinese" or "Oriental" medicine outside of China may also call themselves *eclectic* practitioners because they don't limit themselves to a single approach.

Traditional Chinese Medicine

Traditional Chinese medicine — TCM for short — is a complete medical system that covers physical, emotional, and psychological healing, as well as preventive health care. Whether a practitioner was trained in China or in one of the many schools of TCM elsewhere in the world, you can expect full-scale service that combines a variety of hands-on approaches, plus herbal medicines, exercises, massage, and prescribed lifestyle changes. Treatments aim at restoring (or maintaining) overall health — not wiping out a specific disease or fixing a single broken part.

The five pillars of TCM

Traditional Chinese medicine is said to rest on five pillars, all important parts of maintaining and restoring health:

- **Acupuncture.** In this ancient practice, the healer inserts thin disposable metal needles into key points in the skin and manipulates them. In related variations, the key points can be stimulated with the fingertips (*acupressure* or *shiatsu*) or a weak electrical current or the needles can be warmed first with a burning herb (*moxibustion*).

- **Traditional Chinese herbs.** Despite the word "herbs," these substances are not necessarily plants. As long as they are natural and "whole" — that is, do not involve specific chemicals isolated from plants or synthesized in a lab — they count. Often a combination of different substances, they usually come in one of three basic forms (and there's a lot of *unresolved* debate about which is most effective):

    - Raw (also known as *bulk*) plants that you boil into a tea or soup

    - Tablets, pills, powders, capsules, or tinctures (alcohol-based mixtures)

    - Extracts (concentrated preparations) added to water, teas, or soups

- **Diet and nutrition.** Often a complete TCM treatment plan includes advice about food and diet. Depending on your condition, you may be told to avoid certain foods (such as dairy products or "hot" foods), for example, or to change meal times.

- **Exercise, stress reduction, and lifestyle counseling.** Traditional Chinese exercises and martial arts such as *Qi Gong* or *Tai Chi* are a regular part of the healing and health maintenance process. But these "exercises" involve a lot more than pumping iron. Each is a form of mind-body medicine that uses breathing and postural exercises together with meditation and relaxation techniques. A TCM healer may also tell you how to live your life better, whether by correcting your bad habits or cleaning out "toxins" from your bowels.

✔ **Massage.** Traditional Chinese doctors also use age-old massage techniques (called *An-mo* and *Tui Na)* to relax and heal the body and to release "toxins" from the tissues.

All these pillars spring from the Confucian-Taoist theory that everything — from the smallest atom to the universe itself, and including human beings — must be in balance. The human being is the universe in miniature, basically an ecosystem parallel to the larger ecosystem and just as subject to outside influences. For that reason, relationships are extremely important to health. In TCM, it's just as unhealthy to be in a bad relationship with your community as to have a poor diet or be exposed to a particular disease-causing germ.

You can't avoid a few basic philosophical terms if you spend more than five seconds considering TCM. People can (and have) written books on each one of these terms, debating their exact meanings and trying to explain them to the Western mind — which is no mean feat. In this chapter, we won't even pretend to get into all that. But we will tell you as little — and we mean as little — as you need to know to get the gist of TCM.

If you prefer to skip this section, all you really need to know boils down to this: According to TCM, you won't be healthy unless you have a free flow of "vital energy" (*qi*) throughout your body and a harmonic balance of *yin* and *yang* — the inextricably linked opposite states that make up all things.

Tao — the way of life

Tao means "the way" or "the way of life." It's the supreme guide of human conduct and the sum total of everything you should do to be strong, healthy, good, and anything else your heart desires. It's also the source of harmony throughout the entire universe. According to TCM, health depends largely on your behavior toward the Tao. If you follow Tao perfectly, you can have perfect health and eternal youth. But, of course, no one can follow it perfectly.

Yin and yang — opposites that explain all change

Yin and yang are dual and inseparable powers that regulate everything that exists — and everything that happens in the universe. These linked opposites are sometimes described as negative and positive, female and male, dark and light, motion and stillness, low and high, evil and good, ugly and beautiful, disease and health, death and life, and just about any other pair of opposites you can imagine. In ancient Chinese philosophy, every object and event in the universe consists of both yin and yang. It's the relationship between the two that makes things what they are.

Wit and wisdom from The Nei Jing

Pretty much everything you'd ever want to know about Chinese medicine (and philosophy) is summed up in a classic (and ancient!) book called *The Nei Jing* — or *The Yellow Emperor's Classic of Internal Medicine*. This treatise is supposedly the oldest known medical text on the planet — and the Chinese regard it as the most influential work on earth, bar none.

Whether or not the Yellow Emperor (also known as *Huang Ti*, but this name is harder to remember) was a real person is a hot topic of scholarly debate — which, fortunately, makes absolutely no difference in your decision to use Chinese medicine. Part of the debate is about when this guy, who may or may not have existed, actually lived (and the range is huge!).

Whoever or whatever "the Yellow Emperor" was, the treatise itself is chock-full of useful insights, many of which are just as valid (and used by practicing doctors) today as they were thousands of years ago.

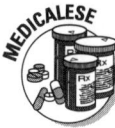

All you really need to know is that health according to TCM requires a perfect balance of yin and yang. Sometimes achieving that balance means increasing *("tonifying")* yin and decreasing *("dispersing")* yang; sometimes it means deciding where the imbalance is and correcting it. A person who lives correctly (that is, follows the Tao) will keep up a perfect balance of yin and yang.

Qi (Chee) — the invisible energy force

Basic to Chinese medicine is the idea of "vital energy" or "life force" — known as *qi* (and pronounced "chee"). If you have *qi*, you're alive. If you don't have it, you're dead. *Qi* circulates through the body and the universe.

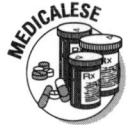

By the way, *qi* is sometimes written out as chi depending on the system used to transform Chinese characters into English; in fact, because Chinese characters don't correspond with the English alphabet exactly, you'll often see the same word written in three or four different ways, with or without capitals, as a compound word or two separate words. We try to stick to spellings most familiar in Western countries whenever possible.

Just as every culture seems to enjoy a version of dough-covered meats or vegetables (samosas, pierogies, blintzes, pastries, burritos, kibbes, Chinese dumplings, and so on — we must be hungry), just about every system of healing includes some version of vital energy, invisible energy force, or animating force (except for mainstream Western medicine!).

The Nei Jing on preventive medicine

"To administer medicines to diseases which have already developed and to suppress revolts which have already developed is comparable to the behavior of those persons who begin to dig a well after they have become thirsty, and of those who begin to cast weapons after they have already engaged in battle. Would these actions not be too late?"

—The Yellow Emperor's Classic of Internal Medicine

An imbalance of *qi* (which is related to an imbalance in yin and yang) underlies all disease. If you have too little *qi*, or if your *qi is* blocked — which is believed to occur from excess stress, lack of exercise, or improper diet — you're said to have a *qi deficiency disease*. This in turn makes you vulnerable to infection, degenerative processes, and other nasties that are characteristic of modern existence. (Interestingly, Western medicine has a long history of theories linking disease to excess or deficient energy, although these theories have been overshadowed by less philosophical explanations in the past century or so.)

Principles for keeping yourself healthy

Buddhist, Taoist, and Confucianist terms aside, TCM can be translated into certain basic principles of health:

✔ **Prevention is key.** Chinese medicine assumes that disease is easier to prevent than cure. In fact, ancient Chinese doctors only got paid if their patients stayed healthy — kind of an early version of HMO thinking! Most practices can be done on a regular basis to keep the system in balance and prevent problems down the line. Even herbs are given more often to balance *qi* or nourish organ networks than to cure specific problems.

The Nei Jing on the environment

"All types of disease may occur when one is over-exposed to wind, rain, cold or heat; also when there is imbalance of yin and yang; or in extreme joy or anger, with irregular eating, undesirable living conditions, or in a state of fright or dread."

—The Yellow Emperor's Classic of Internal Medicine

✔ **Keep up your resistance.** Instead of focusing on combating disease, Chinese medicine focuses on keeping up normal and healthy bodily functions (such as digestion, breathing, and so on). So you're better equipped to keep outside agents from invading — and causing disease.

✔ **Watch the weather.** In Chinese medicine, the human body is a universe in miniature. And like the universe, it's affected by all sorts of outside forces. That's why what you do to keep healthy should vary with the season and the climate. It isn't enough to stick the acupuncture needles in the right place — the process has to be done in the right season and climatic conditions to work right. Plus the exact technique has to be adjusted to the patient's breathing. Too much cold, damp, dryness, heat, wind, and so on can also make you sick. Various diseases are caused by excess heat (such as a skin rash) or cold (such as kidney trouble). Practitioners of TCM also talk about "internal climate" — for example, you may have "excess dryness" inside if you have a disease, such as diabetes, that makes you urinate a lot.

✔ **Focus on overall balance, not symptoms.** In TCM, symptoms indicate what's out of balance in the whole person. Everything is related. So practitioners treat diseases by correcting and rebalancing the flow of *qi* throughout the body, not blasting symptoms.

✔ **Be a partner with your practitioner.** The philosophy behind Chinese medicine often attracts practitioners (especially in Western countries) who think of themselves more as facilitators than powerful magicians or gods. As a result, patients often regard practitioners as partners — or even friends. This cooperation doesn't mean that some acupuncturists won't stick in needles to "cure" you without saying a word — in fact, traditionally, Chinese practitioners were pretty cold fish. And if you're the kind of person who just wants to be "fixed" without putting in much effort, you may want this kind of practitioner.

Visiting a TCM Practitioner

On your first visit to a TCM practitioner, be prepared to answer a bunch of questions about your health and family health history, as well as your lifestyle, diet, exercise habits, emotional state, sleep patterns, bowel movements, and even home and work environments. Your responses will help the practitioner determine *(diagnose)* what may be causing imbalances in your body.

The practitioner will also give you a good once-over to figure out where your imbalance may lie. Practitioners pay a lot more attention to your whole being (including the way you look, feel, sit, speak, breathe, and even smell) than any specific symptom. You may even be asked about your dreams.

The healer will undoubtedly analyze your pulse — and we don't just mean pressing your wrist and counting. TCM healers believe that the pulse has close to 30 different qualities (different rhythms, lengths, thicknesses, and so on) — all of which are based on the way the *qi* is moving through a body.

Many practitioners also examine a patient's tongue. This practice may seem weird. The truth is, though, that mainstream medicine has all but forgotten the many clues to illness that can be read by looking, listening, feeling, even tasting parts of a patient's body (mainstream doctors used to taste urine, believe it or not, to check for signs of what we now call diabetes).

By looking at the tongue's color, coating, texture, shape, dryness, and the like, a TCM healer tries to determine whether you have too much or too little *qi*, moisture, or blood in your system — and even which organ system is at the root of the imbalance. Important clues also come from your eyes, skin, hair, and nails.

After the imbalance and your "individual conformation" are determined, you'll get a diagnosis — perhaps "excess heat in the lungs" or "insufficient *qi* in the kidneys." Then the practitioner will offer a personalized healing program to rebalance your energy. This program may involve a series of acupuncture treatments, dietary and exercise instructions, and perhaps prescriptions of various Chinese herbs.

Because Chinese herbs can be lethal in large amounts or if used improperly, make sure that you take only what is prescribed and follow directions to the letter. And leave the mixing to the practitioner or the herbalist — for this task you definitely need to rely on people who know what they're doing!

You will probably arrange to go back for additional treatments and to allow the practitioner to look for changes in your condition. Make sure that you understand why the particular treatment plan (and number of treatments) is right for your particular problem.

The Nei Jing on thorough examinations

"In order to examine the course of a disease one must investigate whether a man is courageous or nervous or cowardly, and one must examine his bones, flesh, and skin and then one can know the facts of the case which are necessary for the methods of treatment."

—*The Yellow Emperor's Classic of Internal Medicine*

Something This Old Can't Be All Wrong

All this stuff about *qi* and yin-yang can sound like a bunch of gobbledy-gook to Westerners. Did someone just pull it all out of a hat — or is there actually any evidence for it? Well, yes and no. The answer depends on how much you want to count experience as evidence.

A different view of evidence

Much of the theory behind TCM is caught up in early Chinese religion and cosmogony (explanations of the origin of the universe), rather than dissection of the body or formal experiments — not that the ancient healers didn't dissect corpses to learn anatomy or try out their cures on real people. But all conclusions had to fit into the larger system of explanation — the one with Tao, yin and yang, five elements, all that — and flow out of it like a beautiful piece of poetry. Documenting a statement — by saying how many times the result had been seen and under what conditions — in the style of the modern scientific method wasn't required.

But whether the reasons of the ancient Chinese healers convince the Western mind, many of their observations were right on the mark. And today more and more researchers are using conventional scientific studies to document some of the practices (if not the theories that supposedly explain them).

And don't forget history. Nobody's certain when TCM began, but one thing's for sure: 2,300 years of historical records back it up (dating to about 300 B.C.). The story of *The Emperor's New Clothes* notwithstanding, it's hard to believe that so many people over so many years could have been totally wrong. The fact that traditional Chinese medicine continues to be widely used throughout Asia to this day doesn't prove that it's the best system of medicine on earth, or even that it does everything it claims to do — but it suggests that there must be at least *some validity* to it.

The Nei Jing on the mind-body effect

"Those who are about at night have difficulties in breathing emanating from the kidneys. Those whose demeanor is dissolute and licentious get a disease of the lungs. Those who are lazy and full of apprehension and fear have difficulties in breathing, emanating from the lungs. Those whose deportment is licentious and excessive will injure their spleen. . . . Those whose demeanor is immoral and dissolute will injure their hearts."

—*The Yellow Emperor's Classic of Internal Medicine*

More recent (and mainstream) evidence

Qi is invisible, and it flows through invisible channels called *meridians* (see Chapter 15 for more information). This is a big bummer for scientists who want to see, feel, measure, and document *qi*. It doesn't help that the success of some Chinese medicine techniques depends on the skill of the healer or that each treatment is supposed to be personalized — so that the procedure that works for one person won't necessarily work for another.

Claims that Chinese medicine (or any health program) can prevent you from getting sick are even harder to prove — if not impossible. Because you only go around once in life, you can't possibly know whether doing (or not doing) something would have kept you healthier or extended your life span. (Researchers have ways to get around this problem — called retrospective and prospective studies — but they're far from perfect.)

No wonder, then, that most studies so far have crummy methodology and that most of the better studies contradict each other. Even so, for at least some conditions, researchers can see and measure the *effects* of Chinese medicine on specific problems, and on large enough groups of people to convince the statisticians that aren't sold on the "long history" argument. And growing evidence indicates that at least some of the approaches can work (see Chapter 15 on acupuncture and Chapter 20 on herbs).

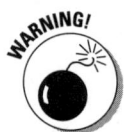

You may hear or read about many other herbs that supposedly help cure cancer or heart disease — but keep your enthusiasm in check. Most, if not all, of these claims are based on studies published in questionable journals. Chinese medicine *can* complement conventional treatments for these conditions, however. Acupuncture, for example, can help relieve the nausea that often accompanies cancer chemotherapy — and boost the power of more conventional antinausea medications.

When to Try Chinese Medicine

Even though Chinese medicine aims at overall health, some aspects of it — particularly herbs and acupuncture — can be used to treat specific ailments. Check out Chapter 15 on acupuncture or Chapter 20 on herbal remedies for more information. Other aspects of TCM — particularly massage therapy and *Qi Gong* — may be particularly useful in reducing stress and anxiety, or just building up your general health and resistance to diseb0e.

You might also consider using Chinese medicine together with other types of medicine — such as mainstream medicine, chiropractic, or naturopathy. That way, you don't miss out on the benefits of any of these approaches, and you still have a way to overcome each of their limitations.

How much will Chinese medicine treatments cost?

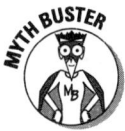

Even though Chinese medicine bypasses the hospitals, expensive tests, and high-tech treatments of mainstream medicine, it's not necessarily "cheap" when it comes to your overall budget. After all, if you're using Chinese medicine to supplement mainstream treatment, the cost is still additional. Plus, you may well have to pay for these treatments out of your own pocket.

Cost also varies depending on the training of the practitioner (M.D.s usually cost more), your location, and the length of treatment. In general, though, expect a first visit to a practitioner of Chinese medicine (or an acupuncturist) to cost from $60 to $110, and follow-ups from $30 to $80. Herbal remedies may run you another $25 a month (though certain remedies can cost double that). Just how many times you'll have to go back depends on your personal treatment program, but if acupuncture is involved expect to be back at least once or twice a week and to need at least six to ten treatments.

Will insurance cover the cost of Chinese medicine treatments?

There's a chance that your health plan will cover acupuncture, at least for certain types of problems (especially drug and alcohol addiction) — but probably only if the procedure is performed by a conventional M.D. Check your plan, too, to see if it covers Chinese herbs. Some people think that coverage may soon expand — especially because the National Institutes of Health (NIH) recently endorsed Chinese medicine for some ailments, and the Food and Drug Administration (FDA) has stopped labeling acupuncture needles "experimental." But we'd be surprised if most insurance companies will cover treatments not done by an M.D.

Possible benefits of Chinese medicine

Chinese medicine is probably most useful in treating: low-back pain; muscle cramps; osteoarthritis of the knee; tooth and facial pain; muscle pain; fibromyalgia; headaches (including migraines); asthma; chronic fatigue syndrome; chronic bronchitis; chronic obstructive pulmonary disease (COPD); Crohn's disease; ulcerative colitis; nausea and vomiting (especially associated with surgery, chemotherapy, or pregnancy); withdrawal symptoms during recovery from addictions; and paralysis related to stroke, head and spinal cord injury, multiple sclerosis (MS), or Bell's palsy.

When Not to Try Chinese Medicine

As with any larger system of healing (including conventional), TCM has both reasonable and not-so-reasonable parts. So instead of embracing or discarding the whole system, the idea is to use expert advice and common sense to find the potentially useful parts — and just say no to the parts that seem foolish or dangerous.

One other thing: If you have a high fever or were just in a car accident, get yourself (or have someone get you) to a conventional emergency room or surgeon. A serious accident or raging infection is not the time to think about *Qi Gong* or herbal teas (although some viral infections, untouchable with mainstream antibiotics, may be treatable with Chinese herbs).

Possible Harmful Effects

All in all Chinese medicine is pretty safe. Acupuncture poses few dangers — if the needles are clean (and since the mid-1990s most acupuncturists in the United States have been trained in clean-needle techniques).

Toxicity from Chinese herbs is possible (though rare) — especially if the herbs are used or mixed incorrectly (you may remember the widely re-ported deaths from overdoses of ma huang — *Ephedra sinica* — in 1996). Watch out in particular for jin bu huan, a Chinese herbal pain-reliever. It contains substances that can cause liver problems and even death — especially in kids.

Keep an eye peeled, too, for Chinese "patent" remedies manufactured overseas, which are sometimes adulterated with lead or steroids. The best way to stay safe is to use these herbs only under the supervision of some-one well-trained in identifying, preparing, and prescribing Chinese herbs.

As with any alternative therapy, however, even the most innocuous tech-nique poses a danger if it keeps you from getting an accurate diagnosis or conventional treatment for a serious illness.

Resources for Finding a Good Practitioner

You may already be using an M.D. — or chiropractor or naturopath — trained in Chinese medicine, or aspects of it. If you're not so lucky, check out local alternative clinics or wellness centers, which often have TCM practitioners working alongside naturopaths, chiropractors, nutritionists, homeopaths, or other alternative practitioners. They can also be good sources of names of reputable TCM healers, if they don't happen to employ one themselves.

Getting the names

If you live in California, Colorado, Florida, New Mexico, New York, Oregon, or Washington, you may be in luck. TCM healers are abundant in these areas. But wherever you live, national organizations of practitioners can give you names of at least minimally competent practitioners in your area as well as more information on standards of competence.

The quickest way to get names is right off the Web — either cruise to the American Association of Oriental Medicine (AAOM) at www.aaom.org for a list of members in your state or to the National Certification Commission for Acupuncture and Oriental Medicine (NCCAOM) at www.nccaom.org/dir.html for practitioners (in the United States and other countries) who are currently certified and active in acupuncture, Chinese herbology, and Oriental bodywork therapy. Or check out the associations listed in the appendix.

Legal requirements to practice TCM and acupuncture vary from state to state (see Chapter 15) — and so do the meanings of the terms "licensed," "registered," and "certified." In some states, only M.D.s or D.O.s can practice acupuncture; in others, you just need to sign a consent form stating that you understand that TCM isn't meant to replace conventional treatment.

To find out your state's requirements (and the local meanings of the terms "licensed," "registered," and "certified") — call the AAOM (see the appendix).

Finding a healer with the right stuff

Don't rely on licenses or registrations to choose a healer. Above all, you want someone who has been fully trained in TCM (unless all you want are acupuncture treatments). Even if an M.D. has been licensed to practice acupuncture, this license doesn't mean that she knows very much about *Qi Gong*, herbal remedies, or the other parts of TCM. She may not even understand all the intricacies of acupuncture.

Any M.D. practicing acupuncture should have at least 200 *hours* of acupuncture training (and many people argue for three times that). Non-M.D.s should have completed at least a two-year course in a recognized acupuncture program and have appropriate licensure or registration. And they should have passed the National Certification Commission for Acupuncture and Oriental Medicine (NCCAOM) exam. Best of all are graduates of one of the reputable schools of Chinese medicine that trains nonphysicians in three-to-four-year programs (right now the United States offers 35 of these programs, some of which have rigorous admission standards and curricula).

Whatever the training, dump any practitioner who doesn't understand the limitations of TCM — one who tells you, for example, that he can reset your broken arm with herbs. The same goes for one who tells you that TCM can "replace" regular medical examinations and treatment for every conceivable problem or who refuses to communicate with your mainstream M.D.

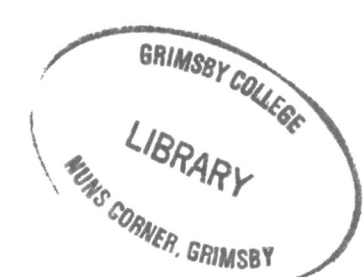
Chapter 10

Trying a Little of Everything: Ayurveda

● ●

In This Chapter

▶ Doshas, prakriti, and other neat ideas

▶ Traditional and clinical evidence for Ayurveda

▶ What it's like to visit an Ayurvedic doctor

▶ When to try Ayurveda, and when to seek another method

▶ Best ways to find a reputable healer

● ●

Ayurveda is a 5,000-year-old system of mind-body medicine from India that includes elements of herbal medicine, nutrition, meditation, stress reduction, yoga, and massage therapy. Actually, Ayurveda is much more than a system of healing — it's an integral part of a larger spiritual system that evolved from the teachings of sages (rishis) in the Himalayas — but many practitioners, especially outside of India, skip the religious stuff. Like many ancient systems of healing, Ayurveda regards disease as an imbalance and offers ways to restore and preserve physical, emotional, and spiritual health by re-establishing the body's natural balance.

Ayurveda's most famous proponent in the United States is Deepak Chopra, M.D. Reading Dr. Chopra is a little bit like reading the ancient Greek doctor Hippocrates (except his text is in English, of course) or even like reading the tracts of the great 18th-century European doctors — and that's not a criticism. These earlier healers were no fools. Even without modern standards of scientific evidence, they had remarkable and often valid insights, even if they had baffling explanations for them. There is more than a grain of truth in what Hippocrates had to say about the four temperaments, and more than a grain in what Dr. Deepak Chopra has to say about the three basic metabolic types.

Even so, practitioners of this old medicine — and its modern-day counterparts that come to us in the form of alternative medicine — sometimes lose sight of what is good in today's "scientific medicine." In particular, they lose sight of the need to distinguish fact from fantasy. The result is lots of advice mingling the two — and little way to know how to untangle one from the other. So — voilà — here's a little untangling.

Doshas and Dr. Chopra

Two main schools of Ayurveda are practiced outside of India. One, Maharishi Ayur-Veda, was started by Maharishi Mahesh Yogi (of transcendental meditation fame) and emphasizes meditation as the key to healing. This for-profit (and highly profitable) group runs its own training programs worldwide and sells an exclusive line of products.

The other branch of Ayurveda — popularized by Deepak Chopra, M.D. — also advocates meditation but not as the most important means to health. It's basically a loosely associated group of healers and health care advocates, many of them trained in India and now based at various alternative medical schools or mind-body centers.

A holistic approach

Chinese medicine and Ayurveda share a lot of underlying philosophy:

✔ **Macrocosm/microcosm.** The idea of a living, breathing, thinking universe is central to Ayurveda. But it's not as revolutionary as some Ayurvedic healers would have you believe. The idea that the universe is one big organism, analogous to all the lowly organisms here on earth, pervades many ancient philosophies and healing systems.

✔ **Vital energy.** Ayurvedic medicine holds that all life is based on an underlying energy or vital force called *prana* — basically similar to the *qi* ("chee") of Chinese medicine. Ayurvedic healers say that this prana is centered in various energy centers called *chakras* that work together to keep the prana flowing through the body — considered essential to the health of body, mind, and spirit. Various massage, breathing, and yoga techniques (with names such as chakral pranic healing, chakra balancing, and chakra yoga) aim to help out the chakras.

Possible benefits of Ayurveda

Ayurveda seems to be most useful in treating allergies, chronic fatigue, rashes, ulcers, indigestion, insomnia, anxiety, and depression. It may also help speed surgical recovery and supplement conventional treatment for serious illnesses such as cancer.

✓ **The unity of body, mind, and spirit.** Most Westerners naturally separate thoughts and feelings from what happens to their bodies, but both Ayurveda and Chinese systems of healing assume that they are inextricably linked. That idea means that you won't heal your nausea or pain until you get your mind and spirit in order as well. This way of thinking may take a little getting used to, because most modern Western thought compartmentalizes body and mind, and often doesn't know what to do with spirit at all.

✓ **Body, mind, and spiritual awareness.** In Ayurveda, these three factors are the holy trinity — and you can't be free from disease unless all three are working right. In other words, your food, friends, family, environment, exercise regimen, sleep, play, and work habits — everything! — affect your health.

✓ **Balance.** If you want to get — and stay — healthy, the key is rebalancing your whole system, not attacking a specific symptom.

✓ **Personal responsibility.** As Dr. Deepak Chopra puts it in his book *Perfect Health: The Complete Mind/Body Guide* (Harmony Books, 1991) "The first secret you should know about perfect health is that you have to choose it. You can be as healthy as you think it is possible to be. Perfect health . . . involves a total shift in perspective which makes disease and infirm old age impossible."

Table 10-1 shows where to find more information on some of the many alternative techniques that derive from Ayurvedic principles.

Table 10-1	Where to Find Information on Alternatives Related to Ayurveda
Subject	*Chapter of This Book*
Massage therapy	See Chapter 16.
Meditation	See Chapter 17.
Yoga	See Chapter 17.
Herbal medicine	See Chapter 20.
Aromatherapy	See Chapter 21.
Dietary changes	See Chapter 22.
Music and color therapy	See Chapter 24.

What's your prakriti?

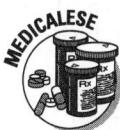

Ayurveda holds that there are five elements in nature and in the body: ether, air, fire, water, and earth. These elements are the foundation for all nature — including human beings. And every part of the human body is the manifestation of one or more of these elements. For example, air is manifested in the beating of the heart and the expansion and contraction of the lungs, and fire is manifested in the digestive tract, body temperature, and metabolism. The five elements also govern the five senses — that is, the ability to perceive and interact with the rest of nature. That's good, because in Ayurveda staying in harmony with nature is essential for optimum health.

The five elements combine to form three basic forces, known as *doshas,* which exist in everything in the universe. Ether and air combine to form *vata,* fire and water combine to form *pitta,* and earth and water combine to form *kapha.*

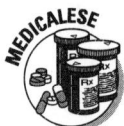

These three doshas — vata, pitta, and kapha — can be found in every person, too, in various combinations. Your particular combination is called your *tridosha* (this term is easy to remember if you recall that "tri" means "three" and that there are three doshas to combine). Everybody is said to have all three doshas in every cell, but your particular tridosha is determined by which one (or combination) dominates.

Often only one of the three doshas dominates, creating one of three basic mind-body (or constitutional) types (which sound a lot like the ectomorphs, mesomorphs, and endomorphs that conventional docs used to talk about):

✔ **Vata types** are enthusiastic, vivacious, imaginative, anxious, quick to learn, and quick to forget. They tire and chill easily, sleep poorly, and tend to have digestive troubles, lower back pain, nervous system diseases, and arthritis. They're often thin, with narrow shoulders and hips.

✔ **Pitta types** are intense, quick to anger, sharp-witted, enterprising, impatient, commanding, orderly, and critical. They tend to have medium and muscular builds, fair or reddish complexions, warm skin, and large appetites, and are prone to heartburn, gallbladder and liver disorders, skin problems, ulcers, and hemorrhoids.

✔ **Kapha types** are relaxed, graceful, slow-moving, tranquil, affectionate, complacent, indecisive, empathetic, and slow to learn but long to remember. They tend to be thickset and gain weight easily, need a lot of sleep and warmth, and are prone to sinus problems, colds, allergies, asthma, and painful joints.

Besides determining your mind-body type, the doshas are also "metabolic principles" that control basic bodily functions. Vata controls movement, pitta controls metabolism (the processing of food, air, and water), and kapha controls structure.

Many people are combinations of types (for example, vata-pitta type), with one type dominant. A few people have nearly equal aspects of all three doshas. Your particular combination gives you a unique *prakriti* — or nature — from birth.

No one dosha is healthier than another. But if you want to feel your best, you have to get your inborn doshas into the best balance possible. In other words, harmonizing your doshas with your inborn nature is the key to health. The job of the Ayurvedic practitioner is to identify both your prakriti and your tridosha and to prescribe treatments that will get them into harmony with each other and with nature as a whole.

The Evidence for Ayurveda

Like much of alternative medicine, Ayurveda sounds a lot like the medicine practiced centuries, even millenia ago — and, in fact, it is. Remember that Ayurveda is 5,000 years old. And as with other older systems of healing (including Chinese medicine), the proof is more in the pudding than in the statistically significant study.

Evidence from tradition — and philosophy

For most of human history, healers — perfectly intelligent and well-intentioned men and women — sat down and thought out reasonable explanations for their observations about sickness and health and then elaborated these thoughts into what seemed like sensible explanations. It's these explanations — plus the fact that this system has stuck around for so many years — that's supposed to make Ayurveda (which is the Sanskrit word for the "science," or "knowledge," of life) worthy of consideration.

Again, these arguments don't necessarily mean that Ayurveda can do everything its proponents say that it can do. But they do mean that this system can't be dismissed without fair trial. The idea that medicine should be based on evidence, actual data, is a relatively new one. Although modern proponents of Ayurveda pay lip service to evidence, the bulk of the system is based on analogies, metaphors, or hunches.

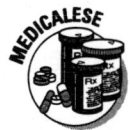

Remember, we don't deny that a great deal of conventional medicine is also based on tradition or wishful thinking. Asthma medicine for kids — most medicines for kids for that matter — have never been tested in clinical trials. The same thing goes for popular heart medications called calcium-channel blockers. The fact is, doctors are often taking risks with unproven conventional medicines. But, at least in theory, the gold standard for a valid practice in conventional medicine is a scientifically valid experiment — preferably a whole lot of them.

The problem is, as with many other alternative and preventive approaches, many Ayurvedic practices are hard to "prove" by standards of conventional medicine. Some Ayurvedic teachings are more like religion than science, too, and have to be taken as a given — the idea that life is not random, for example, or that a guiding intelligence must exist. And who are we to argue with that? This book is not, after all, *Personal Faith For Dummies*.

Clinical evidence

As for published studies, most to date involve herbal products sold by the Maharishi Ayur-Veda followers. So far there isn't any *convincing* evidence that any of these herbs do anything much for humans. That doesn't mean that there won't ever be evidence, of course, but right now it doesn't exist. Some of the studies currently funded by the Office of Alternative Medicine may give us some better answers in a few years.

The evidence for most other Ayurvedic preventive techniques isn't much better, mainly because few studies so far have used a control group. What does seem clear, though, is that a lot of people *think* that some Ayurvedic practices (including yoga and cleansing rituals) are a great way to relax, relieve depression and anxiety, boost energy, improve digestion, and relieve chronic pain. And that's not anything to scoff at.

A few studies also suggest (but don't prove) that yogic breathing may help stimulate the brain and that other yogic practices may help control asthma. Also, numerous studies link meditation (not necessarily Ayurvedic) with improved immune response and reduced levels of stress hormones.

Visiting an Ayurvedic Doctor

On your first visit, an Ayurvedic physician will determine your prakriti or particular combination of doshas (your *tridosha*) by examining your pulse, tongue, nails, eyes, face, and posture — as well as by listening closely to what you say about your eating, working, playing, sleeping, and other lifestyle habits — and assessing the way your voice sounds when you say it. You may also be asked to fill out a written questionnaire.

The practitioner will then give you a customized health plan to help harmonize your doshas. This program involves a specific regimen of herbs, foods, massage, yoga postures (*asanas*), breathing exercises, and meditations. The idea is for you to learn to heal yourself — you don't rely on the healer to do it for you. Your relationship with your healer is vital, but ultimately you're in charge (which is where you want to be).

You will probably be put on a regular regime called a *rasayana. Herbal rasayanas* are mixtures of herbs, fruits, and minerals in various forms to promote good health or treat specific diseases. *Behavioral rasayanas* are customized plans for you to change your lifestyle. Expect to make some basic changes in your patterns of eating, sleeping, working, and exercising.

The first session with the healer may last an hour or so. Weeks or months later the healer will probably want to monitor your progress by conducting much shorter follow-up exams.

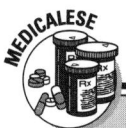

Healing the Ayurvedic way

Ayurvedic healing involves many different techniques. Among the most common are

✔ **Sensory delights.** Because everything you see, hear, smell, taste, and feel can also affect your health, many of the Ayurvedic healing techniques involve surrounding yourself with balms for the senses — including soothing music, beautiful hues, invigorating aromas, and special massages (often with warm sesame oil).

✔ **Diet and dosha.** Ayurveda divides foods into six basic tastes — sweet, sour, salty, pungent, bitter, and astringent — each of which has specific effects on the doshas. That's why Ayurvedic dietary therapy often involves eating specific foods to "pacify" a dosha that is out of balance. If you're a vata type, for example, you may be told to eat more butter and fat (to "pacify" your vata). If you're a kapha type, you may be told to avoid sweets and eat more pungent, bitter, and astringent foods such as greens, spices, beans, and potatoes.

✔ **Marma therapy.** In Ayurveda, internal prana meets the outside world at 107 junctions *(marmas)*. By pressing on these points (which are a lot like acupuncture points), you stimulate the mind-body connection and help balance your doshas. You can get marma therapy at Ayurvedic clinics or learn to do it for yourself. Do you want a quick way to relieve worry and headaches? Try gently massaging the marma between your eyebrows with your eyes closed!

✔ **Yoga asanas.** Various yoga exercises can be used to stretch and activate marma points. Yoga is a set of postures *(asanas)* aimed to integrate mind and body. Ayurvedic medicine usually uses hatha yoga, which stresses physical exercises.

✔ **Meditation.** Meditating is basically a way of focusing on the silence and wisdom inside us by using special chanting or breathing exercises. Because Ayurveda holds that by discovering this inner place we will find the means to health, meditation is an important part of self-healing.

✔ **Breathing exercises.** Breath is supposed to be the bodily expression of the vital energy (prana). Many Ayurvedic doctors recommend a soothing set of balanced breathing exercises (often performed before meditating) called *pranayama*. These exercises help you relax and get in sync with universal energies.

✔ **Detoxification.** One important part of Ayurvedic healing is to rid the body of toxins that can mess up your dosha balance and predispose you to disease. A lot of effort is devoted to purging impurities *(ama)* via the three *malas* (sweat, urine, and feces). In other words, expect talk of steambaths, enemas, laxatives, vomiting, and maybe even bloodletting. Impurities can also be mental, so you may have to purge negative thoughts and feelings, too.

Also expect talk of *panchakarma*. Undergoing this rigorous and intensive purification ritual, in our humble opinion, is kind of like going to a Third Reich spa. To get the ama out, you not only take and inhale medicated oils and undergo oil massages and herbalized sweat treatments, but you have to endure extended periods of fasting, diarrhea, mucous discharge, induced vomiting, and occasionally bloodletting as well. In his book, *Perfect Health: The Complete Mind/Body Guide* (Harmony Books, 1991), Dr. Deepak Chopra recommends that everyone over the age of 12 — sick or well — undergo a week of panchakarma a minimum of once a year. We don't think that it's a great idea for many people.

Expect to pay up to $100 to $150 for the first visit to an Ayurvedic healer, and much less for follow-ups. The cost of the herbs can vary from a few dollars a month to nearly $50. Panchakarma treatments (see the sidebar, "Healing the Ayurvedic way") run the gamut and can be quite pricey, especially if they involve retreating to luxurious accommodations.

Don't expect your insurance to cover these costs unless they were administered by an M.D. (and even then, they may not be covered).

When to Try Ayurveda

Not a lot of hard-core scientific evidence links specific techniques to specific cures, but there's a good chance that some Ayurvedic techniques can boost your energy levels, relax you, and just make you feel better in general. And chances are high that by trying these practices you'll lower your risk of serious illness.

Really, though, asking if you should use Ayurveda (or any larger "system" of medicine) is a lot like asking whether you should consider Judaism, Buddhism, or some other religion. Because we still have a lot more questions than answers about the ultimate superiority of one system over another (and there may never be any answers), you have to decide for yourself if this approach may be worth a try.

If it does sound appealing, just remember this: A lot of Ayurvedic practice may make you healthier in general and may be worth a try for chronic but minor ailments, especially in conjunction with other medical systems.

When Not to Try Ayurveda

If you're expecting to avoid aging or dying, you'd better go elsewhere (whatever popular book titles may suggest). Ayurveda can't give you eternal vigor and life, nor can it cure cancer, diabetes, or heart disease.

Eventually, researchers may find that some Ayurvedic approaches — such as the cleansing and fasting techniques — may help in these (or other) areas. For now, though, Ayurveda basically remains a lifestyle that makes you feel better. Undernutrition (without malnutrition) promises to be the only scientifically validated way to prolong life in mammals (with no proof about human mammals), and even here the jury is still out. Even so, imposing *any* form of discipline on lifestyle and habits may make you feel better.

Like Chinese medicine, Ayurveda is generally not a recommended way to deal with an acute infection — such as pneumonia — or major injury. It can be used to supplement more conventional treatments for serious or advanced disease (including speeding surgical recovery or relieving side effects from cancer therapy), but only under the supervision of a qualified conventional physician.

If you're using herbs from other traditions, don't mix them with Ayurvedic herbs without consulting a practitioner who knows about all of them.

Possible Harmful Effects

Physical side effects from Ayurveda are rare — as long as Ayurvedic treatments don't keep you from having a more serious problem diagnosed. Once in a while, reports reveal side effects from certain Ayurvedic herbs. The FDA restricts some herbs manufactured in India, which makes some sense. Because formulas made by different Indian companies can vary considerably, knowing just what you're buying is difficult.

Ayurvedic medicines containing heavy metals such as lead or mercury may be poisonous (whatever anyone tells you about deactivation through heat processing). Avoid them.

Also be careful not to let the spiritual side of Ayurveda get you down. Much of Ayurveda is uplifting — it's encouraging to hear that people can control their own destiny, for example. But the flip side of this message is that it's your own fault if you get sick — obviously not a very helpful attitude.

Resources for Finding an Ayurvedic Healer

You can live by Ayurvedic principles without consulting an expert healer. Many healers trained in other traditions (including M.D.s, naturopaths, and chiropractors) have picked up Ayurvedic techniques along the way and can practice them competently, too. But if you're going to use some of the specialized herbs or food supplements or want an authentic diagnosis of your prakriti, see a trained Ayurvedic doctor (and tell your regular M.D. as well).

Because the United States offers no licensing system for Ayurvedic practitioners, you have to rely on other credentials. An Ayurvedic specialist trained in India probably knows how to diagnose prakriti accurately. Whatever healers you use, always ask where they were trained, how long they've been in practice, and what experience they have treating people with conditions similar to yours.

For Ayurvedic practitioners and clinics, check with any of the Ayurvedic organizations listed in this book's appendix.

Chapter 11

Looking at the Big Picture: Naturopathy

In This Chapter

▶ What naturopathy is all about

▶ What you need to know about the evidence supporting naturopathy

▶ When you should consider using these practices — and when you shouldn't

▶ How to find a reputable naturopath

*I*f you've ever thought about changing your diet or taking nutritional supplements to lower your risk of heart disease, reduce allergies, or relieve constipation, you already know something about naturopathy. The same is true if you've ever soaked your feet, experienced natural childbirth, or tried relaxation exercises.

Just about anything "natural" you do to help stay or become healthy is part of naturopathy — including herbal treatments, dietary supplements, acupuncture, lifestyle changes, stress management, counseling, hands-on manipulations, homeopathy, hydrotherapy, and electrotherapy. That's because naturopathy, which can often be used together with other systems of healing, is really more of a philosophy than a single set of methods or techniques.

This chapter fills you in on the basics of this optimistic and open approach that in many ways is the most "conventional" way of healing in the world.

Whole-Body Health: Naturopathy Basics

Naturopaths cite a lot of fancy principles (some of them in Latin), but the bottom line is pretty simple: The body has the power to heal itself. The physicians' job is to help keep those natural powers in shape and help them along when necessary.

Possible benefits of naturopathy

Naturopathy includes so many different healing practices that it's used to treat just about any ailment you can imagine. But it's most often used to treat the kinds of conditions that often don't respond to conventional treatments — including allergies, asthma, arthritis, stomach and intestinal problems, depression, insomnia, nausea, high blood pressure, labor pains, gynecologic problems, stress, and chronic pain of every sort. Above all, it's used to help prevent people from getting sick in the first place by helping improve lifestyle habits.

Everything counts in naturopathy

No matter which of the countless approaches are used, every naturopath works according to six basic principles. Many of them are in Latin, a language that appeals to naturopaths — maybe because it reminds people that they're followers of a long tradition.

> ✔ *Vis medicatrix naturae* — **or the healing power of nature.**
> Naturopaths firmly believe in the body's amazing ability to heal itself. For a naturopath, many so-called "symptoms" are nothing more than the body's way of getting rid of some underlying problem. For example, naturopaths (and a surprising number of conventional M.D.s) see fever not as a symptom to eliminate but rather as the body's way of attacking a toxin.
>
> Sometimes nature needs a little help, though — and that's where the healer comes in. If you have a bad cold, for example, a conventional technique would be to clear your stuffy nose with a decongestant. A naturopath, however, would say that the mucus — however unpleasant — is your body's way of bringing in white blood cells to combat the cold virus. Instead of shutting down your own healing powers, why not give them a hand — say by drinking more fluids; stimulating your immune system with vitamin C, zinc, or garlic; or stimulating mucous membranes with salt water gargles?
>
> ✔ *Tolle causam.* Translated from Latin, this phrase just means "find the cause." Naturopaths believe that every illness has some underlying cause — not a germ or physical cause, like conventional M.D.s generally believe — but usually some part of the patient's environment, lifestyle, diet, or habits of living. To cure the patient, this underlying cause has to be found and then corrected.
>
> When conventional medicine aims its guns at symptoms rather than true causes, say naturopaths, it not only messes up natural healing but wreaks permanent havoc. By suppressing symptoms — such as the runny nose of a cold — people train their bodies to be worse fighters in

the future. Some naturopaths say that this indiscriminate battling down of our immune systems with heavy combat gear (including antibiotics) even explains the current preponderance of chronic and degenerative diseases.

✔ *Primum Non Nocere.* All this one means is first, do no harm. This third principle of naturopathy reminds healers to try the least invasive, least risky treatment first.

✔ **Be holistic.** The fourth principle of naturopathy is to treat the whole person — not just the obviously impaired part. Naturopaths see disease as arising from a whole complex of factors — physical, emotional, social, genetic, and the like — so effective treatments should involve all of them.

✔ **Doctors should be teachers.** Naturopaths remember that the word doctor came from the Latin word meaning "to teach" *(docere).* That's why a naturopathic doctor's most important role is training patients to heal themselves. Plus, a good relationship between doctor and patient can help healing along even more.

✔ **Prevention is the best cure.** Naturopaths are even more interested in preserving health than in eliminating illness. That's why they teach people how to keep themselves from getting ill by adopting healthy lifestyle habits (healthy diet, regular exercise, low stress, and so on) as well as how to keep minor problems from getting out of hand.

Two more letters: N.D.

If you find a doctor with an N.D. after her name instead of an M.D., don't worry about needing glasses. Usually these initials mean that the doctor has taken standard premed courses at college and then graduated from an intensive four-year graduate school in naturopathy. As a result, she gets to call herself a "Doctor of Naturopathic Medicine," or N.D. for short.

These programs offer training — both academic and hands-on — in most of the stuff M.D.s learn, including minor surgery and diagnostic testing such as X-rays and ultrasound (although they avoid man-made drugs and major surgery). Plus, they teach the whole range of naturopathic approaches that M.D.s don't learn — not the least of which is the use of diet to treat and prevent disease.

Most naturopaths are pretty well-trained in acupuncture as well as physical manipulation and massage. Partly as a result, naturopathy is rapidly gaining respect in the mainstream. Throughout the United States, particularly the Pacific Northwest, naturopathy is increasingly a regulated/licensed specialty. Some insurers even include credentialed naturopaths as part of their networks and/or pay for naturopathic services.

All this from Lust

Naturopathy can trace its origins to ancient Greek, Indian, and Asian medicine. But its modern "official" version — and current popularity — can thank a German immigrant named Benedict (or Benjamin or Bernard, depending on the source) Lust. Convinced that a water cure had obliterated his tuberculosis, Lust came to the United States in 1895 set to free people from "superstitious" modern methods such as noxious drugs and vaccines. He founded New York City's American School of Naturopathy in 1902 and the American Naturopathic Association in 1919. Lust's ideas spread like wildfire through the 1920s and 1930s, though dazzling feats of conventional medicine led to a temporary lull mid-century. More recent frustration with conventional approaches has revived interest in the kind of nontoxic, natural approaches to health that Lust advocated.

The Evidence for Naturopathy

Because naturopathy is such a mixed bag, it's no surprise that some of its approaches are backed by better evidence than others.

If you start looking into naturopathy, you'll undoubtedly hear many claims that naturopathic treatment can remedy just about any ailment on earth. This includes naturopathic treatment of HIV infection, the use of shark cartilage to treat Kaposi's sarcoma, and the value of garlic oil in preventing blood clots and lowering blood fats.

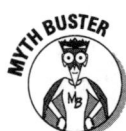

But be careful. The lion's share of the "evidence" for these claims comes from alternative journals such as *Homeopathic Links,* the *Journal of Naturopathic Medicine,* and the *Journal of Orthomolecular Medicine.* These journals have looser standards of evidence (see Chapter 3) than more mainstream journals — so take their conclusions with a very large grain of salt.

Again, we're not saying that natural remedies don't work — far from it. But many of the claims about natural remedies are premature. And we just don't know what, if any, long-term dangers may exist. When we see these studies appearing in *The New England Journal of Medicine* and *The Lancet,* we'll pay more attention.

To be fair, too, some studies of naturopathic remedies have already made it to the big time. Most notable is the ever-mounting evidence that dietary changes can help prevent and possibly even treat various diseases (including heart disease, high blood pressure, and certain cancers). Expect more of the same as results of OAM-funded studies come in (including those from Bastyr University in Washington state, which are evaluating naturopathic therapies for HIV disease).

Plus, many naturopathic treatments (especially the ones involving lifestyle changes) are probably safe and "good for you," even if no one knows for sure whether they'll heal a specific ailment.

When to Try Naturopathy

If you've tried conventional treatments to no avail, you may want to talk to a naturopath about possible natural approaches to your problem. And if you're pretty healthy right now, visiting a naturopath may clue you into how to stay that way.

Visiting a naturopath

Better clear your calendar for your first visit. For those of you accustomed to fifteen-minute, drive-through exams, the hour-or-so session may come as a shock.

Besides doing the usual history and physical, standard lab tests, and maybe an analysis of your pulse or tongue, naturopaths are inclined to (horrors!) get to know you. The idea is to work with you to design a healthier diet, attitude, and lifestyle — plus a customized treatment plan — so the more the naturopath knows about you, the better. And though you're ultimately responsible for your own health and recovery, many naturopaths will continue to be there for you in the form of follow-up visits or even between-visit phone calls.

Detoxification do's and don'ts

Detoxification is a popular word among naturopaths, so expect a lot of talk about getting the toxins and poisons out of your system. Most of this advice sounds pretty convincing — it makes sense that all the pollution, junk food, stress hormones, and so on that bombard you every day leave some kind of residue, even if there isn't a lot of hard evidence showing exactly what it is or what it does. And if "detoxification" just means eating better and reducing stress, it certainly can't hurt (even if the benefit has nothing to do with toxins).

If detoxification means getting your blood leeched out or subjecting yourself to brutal enemas ("colon therapy") or vomiting regimens, though, be careful. Sure, you may be aiding your body's innate healing ability. (After all, our bodies often make us vomit and so on when we're sick, probably in part to get irritants out.) But why subject yourself to such misery for a claim based on so little evidence? The fact is, a properly functioning liver is better than any detoxification program at neutralizing and eliminating most toxins.

Of course, sometimes the body's natural healing powers just can't cut it. In those cases, a good naturopath recognizes when it's time to call in the heavy artillery and send you to an appropriate practitioner.

Considering cost

A session with a naturopath will probably cost you about half of the cost to see an M.D. Of course, you can't really count naturopathy as economical if you have to pay for it yourself (in addition to your regular insurance premiums) or if you're using it to complement conventional treatment.

On the other hand, if you end up healthier in the long run, you may be saving yourself money over time. Plus, some health plans pay for care by naturopathic physicians (and some in Washington state even consider them to be primary care providers — so be sure to check your policy!).

When Not to Try Naturopathy

If you have — or may have — a serious or life-threatening condition such as cancer, diabetes, heart disease, and the like, don't rely on naturopathy alone. Many naturopathic treatments may help improve your response to conventional treatments, minimize side effects to them, or even speed recovery, but they shouldn't be your sole therapy. And, as with most other alternatives, naturopathy is not the way to go for broken bones, surgical emergencies, life-threatening crises, or new, undiagnosed conditions that worry you.

Possible Harmful Effects

Because "first, do no harm" is a main principle of naturopathy, you can feel pretty safe with most of its approaches (assuming that you've seen a conventional M.D. first to rule out a serious condition). Even so, some of the techniques pose potential dangers, especially the ones that involve using large doses of vitamins or poorly understood herbs.

Check out our more specific discussion of any technique you're considering for more details. In most cases, being under the guidance of a qualified naturopath should minimize the chances of serious problems.

The naturopaths who think (or claim) that they can do more than they can probably account for most of the harmful effects and horror stories sometimes associated with naturopathic doctors. If you're dealing with a healer who won't recognize his own limitations or admit a treatment isn't working, it's time to say good-bye — and fast.

Resources for Finding a Good Naturopath

To find a good naturopath, one way to go is to contact the American Association of Naturopathic Physicians (AANP) — see the appendix — for a list of qualified N.D.s in your vicinity. In a growing number of states, qualified includes having a license to practice. The Health World Online Web site also lists requirements of certain states www.healthy.net/legal/regulations/naturopathy.htm.

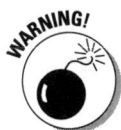

Unfortunately, some unscrupulous "N.D."s out there picked up their credentials at diploma mills — or just added these letters to their names at will. Some of these people even manage to get themselves licensed (sometimes with disastrous results).

So — besides asking the right questions and trusting your gut — make sure that anyone claiming to be an N.D. graduated from one of the four accredited naturopathic medical colleges in North America: Bastyr University in Seattle; Southwest College in Scottsdale, Arizona; National College of Naturopathic Medicine in Portland, Oregon; and The Canadian College of Naturopathic Medicine in Toronto. The Naturopathic Medicine Network's Web site at www.pandamedicine.com/physdir.html offers a list of N.D.s practicing in the United States and Canada. The network states that the list includes only graduates of accredited graduate-level, four-year naturopathic schools. But remember that ultimately it's up to you to check references and credentials.

Another choice (and easier, because you can choose from more practitioners) is to forget about the N.D. qualification altogether. Plenty of competent health professionals (including M.D.s, D.O.s, D.D.S.s, and nurses) practice according to naturopathic principles. If they are qualified by the standards of their own specialty, they may be able to provide fine naturopathic care. But be sure that they have had some serious, documentable training. Having an M.D. degree alone does not qualify someone to practice naturopathy.

Chapter 12

Doing a Lot with a Little: Homeopathy

. . . .

In This Chapter

▶ Understanding the science of homeopathy

▶ Finding out about homeopathy's erratic history

▶ Exploring "like cures like," "less is more," and other amazing ideas

▶ Evaluating the evidence for and against homeopathy

▶ Using homeopathy effectively — and finding out when to avoid it

. . . .

*H*omeopathy is probably the system of healing that baffles conventional doctors most. Frankly, it baffles a lot of alternative advocates, too. The confusion is because it's based on principles that violate every known law of chemistry and physics. And yet, increasingly convincing evidence suggests that it works!

In this chapter, we describe the basics of this 200-year-old system that has persisted despite some pretty unlikely foundations — and premature rumors of its demise. More importantly, we describe what homeopathy may be able to do for you and how to use it sensibly.

The "Science" of Homeopathy

Homeopathy is a system of healing that uses diluted portions of natural substances to cure symptoms of disease — and the more diluted, the better. Remedies aim at revving up an invisible "life force" or "vital energy," which — at first — actually stimulates symptoms. Homeopaths consider symptoms to be good, because they are the body's way of healing itself.

With all the talk about mystical forces, it's no big surprise that many conventional M.D.s dismiss homeopathy as a bunch of bunk. If it works at all, they say, the improvement is only because of the placebo effect (the power of suggestion). But the evidence is beginning to look like they're at least partly wrong. Maybe that's why in virtually every part of the world, homeopathic remedies are an accepted part of everyday health care.

A Long — and Sometimes Sordid — History

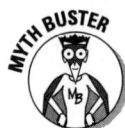

A lot of people think that homeopathy is some newfangled reaction to high-tech medicine. And, yes, homeopathy is a response to technological overkill — not today's overkill, but that of the late 1700s.

Homeopathy was all the rage in Europe and North America during the 19th century. Unlike some other unconventional practices, it was based on a scientific theory, and it tended to appeal to a well-educated and affluent crowd — including the British royal family and various artists, writers, and intellectuals. Many orthodox doctors converted to homeopathy, too, and understandably so. When the alternative was bloodletting, induced vomiting, and massive doses of mercury-laden calomel and other purgatives (often called *heroic medicine*), people didn't need much convincing for homeopathy to be a major threat.

The fight against "heroic" medicine

The complaints homeopaths made about the "raging hurricane" of conventional medicine were amazingly similar to complaints made by alternative advocates today. They must have been pretty convincing, too. Even one of homeopathy's most famous foes, the Harvard physician and poet Oliver Wendell Holmes, admitted in 1860: "I firmly believe that if the whole *materia medica* [conventional drugs], as now used, could be sunk to the bottom of the sea, it would be all the better for mankind — and all the worse for the fishes."

Their incomes threatened, the "regular" doctors resorted to desperate measures to keep homeopaths from stealing patients (not the least of which was creating the American Medical Association). But homeopathy flourished anyway. By the 1880s, homeopathic medical colleges were in most major cities. And by 1900, even the AMA had to acknowledge homeopaths as legitimate doctors. Because around 15 percent of physicians back then were homeopaths, this acknowledgment was probably a smart move.

The fall and rise of homeopathy

Just as many homeopaths feared, though, uniting with "the regulars" nearly wiped them out. As conventional docs laid off the purging and bloodletting and came up with some stuff that actually worked — such as vaccines and antitoxins — the numbers of homeopaths plummeted. By the 1970s, scholars were convinced that the homeopathy business was history — fewer than 100 homeopaths were left in the entire United States, according to Martin Kaufman, "Homeopathy in America," in *Other Healers,* edited by Norman Gevitz (Baltimore, Maryland: Johns Hopkins University Press, 1988), 99–123.

But recently things have started picking up again — big time. Today, the National Center for Homeopathy (NCH) estimates that the amount of money spent worldwide on homeopathy is between $1 billion and $5 billion a year! Most of that money is spent in North America, Great Britain, France, Greece, Belgium, Italy, Australia, South Africa, Russia, Nigeria, India, Pakistan, Sri Lanka, Mexico, Argentina, and Brazil. French pharmacies are required by law to carry homeopathic remedies. Homeopathic hospitals are part of the national health system in Great Britain, and the Food and Drug Administration regulates the manufacture and marketing of homeopathic drugs in the United States. According to the NCH, Americans alone spend about $227 million each year on over-the-counter homeopathic remedies for aches, pains, colds, allergies, and so on — an amount that the American Homeopathic Pharmaceutical Association says is growing at an annual rate of 12 percent.

Homeopathy Basics

If you're thinking that all alternative systems are similar, homeopathy will make you think again. It's based on a refreshingly original and unusual set of ideas:

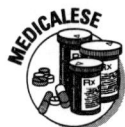

✔ **Like cures like.** Homeopathy is based on the same idea as the hair of the dog: You cure a problem with a little bit of the same thing that made you sick. Specifically, homeopaths take extremely diluted doses of substances that in large doses would produce your symptoms.

Samuel Hahnemann, the founder of homeopathy, called this principle the *law of similars.*

For example, because large amounts of *coffea cruda,* made from coffee beans, leave you wired, homeopaths use minute amounts to treat insomnia. Similarly, because measurable doses of arsenic can lead to massive stomach spasms (or death!), homeopaths use minuscule amounts to soothe cramps.

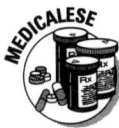

✔ **Nothing may be something.** We're talking about really diluted doses here. So diluted that — from an objective standpoint — you're really taking plain old water, sugar pills, or alcohol. A high-potency dilution can contain as little as one millionth of a drop of the active ingredient!

A standard homeopathic remedy may be made by taking a single drop of a plant substance, mixing it with 100 drops of water, and shaking (this mixture is called a 100-to-1 dilution — or C for short). After that, a drop of this diluted solution is mixed with another 100 drops of water, and shaken again. This process may be repeated 30 or so times (with the last dilution in alcohol). The result is called a 30C dilution because it involved 30 separate 100-to-1 dilutions.

After all these dilutions and shakings, no technology on earth could measure any of the original. No wonder that Oliver Wendell Holmes, in his classic 1842 attack on homeopathy, calculated that by the 17th dilution it would take "ten thousand Adriatic seas" of the remedy to have the slightest effect on a patient. (Holmes also stressed that most patients get better no matter *what* they do — so homeopaths shouldn't give themselves undeserved credit.)

✔ **Water with a memory.** The dilutions have to be shaken, not stirred, so the original substance can leave an imprint of itself on the water molecules — that is, so the water can "remember" whatever was in it before it got so diluted and shaken. In technical terms, the water is said to be *"potentized"* by the original drug. This term just means that it was made more potent, or stronger, than plain old water. Oddly enough, homeopaths insist that the more diluted something is, the stronger it is. Why, they don't know, or claim to know.

To explain how different remedies — that are all basically water — "memorize" different messages, homeopath David Reilly, M.D., of the Glasgow Royal Infirmary uses a snowflake analogy. Even though all snowflakes are chemically H_2O, he explains, each one is unique.

✔ **The healing crisis.** One part of homeopathy that makes many people a little nervous is that you have to expect your symptoms to get worse before they get better. But this "healing crisis" actually makes sense if you truly believe that a symptom is the body's way of healing itself. So when you take a homeopathic cold remedy, expect to sneeze up a storm for a while — presumably the remedy is helping to usher the cold virus out of your body as fast as possible.

✔ **Antidotes.** Some homeopaths say that if a remedy doesn't work, you're just using the wrong remedy. (To skeptics, this is just a convenient excuse.) Others believe that you can also screw things up by taking something that counteracts the remedy — an *antidote*. Coffee, for example, may "antidote" asthma or headache drugs. Other antidotes include electric blankets, dental drilling, X-rays, camphor, mint, prescription drugs, and even acupuncture — which, like homeopathy, also messes around with your vital force, maybe in counterproductive ways.

No diseases, only individuals

According to homeopathy, everybody heals in a unique way. So the way you have a cold is different than the way your brother or friend has a cold. This philosophy is very different from conventional medicine, which lumps sets of symptoms into categories called diseases and then assumes that every-one with the same disease can be treated in the same way.

Of course, by emphasizing the individual, homeopaths make it virtually impossible to prove that what they do "works" by accepted standards of scientific evidence. Saying that everyone's disease is the "same" may not be quite accurate, but it's the only principle that allows doctors to make generalizations — and without generalizations, you can't have science.

Provings

The kind of evidence that homeopaths do believe in are *provings:* Samuel Hahnemann, the founder of homeopathy, did the first provings on himself two centuries ago. He knew that various folk cultures had used cinchona bark (the source of quinine) to relieve symptoms of malaria. So he tried it on himself — and sure enough, he developed symptoms of malaria. He went on to do many similar *provings* on himself, and later on healthy volunteers.

Today, homeopaths still "prove" remedies by giving various substances to healthy volunteers. A drug that makes healthy people cough may be used to cure coughs in sick people. A drug that produces vomiting or nausea may be used to relieve flu symptoms.

Classical versus nonclassical homeopathy

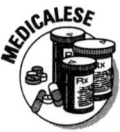

Homeopaths talk about three different kinds of problems: *acute, chronic,* and *constitutional.* Examples of acute problems are colds or flu — stuff that comes and goes pretty quickly. Chronic problems are the long-term woes such as arthritis, fatigue, or sleep disorders. Constitutional problems are also long term, but they have to do with generalized poor health — that is, a body, mind, and spirit that aren't all they could be.

Homeopaths split into two camps according to the way they deal with each of these kinds of problems:

✔ **Classical approach.** This camp basically follows Hahnemann's original premise that everyone gets sick in a unique way. So a classical homeo-path will need to examine you closely to determine a *symptom picture* — which includes your physical ailments (and which side of the body they affect), age, mood, behavior, and so on. Your symptom picture is then matched to an individualized *constitutional remedy.*

Not all classical remedies are aimed at healing both your body and soul. (*Single-remedy homeopathy,* for example, is a variation of the classical approach that prescribes a single remedy for a specific physical problem.) But even here, the emphasis is definitely on tailoring the remedy to your entire system — not just mindlessly matching a remedy to the ailment. A homeopath may need several tries before finding the right remedy. (If more than four are necessary, you should probably go elsewhere.) Finding the right remedy can be so complicated that some homeopaths use computerized databases of cures to help them choose among approximately 2,000 different drugs.

Picking up a vial of "headache remedy" on your own — without really understanding your underlying constitution — doesn't make sense to a classical homeopath. The same goes for the combination formulas you often see in health food stores and pharmacies — you know, the stuff that claims to cure cold and flu symptoms, for example, by combining several different remedies. To a classical homeopath, one remedy is bound to undo the effects of another.

✔ **Nonclassical approach.** If you're buying homeopathic remedies on your own, you're following the nonclassical camp. If you are using this approach, the name of your ailment matters — because everyone with the same ailment uses the same remedy (which is a lot like conventional medicine).

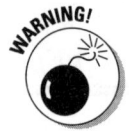

The nonclassical approach is often used by other alternative healers who prescribe homeopathic remedies. If you're using these remedies (or buying over-the-counter homeopathic drugs on your own), though, watch out. If you don't know exactly which remedy is right for you, you could be wasting your time and money.

Evidence That Homeopathy May Work (Sometimes)

Two hundred years of "provings" haven't convinced too many conventional M.D.s that homeopathy works. And, in fact, most of the studies so far have been plagued by lousy methodology.

To be fair, homeopathy is awfully difficult to prove, partly because so much of it depends on the skill of the healer. If a remedy doesn't work, the failure may be because the healer is untalented or inexperienced — and not that the treatment wouldn't have worked if done by the right person. And, again, because the approach is individualized — and what works for one person won't necessarily work for another — it's not well-suited to scientific trials.

Possible benefits of homeopathy

The best evidence so far suggests that certain homeopathic remedies may help relieve allergic asthma, hay fever, migraine headaches, childhood diarrhea, rheumatoid arthritis, fibromyalgia, and trauma — and decrease the duration of labor. But some people swear by homeopathy for almost any common health problem you can imagine.

Even so, at least a few homeopathic remedies have overcome these hurdles. Over the past two decades, several high-quality studies suggesting that homeopathy can work (and work *better* than placebos) have appeared in major *mainstream* peer-reviewed medical journals (the kind that impress conventional M.D.s). A few good studies show that homeopathic remedies can work on animals — who presumably can't be swayed by the placebo effect!

Whether these remedies can work better than conventional therapies remains to be seen. Fortunately, many studies now underway should provide some of these long-awaited answers.

The Good News — It's Difficult for Nothing to Hurt You

Some homeopathic remedies sound like something taken straight from the witches' brew in *Macbeth* — such as the widely available flu remedy Oscillococcinum, which is processed from duck heart and liver marinated for precisely forty days. However exotic, these remedies probably won't do much direct harm, because the amounts remaining in the final solutions are negligible — and possibly nonexistent in any physical sense.

This dilution is a good thing because many homeopathic remedies are made from stuff that's dangerous or deadly in any reasonable dose. We're talking about substances such as snake or bee venom, wolf's bane (aconite), deadly nightshade (belladonna), cuttlefish ink, arsenic, comfrey, iron phosphate, poison oak, and sulphur.

The incredibly small amounts of active ingredients also explain why the FDA has been fairly lenient toward homeopathic remedies — rarely requiring manufacturers to prove safety or efficacy and allowing most of them to be sold without prescription. The FDA probably figures that taking a swig of water, or even alcohol, can't hurt all that much.

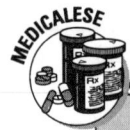

Homeopathy makes the big time

Probably the most influential study on homeopathy appeared in 1997 in the highly respected (and mainstream) medical journal *The Lancet* — K. Linde, et al., "Are the clinical effects of homeopathy placebo effects? A meta-analysis of placebo-controlled trials," *The Lancet* 350 (September 20, 1997): 834–841. This *meta-analysis* pooled results of many small studies. To avoid the big pitfall of meta-analyses, the researchers only analyzed the 89 studies they considered to be of high quality (placebo-controlled, double-blinded, and randomized). The evidence wasn't strong enough to prove that any one homeopathic remedy could successfully treat a particular condition, but it was strong enough to suggest that these remedies may be more powerful than placebos (dummy pills) alone.

A similar meta-analysis appearing in the equally prestigious *British Medical Journal* — J. Kleijnen, P. Knipschild, and G. ter Riet, "Clinical trials of homeopathy," *British Medical Journal* 302 (1991): 316–323 — was a bit more encouraging (though perhaps not as rigorous). It suggested that homeopathic remedies could help conditions including childhood diarrhea, allergic asthma, hay fever, influenza, migraine headaches, and recovery from trauma, plus reduce the duration of labor.

Homeopathic Remedies That May Hurt You (and Why)

The biggest danger from homeopathy comes from using the remedies to treat serious conditions — infections, cancer, and heart disease, for example — that require the guidance of a conventional physician.

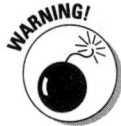

There's one other problem. Because homeopaths believe that you get worse before you get better, you may sometimes have trouble knowing whether or not a remedy is working — or if it's provoking a life-threatening side effect. If you're taking a homeopathic remedy for asthma, for example, more coughing and wheezing could be the first step to recovery. But they could also mean that you end up in the emergency room — or worse.

Seeking the care of a qualified practitioner is a good idea if you're suffering from any potentially serious or life-threatening condition.

Questions to Ask Yourself

Before you experiment on yourself (in true homeopathic tradition!) by reaching for the first intriguing homeopathic drug that catches your eye, we think that considering the questions in the following sections is worthwhile.

Do I want to see a homeopath or just try homeopathic remedies on my own?

A few specific homeopathic remedies have been shown to work for a few specific ailments. But that statement doesn't mean that any old remedy you pick up off the shelves will work for you. The whole idea of homeopathy, after all, is that remedies have to be individualized — which may take a lot of effort to do correctly.

For that individualized treatment, you may want to think about consulting a homeopathic healer. Sure, you can try the extremely diluted stuff sold over-the-counter — at the very least, you're almost certainly safe. (You can also consult nonlicensed people called "homeopathic educators" for guidance on choosing a remedy.) But if you want to give this system a real chance, doing it right may be worth a shot.

What's the best way to find a homeopath?

Of course, finding a qualified homeopath is easier said than done. All sorts of people label themselves homeopaths — ranging from M.D.s and osteopaths to naturopaths, nurses, and even self-trained laypeople. Just who can practice homeopathy, and to what extent, varies greatly from state to state. Plus, there are no national standards (or licensing requirements) to tell you whether self-proclaimed homeopaths are practicing homeopathy the way it's supposed to be practiced.

So what to do? If you're set on seeing a classical homeopath, find someone (M.D., naturopath, or otherwise) who completed one of the five programs accredited by the Council on Homeopathic Education. These programs are the National College of Natural Health Sciences in Seattle; Ontario College of Naturopathic Medicine in Toronto; Hahnemann Medical Clinic in Albany, California; Bastyr University in Seattle; and the International Foundation for Homeopathy in Seattle. Equally excellent is Dr. David Reilly's program at the Glasgow Homeopathic Hospital, which is the most popular continuing medical education program in the United Kingdom. Many other places (some of them decent) teach homeopathy, but you know what you're getting when you use graduates of these particular schools.

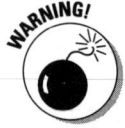

Certification by one of the several groups that certify homeopaths can be a clue to a practitioner's competence. But because no national standards exist, don't rely on this credential alone.

A better option is to contact any of the homeopathic organizations listed in the appendix for a list of qualified practitioners in your area. You can also often get referrals from one of the many local homeopathy study groups that meet regularly to share ideas about homeopathy.

Contact the National Center for Homeopathy (NCH) for a list of a nearby groups. The NCH also provides a *Directory of Homeopathic Practitioners,* which lists only licensed health care providers who dedicate at least 25 percent of their practice to homeopathy. Or go straight to its Internet directory: www.healthy.net/nch/NCHSearch.htm. You can also check the Homepath Home site (www.homeopathyhome.com), which aims to provide links to every homeopathy resource on the World Wide Web.

What's homeopathic treatment going to cost?

According to the NCH, the average first visit to a homeopath lasts an hour and costs $137. Follow-ups usually take under a half hour and cost an average of $55 — but if you have a chronic illness, expect more visits. Many insurance companies reimburse for these services, especially if the homeopath is an M.D. (as many are) or any other kind of health care provider they normally reimburse. Remedies themselves are pretty cheap — usually only $3 to $7 a bottle (and, remember, you usually only need a single dose of a remedy).

What about mixing homeopathic remedies with other alternatives?

Because homeopathy aims at treating symptoms, it's not really a "preventive" form of medicine. So there's no reason not to use homeopathy if you're already using other approaches to get yourself healthy in general. Even if you're treating a specific ailment with a natural intervention (such as massage therapy or bodywork), there shouldn't be a problem — though homeopathic physicians themselves probably wouldn't recommend this approach because they believe that other methods may interfere with the homeopathic remedy.

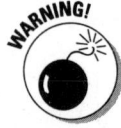

Watch out for antidotes, though. Even some alternative therapies — particularly acupuncture — can counteract a homeopathic remedy. Conventional drugs can, too — especially the ones designed to remove the very symptoms that homeopathic remedies are trying to mimic.

Part IV
Hands-On Approaches

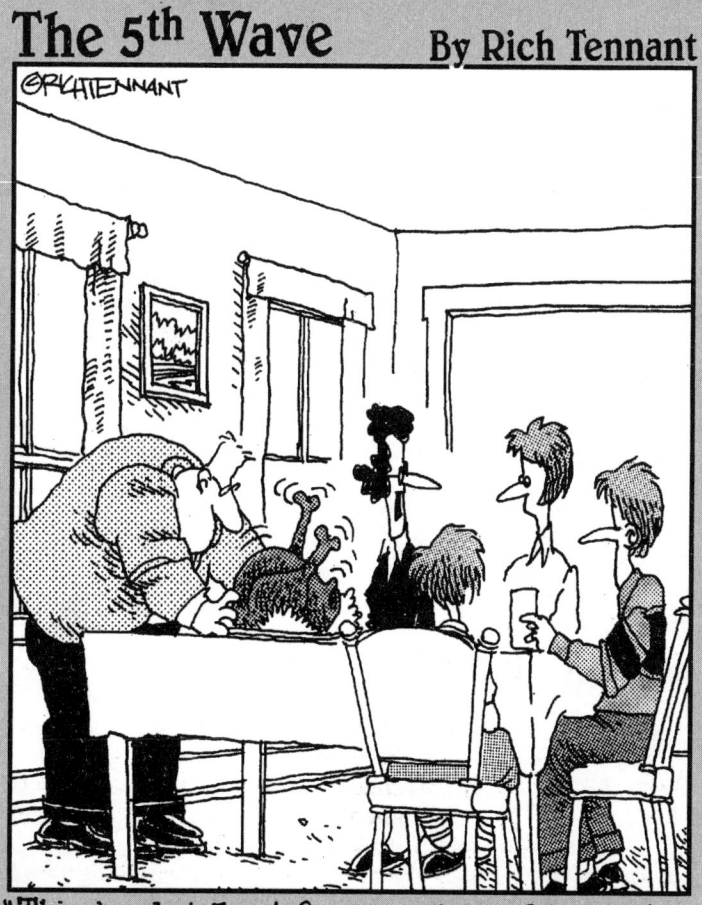

The 5th Wave   By Rich Tennant

"This is what I get for marrying a chiropractor. Every Thanksgiving he's got to align the turkey's spine before he'll carve it."

In this part . . .

We introduce you to alternative techniques that involve moving, shaking, and/or touching to heal the body, mind, and spirit. You can find out how techniques such as chiropractic, osteopathy, and acupuncture may be able to help you, plus you can discover the amazing power of massage therapy and bodywork (including therapeutic touch, polarity therapy, shiatsu, acupressure, Rolfing, and more). We explain when each of these techniques is most effective, how to use it safely, when to avoid it, and how to find a good practitioner or teacher.

Chapter 13

Cracking, Crunching, and Popping: Chiropractic

....

In This Chapter

▶ Finding out what chiropractors actually do

▶ Exploring what naprapathy and applied kinesiology can do

▶ Recognizing when chiropractic can — and can't — help

▶ Finding a good chiropractor

....

*O*ver 40 million people in the United States consulted a chiropractor in the past year alone. If you have low-back or neck pain, you may have thought about joining their ranks, especially if pills haven't worked for you or you don't like the thought of surgery. You may have thought about using a chiropractor to treat other ailments as well — such as headaches, ear infections, and high blood pressure. If so, this chapter is a must.

Chiropractors for much of their history were regarded as quacks and charlatans by the mainstream medical profession — and much of the public. For many years, organized medicine made no bones, so to speak, about wanting to "wipe them out." And, to be fair, some chiropractors were pretty incompetent or poorly trained.

But as good scientific evidence has started to come in, even the most diehard mainstreamers (and insurance companies) are beginning to see that chiropractic has a role in legitimate health care. This chapter tells you what that role is — and what it isn't.

The Good Kind of Manipulation

"Your spine: the key to good health."

—Sign spotted outside a chiropractic office in rural Vermont

We're not wild about the phrase "key to good health" (as if there's only one key). But one thing is for certain: The spine *is* the key to chiropractic.

To a chiropractor, a badly working spinal column is the root of many different ailments. If poor posture, injury, or disease keeps your spinal column from working right, a chiropractor can adjust — or *manipulate* — the areas of malfunction and get them back to work. Some chiropractors do this adjustment with their bare hands using carefully directed and controlled pressure. Others use special tools.

How can a messed-up spinal column affect the rest of your body? According to chiropractic theory, it all comes down to nerves, which (headed up by the brain) are thought to be the body's master controller. When bones in the spine aren't moving correctly relative to each other, chiropractors say that they interfere with the nerves, which in turn, can affect bones, muscles, or nerves elsewhere in the body.

Chiropractic terms in plain English

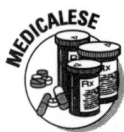

Chiropractors use a lot of esoteric language to describe their philosophy and approach. Fortunately, none of the terms are as complicated as they sound.

- **Diversified technique.** The most common of the many physical methods used to move the spine. This technique has the most science to justify its use in appropriate cases, and produces the familiar "crack" sound.

- **Non-force techniques.** Gentler methods for moving bones. These techniques have little or no science behind them but are often used (and may be worth trying) if a practitioner thinks that more forceful methods may be dangerous.

- **Spinal manipulation therapy (SMT).** The method chiropractors use to get the joints back into alignment.

- **Subluxations.** The term chiropractors use for the misaligned or poorly working joints that underlie many (and, to some chiropractors, all) diseases.

Straights versus mixers

Most chiropractors today don't restrict themselves to spinal manipulation. Instead, they mix in one or more other techniques such as massage, ultrasound, electrical stimulation, hot packs, nutritional counseling, herbal or homeopathic remedies, vitamin therapy, and sometimes (depending on local laws) acupuncture. Many of these *mixers* have even gone on for specialized training (and certification) in other areas of health care.

Mixer chiropractors are undoubtedly the single largest group of alternative-complementary providers in the United States. Mixers are more likely than other chiropractors to

- ✔ Work together with other healers (including physicians)
- ✔ Limit their practice to nerve, muscle, and bone problems
- ✔ Support the use of vaccinations
- ✔ Treat for a briefer period of time

Straight (or conservative) chiropractors tend to do only spinal manipulation. The idea is to boost the body's *innate intelligence* — that is, its intrinsic ability to heal itself. This doctrine, which traces back to chiropractic's originator D.D. Palmer, is not a bad notion to embrace. But it's also a marker for a practitioner less likely to work together with your regular M.D.

Variations on a Theme: Naprapathy and Applied Kinesiology

Chiropractic has inspired some other similar systems of healing. Two you may hear about (especially in certain areas) are *naprapathy* and *applied kinesiology*.

Naprapathy

This offshoot of chiropractic links symptoms to strained ligaments (the tissue that connects and supports bones) rather than irritated nerves. It's used to treat back pain, movement disorders, muscle spasms, and any kind of stiffness that results from bad posture, overwork, bad diet or exercise patterns, or just plain stress.

A *naprapath* or *doctor of naprapathy (D.N.)* gently manipulates the soft tissue around the spine, plus occasionally uses massage therapy and cold, heat, ultrasound, or electricity treatments. The idea is to help the body renew and heal itself. Naprapaths are also big on fixing your diet to help restore your "inner balance," and range of motion training, exercise, and relaxation techniques to help with the outer kind and prevent further problems.

Applied kinesiology

Kinesiology means the science of movement. Literally, all applied kinesiology — *AK* for short — means is using this science to heal the body.

You're not alone — chiropractic treatments are all the rage

The growth of chiropractic has been nothing short of breathtaking in the past two decades (especially in the U.S., where chiropractic originated). Since 1975, the number of U.S. chiropractors has grown by 48 percent, and they are licensed in all fifty states. With 58,000 active chiropractors in practice today, chiropractic is the third largest health care profession in the country. Schools of chiropractic and chiropractic organizations flourish all over the world today.

Chiropractors in the United States see more than double the number of back-pain patients than either orthopedic surgeons or osteopaths, and many more than general practitioners. In fact, several surveys estimate that as many as 15 percent of Americans visited a chiropractor in the past year alone.

In reality, the exact meaning of AK depends on who you're talking to. Some chiropractors and naprapaths describe certain manipulations they use as "applied kinesiology." Other people just use AK as a synonym for the muscle testing performed even by conventional doctors. Still others define it as a way of identifying energy blocks (and we're talking about invisible vital energy — the kind you find in Asian medicine) in the mind, body, or spirit.

But AK is also a system of healing in its own right that was started by a chiropractor back in the 1960s. It uses spinal (and head) adjustments similar to those in chiropractic and naprapathy to strengthen muscles, as well as nutritional counseling, vitamin therapy, acupuncture, or various other supplementary techniques. Because it emphasizes muscle problems, it's no surprise that practitioners often use AK of all sorts to treat sports injuries.

When to Try Chiropractic

If you have new or severe joint pain, be sure to get the necessary bloodwork, X-rays, or other tests to rule out a serious medical illness such as cancer, infections, or rheumatoid arthritis. Ask your M.D. or chiropractor about a good stretching and exercise program, too. In some cases, this program alone may do the trick — and, in any case, you need to move some muscle if you want the effects of chiropractic to last.

After you and your M.D. have ruled out serious conditions and exhausted simpler alternatives, you may consider visiting a chiropractor for any of the following reasons: back pain, neck pain, other musculoskeletal problems.

The evidence that chiropractic can help these problems is so strong that even many mainstream docs would agree with this advice. In fact, in 1994 a federal panel of spine surgeons, back specialists, and researchers published guidelines saying that spinal manipulation can remove acute low-back pain better than most other treatments (they also endorsed pain medications and brief bedrest).

This conclusion thrilled chiropractors. But the findings were not a blanket endorsement of the chiropractic profession. Other professions (such as osteopaths and physical therapists) use the recommended techniques. And the findings were only valid for the first few weeks of acute low-back pain episodes, not for chronic low-back pain or herniated disk syndromes.

Why chiropractic is a good bet for low-back pain

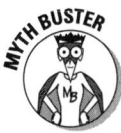

Whatever you may hear, chiropractic is (on the average) no more effective for low-back pain than many other approaches. Lots of backache treatment options work 60 to 95 percent of the time, including bedrest, exercise, painkilling drugs and injections, patient education, and, yes, chiropractic manipulations. But before you get too excited, remember that 70 to 85 percent of all back pain *goes away by itself!* In other words, doing nothing is just as effective — if not more effective — than any of these treatments. (In fact, some of these methods may undermine your body's natural abilities to heal itself; your back just gets better in spite of them!)

So why use a chiropractor (or any other treatment)? Well, mainly because there's more to healing than pain just "going away." You must also count the days of work you missed, the amount of money you spent (or didn't earn), and — above all — your overall "satisfaction" with the experience. When you consider all of these factors, chiropractic wins out.

The fact is, patient satisfaction is driving the move toward chiropractic. Many people prefer the way chiropractors welcome them and explain the nature of the problem and treatment. Patients just trust chiropractors more.

What about physical therapy?

There's no rational reason to use both chiropractic and physical therapy at the same time, said Scott Haldeman, D.C., M.D., Ph.D., professor of neurology at the University of California, Irvine, at a recent conference on alternative medicine. Except for the spinal manipulations themselves, these two fields overlap. Both provider types are competent in treating many musculoskeletal conditions, although (in general) physical therapists may be a bit better with nonspinal problems and chiropractors with spinal problems.

So which one should you use? You have to think about what you want in a healer, according to Dr. Haldeman. Chiropractors can offer you the high-skill manipulation procedure, plus a somewhat higher level of training in diagnosing and treating disease. Plus, although chiropractors ideally team up with your family practitioner, Dr. Haldeman says, they have to take ultimate responsibility for everything they do. Physical therapists, in contrast, are used to practicing under the watchful eye of an M.D.

For moderate to severe conditions, remember to consult an orthopedic surgeon or rehabilitation physician (that is, a specially trained M.D.) before seeking chiropractic treatment or physical therapy.

Can chiropractic help relieve other pain?

In terms of rock-solid evidence, it's too early to determine whether chiropractic can really help relieve headaches, neck pain, dizziness, and other related pains — with one big exception: whiplash. In this case (as with low-back pain), chiropractic can be useful, as can nonsteroidal anti-inflammatory drugs (such as ibuprofen) or appropriate exercises.

Even while you wait for better evidence, though, it's reasonable to try a chiropractor for headaches, upper back pain, or neck pain, especially if nothing else is working and you haven't got a severe condition for which manipulation would be inappropriate.

Can chiropractic cure ear infections, and so on?

You may be wondering whether chiropractic can cure other ailments, for example, ear infections. The answer here — sorry to say — is a big "we don't know." Frustrating as it is, the conclusive evidence just doesn't exist, even though a few promising early studies offer some hope, and good answers may come in the next decade. Sure, anecdotes abound about chiropractic curing ear infections, PMS, asthma, irritable bowel syndrome, ulcerative colitis, and the like. But anecdotes just don't cut it as evidence, because they can be explained away by too many factors — for example, maybe the person never had the problem in the first place, or would have gotten better even without treatment.

A chiropractor *may* be able to offer you treatments other than spinal manipulation to help these conditions, including massage therapy, acupuncture, and herbal remedies. To see if these particular techniques may help your condition, check out the relevant chapters.

What to Expect from Chiropractic

Again, you can't rely on chiropractic alone (we mean spinal manipulations) to treat anything but low-back pain and whiplash, and maybe other back and neck pains and some types of headaches.

Chiropractic is off-limits for fractures and other traumatic injuries, cancers affecting the bones, inflammatory conditions, severe degenerative disease, raging infections, potentially life-threatening conditions, and any condition that may require major surgery. And if there's any chance in the world that your pain may be due to osteoporosis or cancer, get a good diagnosis from an M.D. first.

The pre-treatment exam

Any reputable chiropractor will do the following checks to make sure that spinal manipulations are safe for you:

- ✔ A complete history and physical like the one you'd get from a regular M.D. (including questions about your age, your personal and family health history, and the nature and length of your symptoms)

- ✔ A basic assessment of your joints, muscles, and nerves

- ✔ Tests to rule out cancer or infection and to check for degenerative disease in the spine (the latter doesn't necessarily mean that you can't have treatment but the chiropractor has to know what's going on)

- ✔ Checks for other conditions that could lead to spinal cord problems, especially conditions that involve pressure on or damage to spinal cord nerves that control other parts of the body

- ✔ Signs of significant trauma — such as a fracture or dislocation

- ✔ Signs of psychological, social, or economic issues that may be affecting your pain

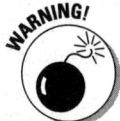

A mainline chiropractor will also happily give your M.D. a report upon request (if not, the refusal is a sign you're in trouble!).

How long will chiropractic take?

Just how many treatments you'll need — and how often you'll need them — is still a matter of big debate. Even so, two widely respected studies (one by the Rand Corporation and one by the State Chiropractic Associations) make basically similar recommendations. First, both studies emphasize that the number and frequency of treatments obviously depends on how bad your problem is. Here are some factors that could increase your treatment time:

- ✔ Symptoms that have lasted more than 8 days
- ✔ Unusually severe symptoms
- ✔ No previous treatment
- ✔ A pre-existing problem in your bones or joints

These studies also gave some ballpark estimates about reasonable length of treatment for acute (short-lived) low-back problems:

- ✔ Most uncomplicated problems should be treatable in about 6 to 8 weeks.
- ✔ Most "complicated" problems (such as a bad sprain in someone who already has osteoarthritis or another pre-existing joint condition) should require about 6 to 16 weeks.
- ✔ You should *stop* seeing a chiropractor if, after 4 weeks, you show no sign of improvement.

Possible complications of chiropractic

Remember — there's no such thing as a completely harmless treatment. Every method that may work also has a potential downside.

Fortunately, most of this downside is relatively minor. The most common adverse reaction to spinal manipulation is a few days of soreness. Occasionally, symptoms will get worse. Rarely, the chiropractor may crack one of the patient's ribs. But it's important to remember that most *careful* chiropractors go through their whole careers without seeing any serious complications.

The more serious stuff (such as certain nerve problems and stroke) are so rare they're hardly worth talking about (especially when you think about the number of people who die each year from taking *prescription* medications!).

If you're taking anticoagulant drugs and need chiropractic treatment for whiplash, make sure that you tell your chiropractor. He or she can then modify the treatment to avert complications that may result from mixing anticoagulants with this therapy.

Four ways spinal manipulation (SMT) may harm you

In some cases, spinal manipulations can

✔ **Aggravate your symptoms.** About one-quarter of people have some kind of scattered spinal pain for up to 2 days after treatment, and muscular aches or spasms for up to a week. Usually these reactions are short-lived and no big deal.

✔ **Produce fractures or dislocations.** This outcome is more serious, of course — but, fortunately, much rarer. Occasionally, some already inflamed tissue may get irritated, too.

✔ **Cause injury to a degenerated disc.** Don't sweat this one too much. Bulging and herniated spinal discs (discs are the spongy cushions between the bones of the spine) are common, even in people with no back pain, and documented injuries to them by SMT are extremely rare.

✔ **Induce a form of stroke called a *cerebrovascular accident (CVA).*** This is the most commonly reported serious complication of SMT, and it seems to occur most often in younger patients (aged 25 to 45).

We don't know how common it is, though, because the studies are so crummy (estimates range from 1 in 400,000 manipulations to 1 in 3.85 million!). What we can say is that even if you have other risk factors for stroke (such as high blood pressure, diabetes, heart disease, migraines, or a history of cigarette smoking or substance abuse), your chances of this side effect are no higher than anyone else's. And remember that CVAs can occur after *any* kind of trauma to the neck — including car accidents, trivial injuries, or just looking at the ceiling, playing tennis, getting your hair washed in the beauty parlor, or doing yoga. Fortunately, they hardly ever do.

Occasionally, there have been miscellaneous reports of other reactions (though no good evidence that chiropractic treatments actually caused them) including perspiration, tremors, chills, fainting, heart palpitations, nausea, menstrual or bowel changes, rashes, bruises, and thyroid problems.

Finding the Right Chiropractor

In nearly every country outside the United States, chiropractic schools are part of the university system and financed by the government. That widely available education gives you a little peace of mind about where your chiropractor is coming from.

What people in the United States have working for them is the fact that chiropractors are now licensed in all 50 states. Every licensed chiropractor must graduate from an accredited college of chiropractic and pass the national chiropractic boards. Most chiropractors have a bachelor's degree before beginning chiropractic school, and some hold an advanced degree, such as a master's degree in nutrition.

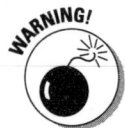

A specialty degree (called a *diplomate*) is one of the many areas chiropractors get extra training in — such as sports injuries, radiology, orthopedics, nutrition, neurology, or internal medicine — and can sometimes be a tip-off to competence. But don't rely on these credentials. Some of the top-notch diplomate training programs are like a real chiropractic residency; others are just a series of weekend training sessions.

Your best bet is to use a chiropractor who has no sanctions against his or her license and a good reputation. And if you're working with a mixer, appropriate training in the other techniques offered is essential. Unfortunately, though, there are no reliable standards above licensure. For more details, contact either the International Chiropractors Association or the American Chiropractic Association, both of which offer lists of licensed chiropractors in specific regions (see the appendix). And, credentials aside, don't forget about trusting your gut!

Be wary of chiropractors who X-ray all patients to check for spinal misalignments. X-rays make sense if a practitioner suspects a fracture or tumor. But some chiropractors use X-rays to look for "bones out of place," a practice that is no longer justifiable.

Getting someone else to pay

More and more health plans in the United States now cover chiropractic services. Many states, including New York, Washington, and Florida, mandate that the health plans in their area cover a certain number of visits to alternative practitioners, including chiropractors, when referred by a primary care physician.

Some health plans that provide coverage in other states are introducing an insured benefit for chiropractic visits, including Oxford Health Plans, Kaiser Permanente of California, and Harvard Pilgrim Health Care in New England. But because restrictions vary a lot — and may involve higher premiums — check your policy (or call your insurer) for details.

Chapter 14

Boning Up on Osteopathy

. . . .

In This Chapter

▶ Why osteopaths are more conventional than alternative

▶ What osteopathy is

▶ How to find a good osteopath

. . . .

*O*steopathy is as mainstream as an "alternative" method can be. It started out pretty radical, but today osteopaths have all the privileges of conventional docs (and equivalent education, too). We're including in this book a brief overview of osteopathy, though, because — despite the camouflage as semi-mainstreamers — osteopaths still uphold an unconventional philosophy of healing that hasn't quite caught on in the world of conventional medicine.

Don't Call Osteopaths Alternative Healers

Many osteopaths like to link themselves with mainstream medicine — and for good reason. Osteopaths have the same education in anatomy, physiology, diagnosis, and treatment — and as much hospital-based training — as M.D.s. They have to pass equivalent board examinations. Plus, they get a little extra schooling in preventive approaches (such as nutrition and exercise) and often in special bone-manipulation techniques.

Osteopathy has less conventional roots. It was developed by Andrew Taylor Still (1828–1917), a midwestern doctor and deeply religious man who claimed (without ever proving it) to be a conventionally trained surgeon. Disillusioned with conventional medicine, Still became interested in the spiritualist healers of the day and set himself up as "A.T. Still, Magnetic Healer." He also started advertising himself as a "bonesetter" (in a day when respectable doctors never advertised) who could relieve pain by manipulating bones. Osteopathy was born when Still discovered that manipulating bones in the spine could also relieve all sorts of chronic ailments.

But some osteopaths are more alternative than others. Today an "osteopath" can fall into one of three categories:

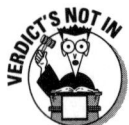

- ✔ **Classical osteopaths.** This now-small group of purists still follow the original principles of osteopathy set out by its founder, pretty much to the letter. That means that they basically stick to manipulative techniques. Classical osteopaths claim that these techniques can help not only musculosketal problems but heart disease, ear infections, menstrual pain, asthma, bronchitis, pneumonia, and various stomach and intestinal woes.

- ✔ **Conventionalists.** Maybe a third of all osteopaths today have essentially *abandoned* the original principles and can't be distinguished from regular M.D.s — except that they went to osteopathy school. Often doctors in this group would have been perfectly happy to go to conventional medical school. But because they got into osteopathy school, they went along for the ride. These conventional doctors in osteopaths' clothing usually do their advanced medical training (internship and residency) at mainstream hospitals and take the same board exams as regular M.D.s (rather than the equivalent osteopathic exams).

- ✔ **Integraters.** Most osteopaths today blend the best of both worlds. Mixing osteopathic manipulative techniques with the more familiar conventional practices, this type of professional is an interesting blend of conventionally trained physician and integrative practitioner.

If you're a little nervous about jumping headfirst into alternative medicine, seeing a good osteopath of this type can be a relatively low-stress introduction to a new way of doing things.

Osteopathy Basics

Osteopathic manipulative techniques (or *OMT*) are supposed to improve posture, make muscles and bones work better, and, as a result, boost the body's innate ability to heal itself. (See Figure 14-1.) Some of these joint-moving techniques are subtle — such as gentle pressing on the head *(cranial techniques)* to improve mental function or relieve headaches. Others can be jolting — such as a sudden blow to the spine to relieve a stiff neck.

How does all this differ from chiropractic? As in real estate, the answer is location, location, location. Chiropractors usually restrict their manipulations to the backbone, but osteopaths may also twist and bend arms, legs, and even the skull. Also, while chiropractors talk about restoring the flow of energy in the *nervous system,* osteopaths are more interested in getting the blood flowing freely through the *circulatory system.*

What osteopathy can do

Anything an M.D. can do an osteopath can do — including performing major surgery, treating emergencies, and prescribing drugs. But the specific bone manipulations that gave osteopathy its name may be particularly useful in treating musculoskeletal problems, including headaches, arthritis, back and neck pain, and various accidental and sports injuries.

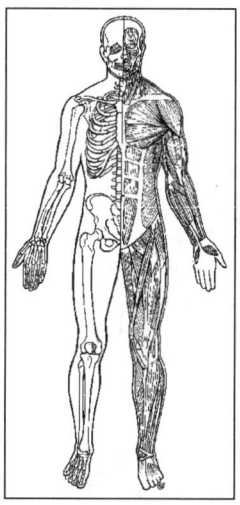

Figure 14-1: Osteopaths believe their manipulations can improve posture, make muscles and bones work better, and help the body heal.

What's osteopathy all about?

There's a lot more to osteopathy than repositioning bones, organs, and body fluids. Certain osteopaths (especially the ones trained at osteopathic hospitals) may also give you a tailored program to improve your diet and exercise patterns, and maybe even prescribe a little acupuncture, massage therapy, or homeopathy. That's because osteopathy — as originally formulated — is based on seven basic beliefs, many of which are shared by other alternative philosophies:

✔ Health is a holistic product of mind, body, and environment.

✔ The body's structure and function are linked.

✔ If a body part isn't working right, it will eventually become diseased.

✔ Blood circulation is essential to healing.

✔ The body constantly readjusts itself to balance weak areas with strong ones.

✔ The body has an innate ability to heal itself.

✔ Prevention is central to health care.

Remember, though, that many osteopaths today practice just like M.D.s. Even osteopathic manipulative techniques (OMT) are now electives in most schools. So if you're looking for an option other than mainstream care, seek out an osteopath who actually studied OMT or who did additional post-graduate training in some alternative discipline.

What's a D.O.?

A D.O. is nothing more than a doctor who got a degree at an osteopathic medical school. The "D" stands for doctor and the "O" for "of osteopathic medicine." A D.O. is as knowledgeable about the human body and what can go wrong with it as an M.D. That's why they get pretty mad when people confuse them with chiropractors, podiatrists, or other health professionals with narrower training — as people often do. According to the American Osteopathic Association, over 40,000 D.O.s practice in the United States, accounting for an estimated 100 million patient visits a year — including many prominent politicians, sports figures, and entertainers.

Resources for Finding a Good Osteopath

Your best bet is probably to start with an osteopath who integrates conventional medicine with osteopathic manipulation. Fortunately, most D.O.s today fall into this category.

You can get a list of osteopaths near you by contacting one of the associations in the appendix. Because all D.O.s have to be licensed and be graduates of an accredited osteopathic medical school, you can feel pretty confident about basic credentials — or at least as confident as with an M.D. But you'll still have to ask (preferably over the phone) about any given D.O.s particular philosophy of practice — and, as always, make sure that you feel comfortable together (see Chapter 6).

Chapter 15

Needling Your Way to Health: Acupuncture

● ●

In This Chapter

▶ How acupuncture works — and what it feels like

▶ What you need to know about the evidence supporting acupuncture

▶ When — and when not — to use acupuncture

▶ How to find a good acupuncturist

● ●

*I*f you're thinking about trying acupuncture, you're in good company. Not only has acupuncture been used as a mainstream therapy for thousands of years in China, but recently it has been attracting many Westerners, too. Millions of people in the United States alone have tried acupuncture to relieve pain that just won't quit. Many others have tried it as a way to avoid surgery or drugs — and to avoid their nasty side effects.

All of this popularity means that acupuncture is getting less "alternative" by the day. Even the U.S. Food and Drug Administration (FDA) recently acknowledged that acupuncture needles are no more "experimental" than surgical scalpels or hypodermic syringes. And the esteemed National Institutes of Health (NIH) declared that acupuncture may effectively relieve pain following dental surgery, as well as nausea and vomiting from surgery, cancer chemotherapy, or pregnancy. They even acknowledged that "the data in support of acupuncture are as strong as those for many accepted Western medical therapies."

Whether acupuncture can successfully treat all the other conditions it's used to treat, however, is still up in the air. This chapter gives you the lowdown on what we know right now — and helps you decide whether you want to try this ancient Chinese technique.

If You're Afraid of Needles, Try Elsewhere

Acupuncture is actually an ancient family of healing methods developed in Far East Asia. The most well-known form involves inserting solid hair-thin needles into key points of the body and manipulating them to relieve pain, promote healing, and improve well-being (see Figure 15-1).

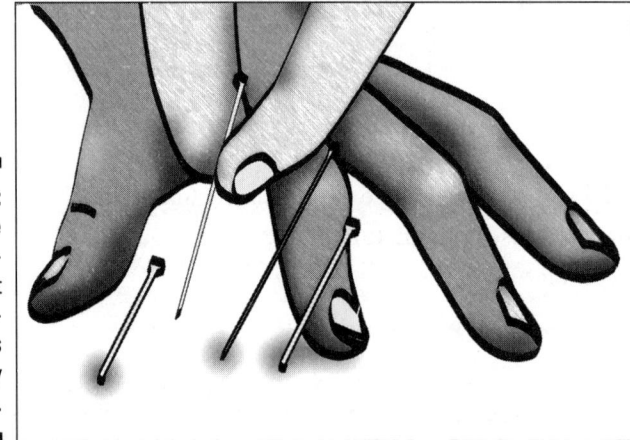

Figure 15-1:
The acupuncturist inserts hair-thin needles at key points.

The very idea of needles — especially shared needles — sends waves of fear through many people. However, most acupuncturists today use sterilized and disposable needles, so there's little reason to worry about infection. Still, if you just can't stand the idea of needles piercing your skin, check out the sidebar, "Needle-free acupuncture — and other variations on a theme," or just head for a different chapter!

To Confucius, Acupuncture Wasn't So Alternative

For centuries, a few scattered doctors and textbook authors in Western countries knew that acupuncture might be useful for treating back pain. But nobody paid much attention until the early 1970s, when a couple of celebrities — including the late President Richard Nixon — visited China. Real credit goes to the late columnist (of *The New York Times*) James Reston's appendix, which happened to act up during his trip to Beijing. Though distressing at the time, this mishap prompted Reston to tell the Western world how acupuncture had helped relieve his post-operative pain.

In the years that followed, the West started waking up to the fact that acupuncture is only "alternative" for those stuck in a Western-focused framework. The fact is, acupuncture has been a *conventional* therapy in China for close to 3,000 years and is one of the main components of traditional Chinese medicine (see Chapter 9).

In China, acupuncture is routinely used to treat everything from flea bites to manic depression. It's used in 40 percent of all surgeries to boost other anesthesia. And the World Health Organization cites over 100 different health conditions that acupuncture can treat.

Meridians and Other Basics

How can sticking a needle in your neck make you healthy? Supposedly that needle unblocks a path of "vital energy" (*qi* in Chinese) that acupuncturists believe flows through your whole body. When this flow gets blocked or unbalanced, you get sick.

To figure out where to put the needles, acupuncturists rely on a dot-to-dot map of invisible channels — or *meridians* — through which the *qi* flows (see Figure 15-2). By stimulating any of the 365-or-so dots, called *acupuncture points*, along this map, acupuncturists can supposedly fix the flow of *qi*.

The reason that a needle in your wrist may affect your lungs is that the meridians connect to various internal organs. The details don't matter — but the idea that everything's interconnected does.

Needle-free acupuncture — and other variations on a theme

All acupuncture is based on stimulating acupuncture points and getting the *qi* back into balance. But acupuncturists use other ways to accomplish this balance besides sticking in needles and twisting them around, including

✔ **Acupressure.** During this needle-free form of acupuncture (called shiatsu in Japan), the acupuncture points are stimulated with finger pressure (see Chapter 16).

✔ **Cupping.** The acupuncturist puts a hot little cup over the acupuncture point or painful muscle, creating a little vacuum to suck out or blow around the *qi*.

✔ **Electroacupuncture.** During this labor-saving technique, the needle manipulations are done by an electric current applied to the acupuncture point.

✔ **Moxibustion.** The acupuncturist burns a powdered herb called mugwort to warm up the needles — or stimulates the acupuncture points directly by burning the herb on or near them.

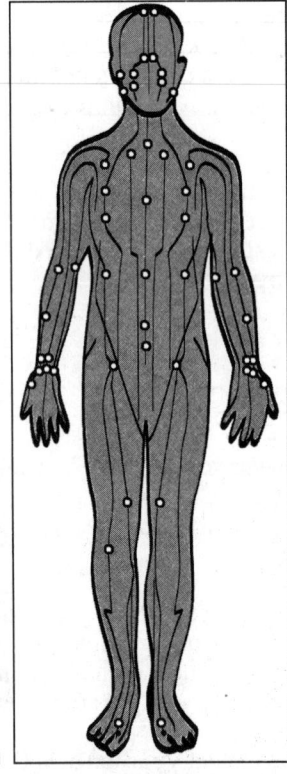

Figure 15-2:
The *qi* (vital energy) flows through the meridians of the body; acupuncture points lie along the meridians.

The Evidence (Or 2,500 Years of History Can't Be All Wrong)

If you don't buy the whole idea of invisible vital energy, explaining just how acupuncture works can be challenging. But whatever the explanation, increasing *scientific* evidence suggests that it does work.

Frankly, the fact that acupuncture works is pretty mind-boggling. To do acupuncture "right," just jabbing the needle in the right spot isn't enough. That kind of approach would be more typical of our Western biomedicine — find what's wrong and fix it. The patient doesn't have to do anything. In traditional Chinese medicine, the needle can't go in until the patient has his or her spirit in order. You also have to adjust the treatment to the season, sun, moon, planets, stars, and atmosphere. The fact that acupuncture works at all is a testament to its power.

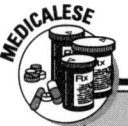

Explaining acupuncture in Western terms

Some scientists think that, at least in some cases, acupuncture needling may stimulate the body to produce natural painkilling chemicals called *endorphins* and *enkaphalins* — which researchers have already isolated from the spinal fluid of patients who received acupuncture treatment. Other scientists think that acupuncture's effects may have something to do with the ability of stimulated muscles and tissues to alter the nervous system, and in turn, affect internal organs such as the gut, bowel, and blood vessels.

Of course, acupuncture doesn't necessarily work for the reasons its advocates say that it works. Sometimes all practitioners have to do is poke some "sham" points anywhere they choose — and patients still get better. This improvement suggests that something is at work that has nothing to do with special acupuncture points. Some acupuncture undoubtedly works because of the power of suggestion, the relationship between the practitioner and the patient, and other mind-body factors. That's why the best studies include a group of people getting "sham acupuncture" to rule out these possibilities. But, hey, if people are getting better out there in the real world, who are we to quibble with the reasons?

The evidence acupuncture does have behind it is a track record of millions of patients treated over thousands of years. And that's nothing to quibble with either.

When to Try Acupuncture

We won't bore you with the many studies showing how well acupuncture can work. What's important to know is that by using acupuncture together with standard therapies for many kinds of discomfort you may be able to

- Reduce side effects of surgery, chemotherapy, addiction recovery programs, and other mainstream treatments.
- Reduce the time and money spent on doctors, hospitals, and drugs.
- Speed your recovery time or the extent of overall recovery.

Possible benefits of acupuncture

Acupuncture can relieve pain after dental surgery, plus nausea and vomiting from surgery, chemotherapy, or pregnancy. It can boost standard therapies for many other conditions, including those for addiction, stroke rehabilitation, headache, facial and neck pain, lower back pain, carpal tunnel syndrome, osteoarthritis, fibromyalgia (general muscle pain), sports injuries, tennis elbow, kidney pain, and menstrual cramps.

Remember that acupuncture is not a therapy of last resort. It's a companion therapy walking hand-in-hand with everything you do. Almost anyone can use it because, if nothing else, it may increase your sense of well-being. But even if it might provide temporary or permanent relief for a specific condition, it's still best to think of it as a way to enhance other treatments and not as a magic cure to be used in isolation.

A Visit to an Acupuncturist

Just what will happen in an acupuncturist's office depends on who you see. Not only do individual styles of practice vary considerably, but treatment should be tailored to your individual complaint and background.

In general, though, you can expect a thorough traditional Chinese medical examination on your first visit — including lots of questions about your symptoms and personality, inspection of your pulse and tongue, and scrupulous observation of everything from the tone of your voice to the tone of your skin (see Chapter 9 for details).

If acupuncture seems like the right course of action, the acupuncturist will ask you to lie on a table, and the needle insertions will begin. Don't let the number of acupuncture points concern you — usually only about ten or so needles are inserted at a time. They are left in place (or manipulated) from a few seconds up to nearly an hour. (If you're getting auricular acupuncture, though, the needle may be taped onto your ear for over a week.)

People tell different stories about how acupuncture feels, just like they tell different stories about how labor feels. In the case of acupuncture, though, the range tends to be less extreme, ranging from mildly uncomfortable to pleasurable rather than from excruciatingly painful to pleasurable. And reports of pleasure are surprisingly common. You may feel a tugging or a vague ache, perhaps even a mild electric shock, but real pain is rare.

If acupuncture hurts, though, speak up! Needles can be moved, but a practitioner can't possibly know to move them unless you say something.

Depending on your particular ailment and the practitioner's areas of expertise, you may wind up the visit with a discussion of possible herbal treatments and various lifestyle changes. And because many acupuncturists work as part of a multidisciplinary team, your practitioner may also refer you to a colleague — perhaps a nutritionist, chiropractor, M.D., or massage therapist — for additional consultation or therapy.

Expect each session to last about an hour and cost between $35 and $80. Some insurance companies will pay for treatments, but only if they're done by a licensed physician. And right now Medicare won't pay a penny.

How many acupuncture treatments you will need depends on how old you are, how sick you are, and how long you've been sick. If you're older, sicker, or sicker for longer, expect more treatment.

As a general rule, though, the standard course of acupuncture therapy usually involves 6 to 8 treatments. That's enough time to know whether it's starting to work. If it does work, it may cost you even more time and money. If it doesn't work, you must go back to the drawing board.

Possible Harmful Effects

In 1997 an NIH panel dubbed acupuncture "remarkably safe, with fewer side effects than many well-established therapies." The needles don't go in far enough to cause problems, as long as the practitioner:

- ✔ Uses "clean needle techniques" to prevent the spread of infection.
- ✔ Stops treatment if there's any sign that acupuncture may be aggravating symptoms or interfering with the conventional treatment in any way.
- ✔ Lets your regular M.D. know that you're receiving acupuncture treatments. If all your caregivers communicate, they can refer you back to each other when appropriate.

Of course, acupuncture (or any kind of therapy) that's done wrong poses a danger — including serious infection and damage to tissues or nerves. That's why using a competent practitioner is essential.

Resources for Finding an Acupuncturist

Make sure that any acupuncturist you use: knows how to communicate with the practitioner who told you what was wrong in the first place, knows his or her limitations, and is extremely well-trained.

Credentials: Which ones matter?

What we mean by "extremely well-trained" isn't what a local licensing board may mean. In some places, you can legally practice acupuncture with no training at all (especially if you're an M.D.!). So at the very minimum, make sure that your practitioner has passed the National Certification Commission for Acupuncture and Oriental Medicine (NCCAOM) exam, which isn't all that hard to do. If you can find someone who has made it through a rigorous post-graduate program in acupuncture (as is now available at Mercy College in New York), all the better.

Obviously you also need to use practitioners who are licensed, registered, or certified to practice in your place of residence. In some states, only conventional doctors and osteopaths can legally practice Chinese medicine; in Alabama, Connecticut, and Illinois, chiropractors are included in this privileged circle. Thirty-six states (at last count) license or regulate the practice of acupuncture by non-M.D.s. Some of these states require acupuncturists to practice under the supervision of an M.D.; others let even untrained people register themselves as acupuncturists. Still other states ask acupuncturists to sign a consent form acknowledging that acupuncture can't replace regular medical care and that patients should consult a licensed M.D. about the condition for which they're being treated.

Where to search for an acupuncturist

For a list of names of qualified acupuncturists and/or the requirements to practice acupuncture in your area, call the American Association of Oriental Medicine (AAOM) or check out their Web site (www.aaom.org). The National Certification Commission for Acupuncture and Oriental Medicine (NCCAOM) at www.nccaom.org/dir.html also puts out an annual *Directory of National Board Certified Acupuncturists.* (See the appendix for details.)

Even the most impressive qualifications mean little if a practitioner gives you the heebie-jeebies. A condescending or cold manner, filthy or smelly office, or surly receptionist can override the finest of pedigrees — and may even make treatment less effective for you. Ultimately, you'll have to make a few phone calls, and even an office visit or two, to see if you like the practitioner's philosophy, personality, staff, and even taste in office furniture. (See Chapter 6 on how to find a healer.)

Chapter 16

Rubbing You the Right Way: Massage Therapy and Bodywork

. . . .

In This Chapter

▶ Discovering some basic information about massage

▶ Discovering the many forms of bodywork

▶ Finding a class or therapist

▶ Doing massage at home — and deciding to go to a professional

▶ Recognizing when massage may be unsafe

. . . .

It's no secret that a good massage can help relax you or uncramp a muscle. More and more studies are confirming that just being touched regularly can boost mental and physical powers and improve quality of life for just about everyone — sick and well, young and old alike. We now know that human beings who don't get touched enough simply don't thrive, physically or emotionally.

Less well-known — but increasingly documented even by mainstream researchers — are all the ways a little "hands-on" can help speed healing, improve thinking skills, and even help relieve pain and other chronic ailments. Study after study is showing that regular massage can even improve your overall health, whether you measure health by how many cups of coffee you drink, how many trips you make to the doctor, how many social occasions you attend, or whatever.

So it's no wonder that massage therapy has been part of virtually every healing tradition known to humanity and continues to be an integral part of medicine in most parts of the world. The glaring exceptions are many modern doctor's offices in the United States — where, often to the doctor's own regret, hands-on therapies have been replaced by technology, and hands-off policies have been encouraged by lawsuits.

This chapter brings you up to speed on what the latest studies reveal about the healing powers of massage and bodywork (a form of massage — even though it doesn't always involve any hands-on at all!). It also gives you the basics about massage therapy and bodywork, helps you decide which approach may be right for you, and shows you how to find a good class or therapist.

There's Nothing Magic about Massage

Massage can make you feel better because it seems to affect almost everything your body does. Massage may improve circulation, bust stress, relieve pain, lower heart rate and blood pressure, reduce swelling, strengthen muscles, promote healing, restore motion to joints, and accelerate basic bodily functions (such as how fast you get rid of wastes).

Credible studies are starting to show that massage may even enhance immune response, perhaps by encouraging the brain to release fewer stress hormones and/or more natural painkillers into the bloodstream.

Massage Basics

When most people think of massage, they're thinking of some version of Swedish massage. This technique — developed in the early 19th century by a gymnastics instructor who cured himself of an elbow problem by tapping on it — was first brought to the United States in the 1850s, where today it's the most popular massage technique.

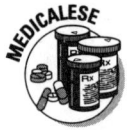

But *massage* is actually a much broader term. It's formally defined as any kind of "systematic manipulation of the soft tissues of the body" (stuff such as muscle and connective tissue). Manipulation can mean any combination of rubbing, kneading, slapping, tapping, rolling, pressing, or jostling, as long as the goal is to make you feel better.

Close to a hundred different techniques fit this definition of massage, most of which were developed in the past 20 years. Many massage therapists use a variety of these techniques. Even so, in this chapter we break these techniques down so you know what you have to choose from. First, we give you the basics of some of the best-known techniques (especially the ones that use the word "massage" in their names). Later, we look at massage techniques combined with various other exercises or approaches, and sometimes classified as bodywork.

Possible benefits of massage and bodywork

Besides helping you relax, soothing sore muscles, reducing some kinds of swelling, and improving general well-being, massage therapy of one sort or another may also help with hypertension, burns, chronic pain (including from arthritis, backaches, and migraines), rashes and other skin conditions, addictions, depression, stress and pain of labor, asthma, and attention deficit hyperactivity disorder (ADHD). It can also alleviate depression and boost self-esteem in people with eating disorders; improve growth and development in premature babies; reduce pain and water retention in women with premenstrual syndrome (PMS); raise blood sugar levels in kids with diabetes; and possibly even boost immune function in people with HIV or cancer.

Bodywork may improve muscle function, expand range of motion, increase balance and coordination, reduce stress, and just plain make you feel better both physically and mentally.

Traditional European versions

The kind of massage familiar to most people in Western countries is based on conventional Western ideas about the body and how it works. These *traditional European versions* of massage include the familiar Swedish massage, plus some of the variations it has spawned over the years.

When you picture a masseuse gliding her hands over someone's back, doing a few karate chops up and down the spine, or kneading a shoulder muscle, you're thinking of Swedish massage (see Figure 16-1). The basic idea is that by stroking and kneading the top layers of muscle, you can rev up the blood flow through the soft tissues. That's why most of the long, gliding strokes are done in the direction of the heart.

Swedish massage and related techniques involve five different kinds of strokes, some of which have formal names in French rather than Swedish for reasons we can't fathom: long strokes *(effleurage)*, kneading *(petrissage)*, friction, vibration, and percussion or tapping *(tapotement)*. These strokes can be gentle, vigorous, or both, and some masseuses throw in a little joint movement as well. The idea is to mimic both active and passive exercise to relax muscles, stimulate circulation, and increase range of motion. Usually the masseuse uses a little oil or lotion to make everything glide a little easier.

Contemporary Western massage

Like traditional European massage, contemporary Western massage is based on conventional Western concepts of human anatomy and physiology. But instead of just aiming to help your body, the "contemporary" techniques also aim to shape up your mind and sometimes your spirit as well. If your massage therapist is using terms such as "personal growth," "emotional release," or "balancing mind, body, and spirit," it's a good bet that she uses some of these techniques.

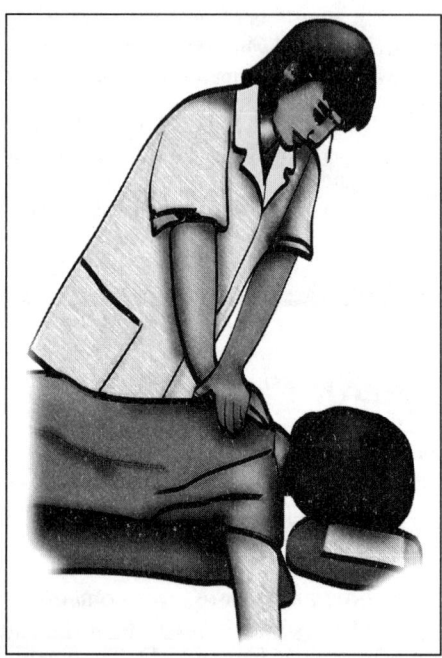

Figure 16-1:
A masseuse gives a Swedish massage.

Contemporary Western massage includes

- ✔ **Deep tissue massage.** This massage takes aim at deeper layers of muscle than Swedish massage by directing strong, slow strokes against the grain of the muscle. Deep tissue massage usually focuses on more specific areas than does Swedish massage — perhaps to speed the recovery of a pulled muscle, relax tense shoulders, or soothe an old injury. You may feel some soreness during or right after the massage, but if it's done right you should feel better than ever within a day or two.

- ✔ **Esalen and Swedish/Esalen massage.** These outgrowths of Swedish massage aim at relaxing the mind and body together to promote overall well-being. Developed at the famous Esalen Institute in Big Sur, California, this method transforms Swedish massage techniques into slow, rhythmic, and hypnotic strokes and combines them with gentle rocking and stretching movements, often to the tune of soothing music.

- ✔ **Manual lymph drainage massage.** The aim is to get the lymph rather than the blood flowing (lymph is a fluid that circulates through the body carrying away debris and bringing white blood cells to sites of infection). Involving light, rhythmic strokes, this method is often used for any condition that blocks the lymph flow, including lymphedema (which sometimes afflicts women after a mastectomy), other kinds of edema (swelling), and certain forms of nerve pain.

✔ **Myofascial release.** During this technique, the therapist uses gentle, prolonged pressure to soften up connective tissue called fascia. Fascia is an interconnected sheet of tissue that surrounds bones, muscles, nerves, and all other internal organs and tissues. Because it runs in one continuous sheet from head to toe, tension in one spot can theoretically cause pain in distant muscles, nerves, and so on. That's why the therapist may work on areas that may seem unrelated to your pain or injury. Myofascial release is often used to treat chronic pain (including headaches) or to restore range of motion (which can be restricted due to whiplash, surgery, or just poor posture).

✔ **Neuromuscular massage, trigger point massage, and myotherapy.** Often used for pain control, neuromuscular massage concentrates finger pressure deep into individual muscles to increase blood flow and release "knots" of tension and pressure on nerves. One form of this kind of massage is called *trigger point massage* because the masseuse works on specific points on the body that "trigger" pain in other areas. When neuromuscular massage is used to control muscle spasms and other muscle-related conditions, it's sometimes called *myotherapy (myo means muscle)* or *Bonnie Prudden Myotherapy* (named after the physical fitness leader who developed this method).

✔ **Sports massage.** Basically Swedish massage for jocks, sports massage uses whatever technique is necessary to get athletes ready for the game — and to make them feel better afterward. One of the most popular of the techniques is *transverse* or *cross-fiber frictioning*, a stroke that is accomplished by pulling the hands across the grain of the muscle without letting the fingers slide across the skin.

Working It Out with Bodywork

Have you ever wondered what all the Feldenkrais, Reiki, *Tai Chi* and other exotic-sounding bodywork courses at the local community center were all about? Have you ever wondered what the beauty parlor's sign for "therapeutic touch" or "shiatsu massage" meant? If so, read on.

Bodywork is everywhere you go today. And despite all the exotic-sounding names for various methods, bodywork is just a form of massage (sometimes without actual skin contact) or movement instruction that aims at both physical and psychological well-being. It's just that the part of the body that gets worked on isn't always the one you might expect. Plus, the explanations for how this stimulation can help vary from one technique to the next. Often too, *bodywork professionals* (which is what these therapists often call themselves) do a lot of talking — because they view education and communication as part of their job.

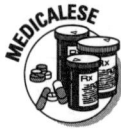

The only reason the term "bodywork" can get confusing is that everyone seems to use it in a slightly different way (without telling you that they're different from everyone else!). Sometimes bodywork just means certain Western-based techniques that emphasize body structure and movement. Technically, these techniques are also called *structural, functional, and movement integration*. Sometimes (as in this chapter) bodywork can also mean certain Asian massage approaches and/or so-called *bioenergetic approaches* such as therapeutic touch and polarity therapy. And sometimes bodywork can mean all of the above, plus conventional massage techniques.

Fortunately, there's no need to remember (or pick!) any formal definition of bodywork. All that matters is getting a basic grasp of what each method is all about — enough to know whether it makes sense for you.

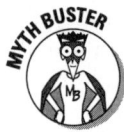

If you have a specific medical problem, particularly past surgery or severe structural problems such as bad arthritis, don't expect bodywork (alone) to cure you. Almost all the "evidence" proving that this stuff does what it claims to do are anecdotes or personal testimonials — "it worked for me." The number of these anecdotes makes it reasonably plausible that bodywork helps some people free up stiff muscles, improve coordination and balance, and just plain relax. But there aren't enough of these anecdotes — and certainly no quality scientific evidence — to prove that any of these techniques can *cure* asthma, endometriosis, hypertension, heart problems, or any other chronic disease.

The bottom line is that until researchers get data from some big, controlled studies, they just won't know for sure all the benefits that may come from these techniques. On the other hand, trying bodywork probably won't hurt you. So if conventional physical therapy or other medical approaches aren't helping, you may want to give one or more of these techniques a try.

Wisdom from the East — Bodywork from Asia

Many bodywork methods are based on ancient principles of Chinese medicine (see Chapter 9), especially the idea that a "vital force" (*qi* in Chinese) circulates through invisible channels (*meridians*) in the body. If this vital force gets blocked or unbalanced, you get sick. Pressing on key points (*acupuncture points*) along these channels helps this vital force flow better. Herbs, acupuncture, and/or stretching exercises may be part of the therapy.

Acupressure and shiatsu

Acupressure is basically acupuncture without the needles. It's a form of massage during which the practitioner uses fingertips or hands to press specific points along the meridians that supposedly affect the flow of *qi* (see Chapter 15 on acupuncture). The idea is that impaired flow of *qi* through the invisible channels can mess up various organs down the line.

Acupressurists sometimes call acupuncture points *acupoints* for short. The 365 acupoints have cool names — such as "Gates of Consciousness," "Sea of Vitality," or "Womb and Vitals" — that usually have something to do with where they are or what they do.

An even older technique than acupuncture, acupressure is mainly used to relieve stress. Even mainstream M.D.s agree that this is probably a good idea, because chronic stress seems to make people vulnerable to illness. Acupressure is also often used to treat the same kinds of conditions as acupuncture (see Chapter 15), only with a less invasive technique — and is commonly used instead of needles when treating children.

Acupressure also has a number of variations:

- ✔ **Shiatsu:** The Japanese version of acupressure. It usually involves deep finger pressure on the acupuncture points. It may also involve pressure on wider areas of the body, with the practitioner using the hands, elbows, knees, or even the feet (making it kind of a "feet-on" therapy).

- ✔ *Tui Na:* Acupressure mixed with other massage techniques, including tapping, vibration, rubbing, and kneading. The idea is to get blood and lymph flowing to move out the debris from the tissues.

- ✔ *An-mo* **(also called An Mo or Amma):** The Japanese version of *Tui Na*. A related technique, called AMMA Therapy, combines bodywork, diet, vitamin supplements, and herbs to treat the emotions and spirit as well as the physical body.

- ✔ *Jin Shin Do* **Bodymind Acupressure:** A trademarked approach to acupressure developed by a psychotherapist. This method emphasizes that tension in one part of the body affects other parts, as well as the feelings and emotions — and vice versa. It involves gentle but fairly deep finger pressure on the acupuncture points for up to 3 minutes to exorcise both mental and physical tension.

- ✔ *Jin Shin Jyutsu:* A "lite" version of acupressure, this technique comes from an ancient Japanese approach and uses much gentler pressure than other forms of acupressure. After analyzing your pulse to see where your energy is blocked, the practitioner gently touches two of 26 specific acupuncture points to clear the passageway.

Self-help: Using acupressure on your own

Almost everyone has tried a little instinctive acupressure on themselves just by pressing a throbbing spot or rubbing an ache. The ancient Chinese eventually figured out — probably by trial and error — that massaging one area of the body sometimes helped problems in distant areas.

To relieve arthritic pain in the elbow or shoulder, for example, try bending your right arm toward you at the elbow palm down and pressing your left fingers into the spot just where the crease inside the elbow ends. This spot is called "Crooked Pond." Do the same for your left elbow.

To relieve pain and inflammation in the hands, arms, shoulders, or neck, try placing your thumb into the webbing between the thumb and index finger of the opposite hand and pressing for a couple of minutes toward the index finger bone while breathing deeply. This spot is called "Joining the Valley." Because some people say this exercise can induce labor, it should be avoided by pregnant women.

If this kind of self-help appeals to you, you don't need to master every single trick developed over thousands of years. Instead, you might try taking a class in *Acu-Yoga* or *Do-In*. Acu-Yoga combines finger pressure with whole body postures, meditation, and stretching and breathing exercises. Do-In is similar but also adds more vigorous ways to stimulate the acupuncture points.

Qi Gong

Qi Gong (chee gong) is an ancient Chinese technique that combines physical exercise with self-healing. During 20- to 40-minute daily practice sessions, you perform a set of slow, choreographed movements while breathing slowly and visualizing the *qi* coursing smoothly and steadily through your body.

The idea is that by directing your *qi* properly you may be able to improve specific health problems as well. Whether or not this premise is true remains to be seen — but there's no question that many people find *Qi Gong* a good way to relax and keep limber, and that's nothing to scoff at.

In China, where *Qi Gong* is extremely popular, *Qi Gong* masters actually appear to direct the flow of *qi outside* their bodies — using it to move balls and other external objects across the room or making people lose their balance without touching them! Even the most skeptical witnesses — including Western-trained scientists and television crews — haven't been able to explain these events away.

Tai Chi

Like *Qi Gong,* this balance and flexibility technique (sometimes transliter-ated as *tai ji*) blends exercise with attempts to get the vital energy back on track. You work your arms through a series of slow, controlled, and continu-ous circles while shifting your weight from one foot to the other.

Like *Qi Gong, Tai Chi* is a blend of physical and mental exercises that is becoming increasingly popular outside of China. In the United States alone, just about every community center and college offers classes, allowing many people to make *Tai Chi* a regular part of their exercise routine. In China, though, many people do *Tai Chi* on their own; in fact, if you stroll through a park just about any morning, you can catch individuals standing on their own, rolling their arms and intensely posturing themselves into various *Tai Chi* positions.

A lot of people claim that *Tai Chi* may provide the same cardiovascular benefits as strenuous exercise without putting the same strain on the heart — and evidence for these claims is starting to roll in. *Tai Chi* may also reduce symptoms of Parkinson's disease and help prevent falls in the elderly. A few studies have already shown that *Tai Chi* can improve breathing, reduce stress, lower blood pressure, and improve balance — although whether it can do these things any better than other techniques remains to be seen. But, if you want to de-stress and prefer *Tai Chi* to reading or meditating or if you want to improve your cardiovascular health and prefer *Tai Chi* to walking, go for it.

Bodywork of the Non-Asian Variety

A newer form of bodywork grew up outside Asia over the past hundred years or so. Many of the techniques are named after the innovative individu-als (physicists, dancers, acrobats, engineers, doctors, nurses, even actors) who developed them, often in an attempt to cure their own disabilities.

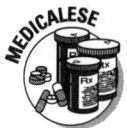

Some people consider these techniques to be examples of contemporary Western massage others call them structural, functional, and movement integration. However you categorize them, all these approaches manipulate soft tissues and/or correct unhealthy patterns of movement by trying to get the body's structure, function, and movement in sync.

Alexander technique

The Alexander technique requires that you work with a private teacher to discover — and, ideally, change — certain unconscious patterns of thinking that have been deforming the way you move and hold your body. Once you're aware of these unhealthy patterns, you can change the way you move and become more graceful, balanced, coordinated, and relaxed. Ideally, you'll also be in less pain. Getting your head, neck, and back into proper alignment are particularly important.

This process usually takes many months of lessons (and both verbal instruction and hands-on guidance). You relearn basic movements such as sitting, walking, and getting up from a chair, and then you must coordinate these movements with what's going on in your head.

Developed by a Shakespearean actor in the late 19th century, the Alexander technique has long appealed to performers and various other celebrities, all of whom were convinced that it could help relieve a Pandora's box of woes — including asthma, depression, exhaustion, muscle pain, tension headaches, ulcerative colitis, and ulcers.

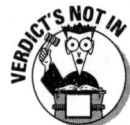

The killer evidence for these claims is still woefully inadequate. But if you're looking for a way to improve your posture and/or relieve symptoms of any stress-related pain (including tension headaches, whiplash, muscle spasms, or chronic back or neck pain), the Alexander technique can be worth a try.

Rolfing (structural integration)

Rolfing's all about *fascia*, the connective tissue that binds and connects all the structures inside your body — organs, bones, blood vessels, nerves, you name it. If you've ever seen the thin whitish stuff surrounding a piece of steak, that's fascia. Fascia comes in the form of a single tough sheet that connects everything from head to toe. This interconnection means that if the fascia gets thick or tense in one area of your body, it could pull on muscles, bones, or nerves somewhere else.

This ability of fascia to affect distant areas of the body gave biophysicist Ida Rolf an idea for helping people with chronic pain and tension. Rolf believed that injury, chronic stress, or emotional trauma could make fascia thicker and stickier. To restore freedom of movement and better align the head, shoulders, thorax, pelvis, and legs, she designed various manipulations to stretch tight and thickened fascia — and Rolfing was born.

This realigning sounds like it could hurt — and, in fact, it can. Rolfing has the reputation of generating the kind of pain that only a masochist could love. And the truth is, because being "Rolfed" involves deep-tissue work, it can be painful. But in the long run, it does seem to help many people relax and move more comfortably, and, in some select cases, may even increase the range of motion of shoulders and other joints. Not a lot of hard-core evidence shows that Rolfing can reduce pain, boost energy levels, or just plain make you feel better — but many people swear it has helped them.

One appealing feature is the predictable length (and therefore cost) of the program. Usually, Rolfing involves ten sessions, which last 1 or 2 hours each and occur a week or 2 apart. Sessions are usually a bit pricier than a massage, often $75 to $100 an hour or more.

Hellerwork

This form of bodywork was developed by an aerospace engineer at NASA named Joseph Heller in the late 1970s. Like so many other bodywork techniques, his version grew out of Rolfing (see the preceding section).

Both of these techniques use deep-tissue massage to rout out pain and tension. But Hellerwork comes with some emotional counseling, too, plus instruction *(movement education)* on how to do certain exercises to ease everyday movements (the latter are now included in Rolfing programs as well). You often get to use before-and-after videos to see your progress.

Although most forms of bodywork can go on indefinitely, you know what you're getting into with Hellerwork: precisely 11 sessions, each one devoting about an hour to bodywork and another half hour to movement education. These sessions run about $60 to $120 a shot.

Aston patterning

Aston patterning was developed in the early 1970s by dancer Judith Aston after she was treated for a back injury by Ida Rolf, the developer of Rolfing (see the section, "Rolfing"). Its basic aim is to enhance overall well-being by making it easier and more comfortable to live, work, and play — although proponents also claim that Aston patterning can relieve pain and fatigue, plus improve strength, endurance, and balance.

Aston patterning is more individualized than many other forms of bodywork. You work one-on-one with a trained teacher who evaluates your way of moving and helps you figure out ways to improve your posture and move more efficiently. The solution usually involves numerous sessions during which you do exercises to relax your body and improve fitness, get special deep-tissue massages, or even discuss ways to make your particular home and work environments more conducive to comfortable living.

Feldenkrais Method

The Feldenkrais Method trains people to move more easily by increasing flexibility, coordination, and range of motion. Developed by a Russian-born physicist (and jack-of-many-trades), Moshe Feldenkrais, it can be particularly

valuable for people who find it difficult to move some or all of their bodies —
including people who've experienced stroke, cerebral palsy, spinal cord
injury, or multiple sclerosis.

Most people start Feldenkrais with a set of movement lessons called *Aware-ness Through Movement* (or ATM). The teacher talks you through a series of
easy movements (such as reaching, bending, and walking), and you focus on
what various parts of your body are doing as you move them.

A more hands-on form of Feldenkrais is called *Functional Integration* (FI).
The teacher gently manipulates your muscles and joints as you move
various body parts, trying to get a sense of the tension and other problems.
You then work together to rediscover more efficient ways to move. Both
ATM and FI emphasize head position above all.

Is Feldenkrais more effective than other forms of bodywork — or more
conventional exercises? There aren't enough convincing studies yet to say
for sure. But many people swear by it as a nearly risk-free way to relieve
chronic pain, defuse stress, and improve overall balance and coordination.

Pilates/Physicalmind Method

Developed during World War I by German-born Joseph H. Pilates (pro-nounced puh-LAH-teez) while he was helping soldiers recover, the Pilates
Method involves a series of precise and controlled movements that can help
people recover from muscle strains. Today, it's mainly used as a body
conditioning method that aims to boost flexibility and strength without
adding muscle bulk. Fans include dancers, athletes, and fitness buffs of all
stripes.

The Pilates Method is more than just exercise. You're supposed to get your
mind hooked into whatever your body is doing as you move, to get a better
understanding of how your muscles work and how you can control them.
Emphasizing this idea is the Physicalmind Method, a variation of Pilates that
developed largely due to a legal battle to control the "Pilates" name. The
Physicalmind Method involves essentially the same exercises as Pilates,
only with a bit more focus on the body's position while going through the
motions.

Both the Pilates Method and Physicalmind Method have to be done under
the supervision of specially trained teachers. They also have to be done
using unique pieces of exercise equipment that no one's going to have
around the house. Expect to go back for 20 or 30 sessions before seeing
results.

Tragerwork

Tragerwork owes its existence to an M.D., Milton Trager, who also happened to be an acrobat, boxing trainer, and a devotee of the Maharishi Mahesh Yogi (see Chapter 10). It's supposed to be particularly effective for people with various neuromuscular disorders (including spinal cord injuries and multiple sclerosis), and possibly even for lung disorders such as asthma. Tragerwork is also known as the *Trager approach, Trager psychophysiological integration,* or just plain *Trager.*

A Tragerwork therapist tries to relax you and increase your range of motion by combining light massage strokes with gentle rhythmic bouncing, shaking, and rocking movements of your trunk and limbs. Afterward, the therapist also shows you how to use a system of self-directed movements called *Mentastics* geared to enhance the feelings of freedom and lightness you felt during the hands-on portion.

Sessions generally run an hour to an hour-and-a-half. As with Rolfing and Hellerwork, each session builds on the next. Tragerwork, however, doesn't predefine the set of sessions.

Cross-Cultural Approaches to Bodywork

Some forms of bodywork are based on the idea that a life force or "vital energy" runs through and surrounds the body. This energy is similar to the *qi* of ancient Chinese medicine, but most of these methods were developed in recent years outside of Asia. All the methods try to mobilize the vital energy with some combination of breathing exercises, massage, and "talk therapy" to release repressed emotions.

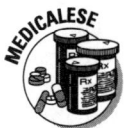

Because of the central role of vital energy, these approaches are sometimes called *bioenergetics.* Other names that get bounced around are *energy medicine* and *biofield therapeutics.* But, again, names and categories don't matter. All that counts is what each individual method claims to do.

Therapeutic touch

Therapeutic touch, which is essentially touch-free massage, is taught at over 100 prominent medical and nursing schools and is used around the world to treat problems ranging from cancer to burns. Healers say that they "manipulate" a patient's energy field merely by passing their hands over the patient's body and feeling compassion for them. This method was developed in 1972 by Dolores Krieger (an emeritus professor of nursing at New York University) and a healer by the name of Dora Kunz.

Recently, alternative medicine in general got a slap in the face when headlines all over the United States announced that a fourth-grade girl had "proved" therapeutic touch to be a bunch of bunk.

Aided and abetted by her nurse mother, inventor father, and a self-proclaimed "quack-buster," 9-year-old Emily Rosa designed a simple study to determine whether these claims could really be true and published the results in *JAMA — The Journal of the American Medical Association* 279,13 (April 1, 1998): 1005–1010. Perhaps because she was an innocent little girl, she was able to do what no one had been able to do before: Get 21 different practitioners to agree to be tested.

Emily simply set up a cardboard screen separating her from a blindfolded healer, who put his hands through two small holes to her side of the barrier. She then randomly placed her own hand over one of the healer's hands and asked him to tell her whether her hand was near the healer's left or right hand — something that should have been obvious to anyone who could detect her "human energy field."

As it turned out, during 280 tests, the 21 practitioners got the answer right only 44 percent of the time — which is even less than the 50 percent probability if the healer had just guessed!

Practitioners of therapeutic touch aren't convinced that this experiment means much. They insist that they can feel unbalanced spots in a patient's energy field and can cite countless anecdotes about how it has worked to cure a host of conditions including burns, ulcers, infant colic, Alzheimer's disease, and even cancer. For all the hype the *JAMA* study got, it doesn't invalidate the countless experiences of the 47,000 practitioners worldwide who've been trained to use therapeutic touch. Of course, therapeutic touch may work for reasons other than the manipulation of human energy, but if it works, it works.

Someone needs to test therapeutic touch in a real-life situation, because part of the effect may come from some holistic interaction between a healer and a patient — rather than a perfectly healthy hand of a 9-year-old skeptic. In any case, this study doesn't invalidate "all" of alternative medicine in one fell swoop.

What's in a name?

The term "therapeutic touch" seems to have two meanings depending on who you're talking to. Some people use therapeutic touch to mean the vague healing power that comes from massage, hugs, and general human contact. Other people use the term to mean a specific kind of bodywork during which a therapist manipulates a patient's invisible energy fields by moving her hands over them without actually touching the patient.

Polarity therapy

When you receive polarity therapy, you become a human magnet. According to this method, which was developed in the 1920s by Randolph Stone (a chiropractor, osteopath, and naturopath), specific points on the body are believed to hold either positive or negative charges, which drive electro-magnetic currents in and around the body. When you get stressed, injured, or exposed to powerful electromagnetic fields, these currents get out of whack — and you feel sick.

If you get into polarity therapy, you'll hear a lot of Dr. Stone's personal rendition of biophysics and philosophy — based largely on Asian ideas about the five elements, yin and yang, and all that jazz (see Chapter 9). But all you really need to know is that a polarity therapist aims to balance your energy field and restore structural balance by placing his hands on electri-cally charged strategic points to release the energy current they control.

Part of the therapy may also involve massage, breathing exercises, encour-aging words *(polarity verbal guidance),* simple stretches, reflexology (see the upcoming section, "Reflexology"), or even hydrotherapy. Sometimes, the therapist also works in some dietary and nutritional counseling (based on principles of traditional Chinese medicine) as well. The goal is to leave you invigorated and refreshed — in body, mind, and spirit.

Given the evidence right now, it's highly doubtful that polarity therapy can cure a specific, serious illness. But it has the potential to relax you in the same way as a good massage. And for some people, participating in the whole gamut of the polarity therapy experience is a meaningful way of life.

Reiki

Reiki is the Japanese word representing the universal life force or energy. (*Rei* means universal and *ki* is the Japanese version of the Chinese *qi*). Reiki is a way to activate this life force and get it to work in healing your body, mind, and spirit.

The idea is that Reiki energy flows into the practitioner's head and through his or her hands into the energy field of the client's body. This energy is so strong that it can flow right through the air and clothing — no touching required! Or you can take a Reiki class to find out how to reconnect to this energy source on your own and discover basic hand positions for treating yourself and others. You can even find out how to practice "long distance healing."

Does this stuff really work? So far the only real evidence is anecdotal — which doesn't mean too much. But, like most forms of bodywork, it can probably help relax you at the very least, and maybe even open your mind to healthier ways of looking at the world.

Reflexology

In reflexology, the feet come first. Actually, this method is a lot like acupressure (see the earlier section, "Acupressure and shiatsu") because it's based on manipulating key points to balance natural energy flow. But unlike acupressure and shiatsu, reflexology is a rather new idea that developed outside of Asia. The earliest version was called "zone therapy" and was brought to the United States from Europe in the early 1900s.

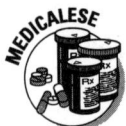

Instead of using the theory from traditional Chinese medicine to explain how balancing the energy flow can work, reflexologists are more likely to talk about "reflex" nerve pathways throughout the body and to call the key points *cutaneo-organ reflex points*.

Reflexologists map spots on the sole of the foot to particular organs, glands, and other body parts. Supposedly, pressing on the right spot on the foot can cause a reflex reaction in the corresponding body part. For example, pressing the ball of the foot can help problems in your heart or lungs. Now and then, practitioners may manipulate trigger spots on the palms or ears as well.

Reflexology can help you relax (like any foot massage) and may give you a sense of well-being. Whether or not it can really relieve pain in distant organs or help with specific medical or psychological problems still needs to be proven — although plenty of anecdotal reports claim cures for hypertension, PMS, anxiety, diarrhea, acne, psoriasis, migraines, chronic pain, and so on.

Should You Visit a Professional?

You can learn many forms of massage at home with a partner. With a little practice, you'll begin to sense areas of muscle tension and discover just how deep and hard to press. Plus the sense that someone cares for you (no small part of massage) can be greater when the person doing the massage truly cares!

Even so, it often pays to have at least a session or two with a qualified therapist to find out the basics of whatever technique you want to try. And if you want to try one of the more exotic and highly skilled forms of massage or bodywork, or if you're suffering from a chronic illness, you should almost certainly seek out a professional.

Seeing a professional

A good massage therapist will tailor the therapy to your particular needs. So before hopping up on the table, expect a little conversation about your medical history and current state of health.

That's the hard part. Getting the massage is easy, because (at least in more conventional forms of massage) you just have to lie in a quiet room occasionally doing what the therapist asks you to do. Usually the first thing she'll ask is that you remove your clothes and cover yourself with a large sheet or towel. Nothing to be modest about here, because only the area of the body being massaged will be uncovered. Getting your clothes out of the way is a good idea, though, both for comfort and to prevent stains left by certain massage oils.

Most sessions last 60 to 90 minutes and cost around $30 to $60 an hour, although more specialized techniques (especially bodywork) can run more. Of course, cost is considerably higher if you're making massage a regular part of your life or if you're participating in a program that requires returning for multiple sessions. Chances are fairly slim that your insurance company will pick up even part of the tab, although there's a bit more hope if your M.D. referred you to a licensed massage therapist.

Avoiding the cranks

Saying that you're visiting a "professional massage therapist" can widen a few jaundiced eyes — and inspire questions about just what part of your body is being massaged. And, of course, some massage parlors are little more than fronts for establishments of ill-repute. That's one of the reasons (besides setting minimal standards of competence) that national certification programs and state licensing for massage therapists can be reassuring.

One of the best ways to find a good therapist is to ask your regular M.D. or another trusted health practitioner to recommend one. A friend's recommendation can also be valuable, although you'll have to do more checking into credentials. You can also contact the American Massage Therapy Association or the National Certification Board for Therapeutic Massage and Bodywork (NCBTMB) for lists of qualified therapists near you (see the appendix for details).

In any case, make sure that your therapist is up-to-date in certification, has all appropriate licenses for your locality, and has adequate malpractice/liability insurance. Your massage therapist should have at least 500 educational hours from a program accredited by the Commission on Massage Therapy Accreditation. This commission helps assure that so-called therapists not only understand massage theory and technique but also know something about how the body works, how to help the body when it doesn't work (first aid and CPR), and how to handle patients who can't or shouldn't be using massage — in terms of medicine, ethics, and law.

How to make the most of a massage

You don't need to let common myths and fears stress you out about the massage that's supposed to relax you. Keeping the following points in mind can help:

✔ Be sure that you feel comfortable with your therapist. Getting touched is fairly personal, and you should feel safe in the process.

✔ Let the therapist know what you want — or ask for help deciding. Is your main goal to relax, or is it to relieve a specific injury or pain? How heavy or light should the pressure be?

✔ Ask the therapist to avoid sensitive areas. If your right shin is tender, there's no reason it has to be massaged (unless you and the therapist think a massage may help heal it). And if you're embarrassed to have anyone touch your neck or right knee or whatever, speak up. Well-trained, professional massage therapists should have a very good sense of clients' personal boundaries and will take these issues quite seriously.

✔ Take off only the clothes you feel comfortable taking off.

✔ Prepare to relax. It's usually a good idea to avoid eating a heavy meal right before a massage. Some people find it helps to take a shower or bath right before the massage.

✔ Speak up if something hurts or tickles. Sometimes a massage can cause temporary discomfort, especially if it involves working on sore, damaged, or tense areas. You may even feel sore in these areas for a day or two after a massage, just like underused muscles can feel sore after unfamiliar exercise.

✔ Speak up if you're sensitive to the aroma of the oil or just can't stand that soporific music in the background. You're the client.

✔ Remember, though, that speaking up has its limits. Focus on your breathing and the soothing hands, the soothing oils, and the relaxing music.

✔ Leave time to savor the results. Jumping back into your business suit and hailing a taxi may be unavoidable, but ideally you should leave yourself a few minutes to enjoy. Meanwhile, drink lots of water, which supposedly keeps the circulation flowing (and is actually a good idea for everyone, as long as you don't have a problem with congestive heart failure).

Don't let the initials L.M.T. (for licensed massage therapist) snow you. These initials have nothing to do with an academic degree. The same is true for most other initials you may see after a massage therapist's name. The best credential of all has no initials attached to it. It simply comes from meeting the NCBTMB's relatively high standards, including passing a national certifying examination, taking continuing education courses, and holding a state license if required. (Some therapists will use the initials N.C.B.T.M.B. to show that they've met these requirements.)

Judging the quality of a bodywork professional can be a bit trickier and is often a matter of intuition. You're best off looking for a therapist who has national certification in whatever kind of bodywork he or she claims to do.

Fortunately, you can get some help here (at least in the United States) from the NCBTMB, which now offers certification in various forms of bodywork — including polarity therapy, reflexology, Rolfing, and shiatsu.

Another option is to take a class in one of these methods at a local community center, hospital, or college. Often the people teaching these courses have private practices — and attracting potential clients is one of the reasons many of them teach the courses. They can also refer you to colleagues. Check out this book's appendix, too, for the names of national associations dedicated to various forms of bodywork. These groups can not only refer you to qualified local practitioners, but will often fill you in on just how much training and experience you should expect in a practitioner.

Trying massage at home

You don't need a professional to benefit from massage. In fact, because giving someone else a massage can actually benefit *you*, working with a friend or loved one can offer real advantages. For example, some evidence shows that giving someone else a massage can be even better for depression than receiving a massage!

Dozens of books and tapes explain how to perform various techniques, and good massage therapists can give you tips as well. Here are a few other tips that should help make the experience more pleasant:

- ✔ Take off all rings and watches and clip your fingernails before giving anyone a massage.
- ✔ Experiment with the right degree of pressure — too much can damage the muscles, too little can just tickle.
- ✔ Use your whole body weight and not just finger or hand pressure.
- ✔ Avoid open sores or injured areas.
- ✔ Use light, vegetable-based oils or lotions to smooth the way. You can usually count on products that are specifically labeled "for massage."
- ✔ Make the atmosphere as pleasant and peaceful as you can — with soft lighting and relaxing music if possible.

Massage can work for you even when you're alone. Most people automatically rub a sore spot or tense muscle — sort of an instinctive self-massage. Others have discovered the joy of a scalp massage during a shampoo. But dozens of other self-help tricks can come in handy when a headache overtakes you at the office or you need to soothe those aching feet.

For a headache, for example, try making small circles over your entire scalp with your fingertips, moving the top layer over underlying layers. Or try cupping both palms over your eyes and making light circles in both directions just under the eye sockets with the heels of your hands. For a muscle cramp, press your fingers into the tight knot at the center of the muscle and gently knead while you try stretching the muscle out with your other hand.

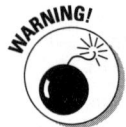

Remember that all home massage can be worth a try for minor, temporary conditions or simply as a pleasurable experience — but if you suspect that you may be suffering from a serious disease, or if the pain is extreme or unfamiliar, check with an M.D.

Can a Massage Ever Harm You?

Massage strikes a lot of people as harmless, but it's actually a powerful tool (if it weren't, how could it help all those ailments?). And it follows that a procedure that has so much power to do good can also — if used inappropriately — sometimes have the power to cause damage. This potential for harm is all the more reason to see a therapist who knows what she's doing — and we don't just mean knows how to give a good back rub. A qualified therapist not only knows a good deal about the human body, how it works, and what can go wrong with it, but above all is willing to tell you when massage is inappropriate or dangerous.

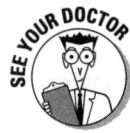

If you may have a serious or chronic illness, never use massage without first consulting an M.D. You should also generally avoid using massage on inflamed, burned, or otherwise injured areas. And because massage works by promoting blood flow, it can potentially spread certain problems throughout your body. You should almost always avoid massage therapy if you have an infection, cancer, swelling (edema), or a blood clot (except under the supervision of a highly skilled physician). People with high blood pressure, an enlarged liver or spleen, or peptic ulcers should also avoid abdominal massages. And pregnant women should stick to well-trained, professional massage therapists who are familiar with pregnancy massage.

Finally, as we keep saying, massage and other alternative treatments can be dangerous if they keep you from getting a valid diagnosis.

Part V
Mind-Body
Medicine

The 5th Wave   By Rich Tennant

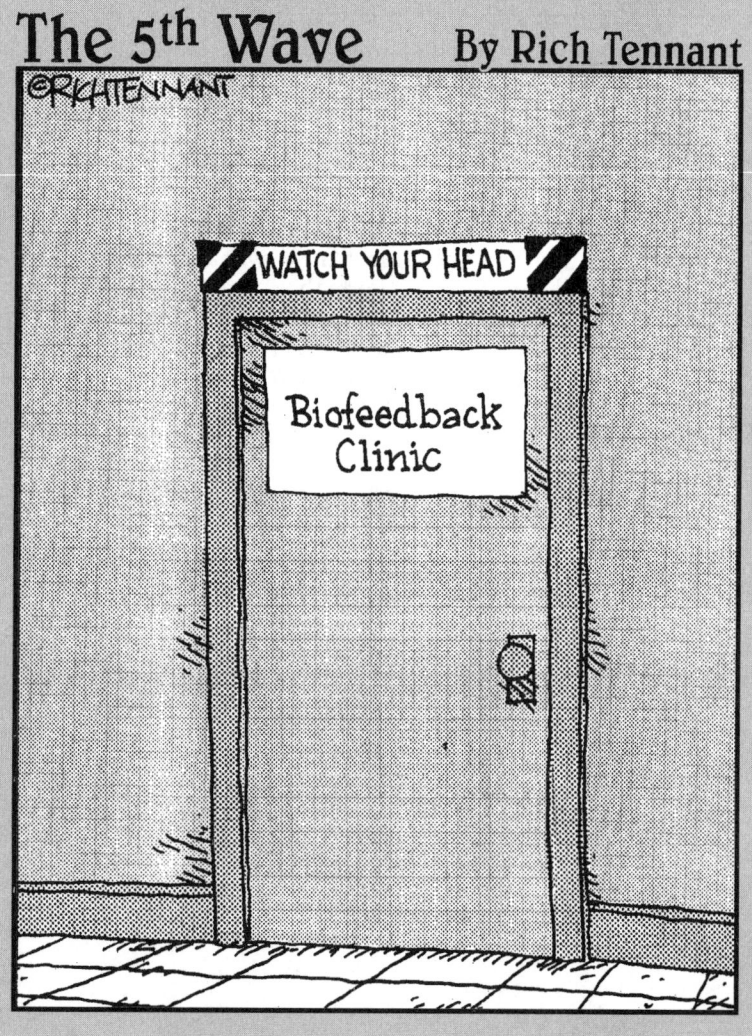

In this part . . .

Pretty much everyone today (even mainstream scientists) will acknowledge that your thoughts and feelings can influence the way your body works. This so-called mind-body effect is at the heart of alternative medicine. Admittedly, scientists know even less about how the mind can affect the body than they know about how the body can affect the mind. But, fortunately, they already know plenty. That's what this part is all about. Here you discover many effective (and often easy and low-cost) approaches that rely on the mind's power over the body — including relaxation methods, meditation, yoga, hypnosis, guided imagery, biofeedback, and even the power of prayer, positive thinking, and a little laughter.

Chapter 17
Finding Ways to Relax

• •

In This Chapter

▶ Ways stress can make you sick

▶ Cheap and simple ways to relax

▶ The relaxation response — the body's natural stress buster

▶ Meditation — including Zen, transcendental meditation (TM), and progressive muscle relaxation — demystified

▶ Yoga — a moving form of meditation

• •

The "mind-body" effect sounds mystical, almost supernatural. But most people have an instinctive sense of how to use it — often without even realizing it. One of the best examples is the way relaxation techniques — such as deep breaths, mental exercises, or just taking a "time out" — can make you feel better.

Of course, it's nice when scientific studies confirm stuff that you've suspected all along. In this chapter, we fill you in on exciting discoveries about the way stress (and the lack thereof) can affect your health — and about how getting some of the stress out of your life can help relieve many different ailments. We also describe some simple and cheap relaxation methods — many of which you can do on your own — to make yourself feel better and keep yourself that way. Plus, we demystify the most popular meditation and yoga techniques and let you know how they can help relax you and improve your health.

How Stress Can Make You Sick

Many people believe that we live in the most stressed-out time in human history. Crowding, crime, competition, pollution — wherever you want to put the blame, stress is everywhere. Whether our lives are really worse than ever is debatable. But there's no question that people are getting stressed out about their excessive stress, especially as study after study links it to a Pandora's box of ailments, including heart attacks, strokes, hypertension, infections, weakened muscles, impaired memory, immune disorders, and maybe even cancer.

Of course, stress gets a bad rap in our society. Some stress is downright desirable. When you get stressed (physically or emotionally), your body goes into a *fight-or-flight* response producing "stress hormones" that make your heart and breath rate soar, your blood pressure jump, and your muscles tense. This response evolved for good reason. When a saber-tooth tiger (or the modern-day equivalent) is chasing you, you probably want your heart pumping and your hormones racing.

Many people find that so-called positive stress motivates them to work and create. Others find a little stress now and then — from bungee jumping, challenging authority, or whatever — makes life exciting, or even worth living.

But there's no question that a lot of stress is destructive, especially when it hangs on hour after hour, day after day. We're talking about stress from humiliating and demoralizing work and family situations, and the all-too-familiar stress from modern existence — crowded cities, constant rushing, overbooked schedules, urban jungles, that kind of thing.

When stress hormones course through your bloodstream all the time, they start to push your organs to the breaking point. The result can be a whole host of "stress-related" diseases, including gastrointestinal problems, insomnia, headaches, chronic anxiety, and depression. Over time, stress can aggravate asthma, back pain, chronic fatigue, and hypertension, and it may even increase the risk of heart disease, weaken the immune system, and wear down every system in the body.

Don't blame it on modern life

Although people blame the modern rat race for their stress problems, stress and anxiety have always been a part of human existence. Frequent threats of war, violence, famine, and disease stressed out many of our ancestors — and healers assumed that part of their role was to help destress their patients.

True, Western doctors in modern times have generally separated the mind from the body (17th century philosopher Rene Descartes — of "I think, therefore I am" fame — usually gets credited, or blamed, for sparking this idea). Modern Western physicians have tried to heal by focusing on physical problems rather than attitude. But for millenia, many other cultures — including Chinese, Indian, African, and Native American — have included techniques to relax the mind as part of their healing traditions. Perhaps Western medicine would have been better off if Monsieur Descartes had said, "I take breaks from thinking, therefore I feel better."

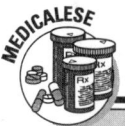

Psychoneuro — WHAAAT???

Not so long ago people who talked about the mind-body connection were viewed as mystics at best. Just about everyone accepted that the mind had some control over the body. (When you feel sad, tears well up in your eyes, for example.) But because no one had the slightest idea how this process happened, scientists dismissed the idea that feelings can control physiology as scientifically empty.

In the past decade, however, evidence has started accumulating that even the most staid researcher could love. The field is called *psychoneuroimmunology,* which is a fancy way of saying that scientists in this field look at the way mental states, the nervous system, and the immune system communicate and relate to each other.

By measuring levels of hormones and other substances in the blood, investigators in this field are beginning to link changes in emotions with measurable changes in the nervous and immune systems. One landmark study showed that practicing a series of relaxation techniques increased activity of natural killer cells (which attack invading microorganisms). Other studies suggest that stress increases the odds of developing colds or other diseases.

So far psychoneuroimmunology hasn't *proved* that relaxing — or changing your attitude in any other way — can cure diseases. But it has already gone a long way toward convincing skeptics that the mind and body are inextricably linked and that a positive mental attitude can help keep people healthy — even if the scientific understanding of just how remains primitive.

Whether practicing a relaxation technique for 10 to 20 minutes a day is enough to reverse symptoms of stress-related ailments remains to be proved. But there's little doubt that it can, at the very least, help you minimize the negative stress in your life, which in turn can leave you feeling alert, self-assured, and more in control — all feelings that can contribute to good health and help minimize symptoms of disease.

How to Find a Personal Stress Management Strategy

Unlike *Tai Chi,* massage, hypnosis, biofeedback, and many approaches to health that include mind-body effects, you can often get the health benefits from relaxation without any special guidance, fancy equipment, or even a partner. The key is finding a stress management strategy that works for you.

Here are a few approaches that may help you get the stress out of your life:

- **Take care of yourself.** If you eat a balanced diet, get enough sleep, exercise regularly, control caffeine and alcohol consumption, and the like, stress just won't bother you as much. "Nourishing" yourself with a little joy, fun, and creativity can help, too. Though often difficult — too many people put themselves last on their own priority lists — making sure that your basic needs are met and taking charge of your own health can go a long way toward making you stress-proof.

- **Try meditation, hypnosis, or other relaxation techniques.** Sure, taking a new class or reading about these methods can create more time pressure. But many people find that making some time for themselves leaves them so refreshed that they consider the pressure a small price to pay. If you can, try to include some kind of relaxation in your daily routine — meditate, listen to pleasing music, take up a hobby, or do whatever floats your boat.

- **Consider taking a time-management course — or at least re-evaluate your priorities.** Even if you don't sign up for a formal class, decide which parts of your life really matter. Chances are good that at least some of the time pressure you're feeling is due to tasks that you don't really have to do. Maybe doing the dishes right after dinner isn't so important. Maybe you can live with the dust bunnies under the couch. Maybe you don't need to fix that crack in the ceiling by tomorrow night.

  Put the activities that make your life meaningful at the top of your list — and don't sweat it if the less important stuff doesn't happen. The only one who thinks that you have to be perfect is you — so let up on yourself. (If anyone you know *does* think that you have to be perfect, be sure to put him or her at the bottom of your priority list.)

- **Take time out from — or avoid — high-conflict situations.** It's not always possible to bury your head in the sand, of course, but when the tension is getting out of hand, try to pull over, walk away, or regroup.

- **Don't discount socializing.** When you have solid and open relationships with friends, family, and coworkers, life looks a whole lot better.

- **Do everything you can to make your surroundings safe, clean, and quiet.** If your physical safety is threatened at your home or work or if your environment is uncomfortable, you're bound to be stressed. That's why surrounding yourself with things that make you feel calm and relaxed makes sense. True, you can't always get rid of the smoke pouring out of the next building or the obnoxious boor in the next cubicle. Still, you may at the very least be able to try a white noise machine, earplugs, a better chair or posture, or a relaxing wall hanging.

  In some cases, changing jobs or even homes can help. Major changes aren't always practical, of course — but if your physical safety or health is threatened, extraordinary efforts to change may be worthwhile.

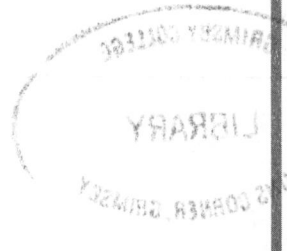

✔ **If all else fails, try changing your thinking.** Realize that you don't have to be a superhero. You don't have to solve the world's problems (or even all of your own!). Open your mind to other ways of solving problems. Learn to recognize and accept your feelings and express them to sympathetic friends. Realize that you do have the power to change yourself. As good old Marcel Proust put it: "The true voyage of discovery lies not in finding new horizons, but in having new eyes."

✔ **If you need help making these changes, join a formal stress-reduction program and/or an assertiveness training course.**

We're well aware that all these strategies are a lot easier to say than to do. Frankly, trying to write this chapter with a deadline gun to our heads makes it rather difficult to practice what we preach! Even so, you may find that merely reading (and writing!) this kind of advice has a kind of calming effect, and reading it often enough can help motivate even the most stressed-out individual to make some changes in the right direction.

How to Use the Relaxation Response

The relaxation response is based on the exciting discovery (championed by Dr. Herbert Bensen of Harvard's Mind/Body Medical Institute) that the body can destress itself. When you're stressed, the fight-or-flight response makes your stress hormones start raging and your heart start pumping rapidly. The relaxation response is basically the opposite.

The idea is that getting yourself in a relaxed frame of mind — usually by using meditation — can transform the body's basic operations (metabolism). Merely by repeating a word, phrase, thought, or even a physical motion, you can rid your mind of distracting and troublesome thoughts and — voilà — breathing eases, muscles relax, oxygen intake decreases, brain wave patterns slow, and (in some people) blood pressure drops. Most impressive of all, blood levels of *lactate* (a chemical associated with anxiety) plummet.

The relaxation response can help you with any disorder that is aggravated by stress. To make it happen, you have to find a technique that puts you into a tranquil state. Here's one way that works for many people (it can be done without formal training — and done just about any place, any time):

1. **Arrange a short period of time every day when you know you will not be disturbed.**

2. **Find a comfortable sitting position, close your eyes, and breathe slowly.**

3. **With each exhalation, repeat a word or phrase that comforts you.**

This *focus word mantra* can be anything that calms you: a nonsense phrase, a concept (such as "calmness" or "peace"), words from your religion, or perhaps the name of a place that makes you feel relaxed (maybe someplace like Bali or Cozumel — Las Vegas probably isn't the best choice for most people).

4. **Relax, but vigilantly banish all distracting or judgmental thoughts.**

5. **Open your eyes for the last minute or two but continue sitting and repeating the focus word and breathing slowly.**

Some people prefer to use more formal techniques of meditation to get the relaxation response going (see the next section). Other people make it happen with bodywork, hypnosis, or guided imagery (see Chapters 16 and 18). For still other people, simply praying can do the trick (see Chapter 19). Whatever method or methods help you get distracting, aggravating thoughts out of your mind will do.

How to Meditate on a Theme

Most people instinctively know when it's time to take a break. Whether it means walking away from a fight or finagling a two-week vacation, most people feel better if they can temporarily remove themselves from overwhelming aggravations and hassles.

Getting away from stress is what meditation is all about. Even better, meditation allows you to get away without booking a flight to Maui. Forget the intimidating language associated with certain techniques, the ones that can make meditation sound like something you need extrasensory perception to do. The truth is, meditation involves nothing more than a quick way to take your mind away from troubling and stressful thoughts — and getting it into the here and now where it can focus on itself and itself alone. You end up being a lot more relaxed — and probably feeling a lot better about your life. You may also end up feeling better physically.

Yes, you can meditate

Meditation doesn't have to be an exotic ritual. Just about every major world religion includes some form of meditation, running the gamut from simple breathing exercises to transcendental meditation (TM) to methods with exotic names such as vipassana and autogenic response.

Whatever the name, though, almost all forms of meditation are merely ways to get the relaxation response going (see the section, "How to Use the Relaxation Response"). Some forms of meditation involve elaborate ways to focus on your breathing *(breath awareness meditation);* others feature complex physical movements or chants to do while you focus. But all meditation methods aim to leave you with a sense of peace and tranquility by getting you into a "state of being" in which all your attention is focused in a single comforting place — away from trivial day-to-day concerns.

Meditation is great because you can do it on your own — just about any place and any time. But you may find it easiest to start by checking out the breath-awareness and other "focus" techniques that have worked for other people. Descriptions of these techniques are abundant in many popular books and tapes.

Zen, mindfulness, and other stress-busters

You can also jumpstart the relaxation response with more formal meditation techniques. Although you can do some of these at home (with the help of a few books or tapes that talk you through the steps), we recommend that you start out by consulting a qualified instructor (see the section "How to Find a Meditation or Yoga Class"). Besides helping you make sure that you're doing the techniques right, you may find that a soothing voice guiding you along is therapeutic in and of itself.

Tips for successful meditating

Whatever meditation technique you try, you'll have a better experience if you:

✔ Minimize potential distractions before you begin. In other words:

- Turn off the phone (or turn on the answering machine).

- Make sure that the kids and pets are accommodated.

- Open a window or readjust the thermostat if necessary.

- Go to the bathroom.

✔ Make sure that you're wearing loose and comfortable clothing.

✔ Wait at least half an hour or so after eating.

✔ Stop if you feel uncomfortable or disoriented.

✔ Go easy on yourself. The idea is not to be the best meditator around or to achieve perfect peace on your first try. Making meditation work for you can take many practices, especially if you expect it to alleviate specific physical ailments. But don't despair. With every (imperfect) effort, you'll find yourself more and more relaxed.

Many of these techniques take only 15 to 20 minutes a day — including a few minutes of calm before getting up and going back to stressland. If you're pressed for time, don't despair: even taking 5 to 10 minutes at the beginning is better than nothing.

You can try these techniques in whatever position is comfortable for you, but one word of warning: If you tend to doze off easily, try not to lie down or close your eyes.

Here are some more formal meditation techniques you may run across:

- ✔ **Zen.** If you're into Zen Buddhism — a religion that includes various meditative practices on the road to total fulfillment and enlightenment — you're bound to come across some breathing exercises that sound a lot like those we describe as ways to get the relaxation response going: Get comfortable, breathe deeply, and focus on the sound and flow of each inhalation and exhalation while tuning out distracting thoughts. In fact, the simple breathing exercises used in basic relaxation and meditation exercises come right out of Zen practice.

  According to Zen (which is the Chinese word for "meditation"), you can get rid of your anxiety by sitting comfortably without thinking anything at all. To experience Zen fully, though, you can't just aim to cure your chronic back pain; you have to buy into an entire religion/philosophy that helps you see the world in a whole different way.

- ✔ **Transcendental meditation (TM).** Popularized in the West by Ayurvedic medicine's Maharishi Mahesh Yogi (see Chapter 9), TM is a simple meditation practice that can profoundly relax you. Rather than concentrating your mind (and trying to control it) or focusing your attention on something tranquil, the idea is to repeat your mantra while letting your mind drift naturally and effortlessly into a heightened state of awareness — which the TM folks call *cosmic consciousness*. During this state, your mind grasps its connection to everything in the universe and understands its "infinite potential." This state is supposed to be not only relaxing but blissful.

  Because it supposedly gets your mind in tune with every possibility in the universe, proponents say that TM can make you healthier than other forms of meditation — and they can cite countless studies to prove that it is particularly good at curing insomnia, reducing anxiety and depression, improving memory and intelligence, expanding creativity, and even extending lifespan. TM is supposed to make you feel better about yourself, get along better with others, and just be a better person. Unfortunately, most of the grandiose claims are supported only by studies done by the Maharishi and his followers, which makes them somewhat suspect. At this point, it seems fairest to say that TM can bust stress at least as well as any other form of meditation — and so lead to changes in basic body operations that can help make or keep you healthy.

✔ **Progressive relaxation.** The idea is to discover how it feels to relax your muscles in isolated areas of your body — eyes, forehead, mouth, shoulders, arms, fists, abdomen, thighs, calves, feet, toes, and so on. Usually you lie down and focus on a single body part or muscle group. While taking a deep breath, you tense that area and slowly relax it as you exhale. You might start by squeezing your eyes shut for about 5 seconds, for example, and then gradually relaxing them. Then you can alternately purse and relax your lips, furrow and smooth your brow, shrug and unshrug your shoulders, and so on. To make sure that you cover everything, start with areas in your head and move down to your toes — or vice versa.

With a little practice, you can soon know how to relax your entire body at will and to relieve headaches and stress-related tension in specific muscles.

✔ **Autogenic training.** According to this technique, your mind gets your body to do what it wants by believing that the body is already doing it. The idea is not to order your body around but just to pretend that certain parts are relaxed, heavy, light, warm, cool, or whatever you want them to be. Eventually, your thoughts become self-fulfilling.

For example, you may silently tell yourself that your breathing is deep, easy, and calm or that you can feel your tension dissolving. Or you may imagine waves of tranquility rolling through each body part in succession. You can then focus on specific body parts, and with each slow breath tell yourself how relaxed its muscles feel.

✔ **Mindfulness (also known as vipassana).** This technique relaxes you by helping you focus on the essentials. Like autogenic training, it's a laid-back approach during which you accept what your body is doing without any kind of judgment or analysis. But instead of telling yourself that each body part is relaxed, you simply breathe deeply and observe what is happening to it — while gently escorting all other concerns and thoughts from your mind. Some people use this technique while exercising or while bending or tensing specific muscle groups.

✔ **Body scanning.** This technique is essentially a more systematic form of mindfulness. You let your mind slowly "scan" down each part of your body from head to toe, stopping at each point to observe what's going on there. You often start by observing your breathing. Again, the idea is not to judge or analyze but simply to note what is happening.

How to Meditate with Your Body — Yoga

Some people think of yoga as sitting with your ankles wrapped around your neck. But actually this and other less taxing postures are all part of an ancient Indian system of philosophy that combines physical and breathing exercises with ethical guidelines, dietary restrictions, and meditation techniques. And you can benefit from them without buying into the philosophy or having rubber limbs!

The yogic philosophy holds that body, mind, and spirit are united. (In fact, the word yoga comes from the Sanskrit word for union.) According to this system, people get sick when they lose their natural balance. The various body postures, breathing exercises, and relaxation techniques taught in yoga classes are all aimed to get — or keep — body, mind, and spirit in sync. In more mundane terms, yoga can also help keep you fitter, more limber and relaxed, and maybe even help lower your blood pressure to boot.

What yoga can — and can't — do for you

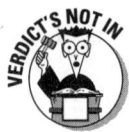

Plenty of anecdotes — and questionable scientific studies — claim that practicing yoga of one sort or another can help alleviate a whole host of serious ailments including asthma, diabetes, heart disease, chronic back pain, hypertension, and mental sluggishness. And a recent study in the prestigious medical journal *The Lancet* suggests that deep, slow ("yogalike") breathing can reinvigorate people with chronic heart failure — help them breath and exercise with greater ease. See L. Bernadi, et al., "Effect of breathing rate on oxygen saturation and exercise performance in chronic heart failure," *The Lancet* 351, 9112 (May 2, 1998): 1038.

These claims may have some validity, but so far there's just no convincing scientific evidence that yoga works any better than any other approach — or even any better than doing nothing. For the time being, the fact that many people insist that yoga makes them hurt less and feel better is still enough to make this generally harmless pursuit worth considering.

At least you can count on yoga as a great relaxer — and probably a good way to help dispel negative emotions such as anger, fatigue, depression, and anxiety. It can also help keep your body strong and limber in a way that's easier on you than aerobics and other heavy-duty exercise. You can get these benefits whether you go to class once a week or every single day (as many people do).

Hatha yoga

Most likely, any yoga class you take (and plenty of them are around) will involve some form of *hatha yoga*. The most physical form of yoga (and just the first in a series of steps toward reaching a higher state of consciousness), hatha has you go through a series of body positions and movements (*asanas*) that involve a lot of stretching and holding, plus a lot of breathing exercises (*pranayama*).

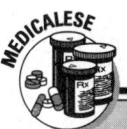

How do you take your yoga? Astanga, Kundalini, and other yoga flavors

As yoga gains in popularity, finding a class in just plain "yoga" or even generic "hatha yoga" is getting harder. More often than not, the class has a more esoteric name. Some of these styles are more technically demanding or spiritually-oriented than others. Following are the ones you're most likely to come across:

✔ **Astanga.** Technically, this form of yoga (also known as *eight-step* yoga) is designed to move you from "ignorance to truth" by combining self-control and ethics with body postures, breathing exercises, and meditation. But most classes boil down to having you move seamlessly through a series of asanas. If you're looking to lie back and reflect on the nature of the universe, try elsewhere: Astanga is as strenuous as yoga comes, and you can expect to work up a real sweat.

✔ **Integral.** This is a gentle form of yoga that emphasizes breathing exercises and meditation as much as the traditional postures.

✔ **Iyengar.** A rather technically demanding (and increasingly popular) form of hatha yoga, Iyengar asks you to concentrate — hard! — on the precise alignment of your body, sometimes using props such as blocks and belts.

✔ **Kripalu.** The most low-key form of hatha yoga, Kripalu emphasizes quieting your mind and developing a better awareness of your mind, body, and spirit. Staying within your individual limits, you work on coordinating your breathing and movement.

✔ **Kundalini.** This form of yoga aims to enlighten (and heal) you by helping you control the release of dormant energy that supposedly lurks at the base of your spine.

✔ **Power yoga.** This term is used to describe classes that are fairly similar to Astanga yoga (and that means a heavy-duty workout!), except that the series of asanas varies from class to class.

✔ **Sivananda.** Developed by a yoga teacher about 40 years ago, Sivananda involves a structured set of breathing and relaxation exercises, plus classic postures. Sivananda is based on five principles: proper exercise, proper breathing, proper relaxation, proper diet, and positive thinking.

✔ **Viniyoga.** This relatively gentle form of yoga tailors poses to your particular abilities. Usually, the goal is to flow from one position to another, with emphasis on coordinating the breathing to each movement.

Breath is key to yoga because each breath is *prana,* the Sanskrit word for the universal life force (the same stuff the Chinese call *qi*). Yogic breathing involves deep, slow breaths that start in the belly and completely fill the lungs.

The asanas are designed to help you balance opposites: stillness with movement, forward with backward, inhaling with exhaling. Probably the most famous asana is the lotus — the one during which you sit like a pretzel with your left ankle on top of your right thigh and your right ankle on top of your left thigh (see Figure 17-1). Also popular is a series of asanas called the "sun salutation" that is often used as a warm-up — and is not all that different from good old-fashioned calisthenics.

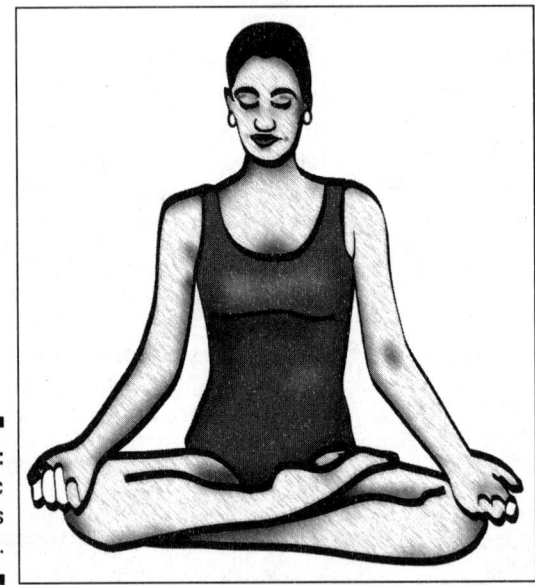

Figure 17-1:
The classic lotus position.

Expect your instructor to remind you to "stay completely present" or to "let yourself be empty." You may well do a little Sanskrit chanting (or throat rumbling — *ujjayi breathing*) along the way, too. In any case, the idea is to find ways to center your mind on your inner being — and expel superfluous thoughts that stress you out.

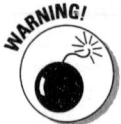

The best way to do yoga — at least at first — is under the supervision of a well-trained instructor who makes sure that you warm up properly and that you're ready to tackle the more advanced positions. Pregnant women should make sure that the instructor is gearing the class to poses that are safe during pregnancy. And, as with any exercise program, checking with your doctor before trying yoga is a good idea, especially if you have — or may have — a pre-existing health condition.

How Meditation or Yoga May Be Risky

Meditation is basically a harmless activity, but its intensity can freak some people out. (It may even provoke psychotic episodes in people suffering from certain mental illnesses.) Also, people with serious heart, lung, bone, or muscle problems should avoid the more pumped-up forms of yoga and the ones that require inverted poses.

 If you find yourself dizzy or disoriented, stop what you're doing. You may also find that it helps to open your eyes now and then and focus on a familiar object. Or try meditating while you walk or do some other relatively mild exercise (as long as you're in a safe environment where "spacing out" for a few minutes won't endanger your life!). If all else fails, consult a qualified instructor.

How to Find a Meditation or Yoga Class

Some forms of meditation are easy enough to figure out on your own. (Some people even do them instinctively.) But if you want to explore the more esoteric forms, you may need a little instruction. You might just want a little group support for any sort of meditation, or you may find that taking a class makes devoting 20 minutes of your life to this activity much easier.

 Finding a class or private instructor is a cinch almost anywhere because meditation and yoga are hot these days. Good places to start are local community centers, hospitals, and health clubs. If you live in a relatively big city, you can probably find free resource guides (often available at health food stores and other "alternative" hang-outs), which list more yoga and meditation classes than you could try in a lifetime, as well as courses on *Tai Chi, Qi Gong,* Ayurvedic cooking, and related pursuits.

 If you're not into lots of Sanskrit-speak and esoteric Hindu philosophy, check out a yoga class at your local YMCA, hospital, or health club. These classes tend to be more down-to-earth than the ones offered at dedicated yoga and "mind-body" centers.

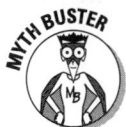 Unfortunately, distinguishing legitimate from dubious courses is sometimes difficult. Without national standards for meditation or yoga instructors, and so-called certification doesn't mean very much. Plus, the resource guides in particular are notorious for mixing ads for straight-shooting classes together with classes in tarot, astrology, and palm reading. They often include mysteriously named classes (often involving words such as "peace," "miracles," and "energy") that are the instructor's idiosyncratic way of describing what most people call yoga, meditation, acupressure, and the like.

So before signing up for a session with the "dynamic Swami" or 6-week classes that promise to "slow the aging process through nutrition, yoga, meditation, detoxification, and cleansing," make sure that you talk to some satisfied former clients and see whether you trust their enthusiasm. If the course is on a technique you've never heard of before, ask for a clear explanation of what it is and how it's related to a concept you *have* heard of. And find out how much you'll pay and just what you'll get for your money.

Above all, remember that any instructor who bad-mouths conventional medicine or won't talk to your M.D. about any pre-existing condition is bad news.

How to Keep Expectations Realistic

Don't expect meditation, yoga, or any other relaxation techniques to change your life overnight. Learning how to relax can take weeks or months of regular practice, and it can take just as much time for the relaxation response to produce noticeable changes.

Don't expect a relaxation technique to cure your ailment or serve as a substitute for other medical care, either. Helpful as it may be, relaxing alone is no remedy for cancer, AIDS, hypertension, or other serious conditions — although it can significantly alleviate symptoms of stress-related disorders. On the other hand, if you incorporate the relaxation response into your life, your symptoms may let up, you may start needing less medication, and you'll almost certainly feel better overall.

Above all, don't let the effort to relax stress you out! Too many people take to relaxation with the same intensity of effort they've poured into their careers, educations, and other achievements. Obviously, this approach is counterproductive.

If your efforts to relax are just adding anxiety to your life, by all means stop them and find some other activity that works for you. For some people, a more individualized approach may work better — perhaps gardening, playing a musical instrument, taking a walk, soaking in the tub, singing silly songs, even vegging out in front of the television. (Stay away from the news though!)

As long as your mind is focused only on your current activity, the relaxation response can kick in. Don't worry about impressing other people with your exotic methods; just find some activity to do every day that shifts your attention away from everyday concerns.

Chapter 18

Focusing on Hypnosis, Guided Imagery, and Biofeedback

• •

In This Chapter

▶ Discovering what hypnosis and hypnotherapy can — and can't — do

▶ Using your imagination to improve your health with guided imagery

▶ Controlling your body with your mind using biofeedback

▶ Deciding when to try these techniques and knowing their potential risks

▶ Finding a qualified therapist

• •

*T*his chapter reviews the benefits of three amazingly powerful approaches that put your mind in the driver's seat: hypnosis, guided imagery, and biofeedback. You can find out how each of these mind-body approaches can help you heal — just by thinking healing thoughts! You can also find out just when each one of these approaches may be right for you, the pros and cons of each, and the best way to get some help in using them.

Forget Svengali — Hypnosis Is Real

Hypnosis is a way to get yourself into a trancelike state during which you're susceptible to the power of suggestion, usually a therapist's suggestion. Getting through to this suggestible part of yourself can be a powerful way to break yourself of bad habits and irrational fears, manage pain, and relieve a variety of ailments.

Hypnotism puts you into a state of "focused concentration," during which you're vaguely aware of your surroundings — you just don't care about them. There are different stages of hypnosis, some deeper than others. But when you're in any of them, your imagination is open to suggestion.

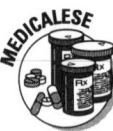

The suggestions made to you while you're hypnotized are part of *hypnotherapy*. This term, sometimes used interchangeably with hypnotism, simply describes the stuff that is suggested to you while you're hypnotized to help make you better after the session is over. Often the suggestions are images — picturing your arm going numb, picturing yourself relaxed — rather than orders to "stop hurting." (See the section "Using Guided Imagery: When Wishful Thinking Works," later in this chapter.)

Over the years, hypnotism has had a rather seedy reputation. This bad rep can be traced back to the late 18th century, when Franz Mesmer, the guy who introduced hypnotism into medicine, got himself kicked out of France for his fraudulent healing practices. Hypnosis was soon discovered to have genuine healing potential, but it was exploited by enough crackpots and vaudeville magicians to stay associated with superstition and evil for a long time. (Just think of all those movies with the mad scientist brainwashing victims!)

Today, though, hypnosis is about as mainstream as an alternative therapy can get. It has been recognized as a valid medical therapy since 1955 in Great Britain and since 1958 in the United States. Many mainstream doctors (particularly anesthesiologists and surgeons) are trained in hypnotherapy, as are a good number of dentists, psychotherapists, and nurses.

So why is hypnosis still considered alternative? Partly because it doesn't work for everyone (as if all mainstream therapies do!). But largely because no one really can explain how it works. Experts even debate whether hypnosis produces an altered state of consciousness at all. Right now, investigators are scrambling to get some of these answers, and already a few theories are floating around. But for now the whole business is still pretty much a mystery.

Even so, many mainstream health practitioners are willing to accept (and use) hypnotherapy because it happens to help their patients. They rest their case on many solid studies that show what hypnotherapy can do — even if researchers don't yet understand how.

Good candidates for hypnosis

If you're trying to lose weight, stop smoking, control substance abuse, or overcome a phobia, hypnosis may be worth a try. And if you're unhappy with your current treatment for warts or other skin conditions, asthma, nausea, irritable bowel syndrome, fibromyalgia, migraines, or other forms of pain, discuss the possibility of hypnotherapy with your M.D.

Hypnosis can work for almost anyone, though some people have an easier time than others. If you're lucky, you'll be one of the few people (about 5 to 10 percent of the population) who is highly susceptible to hypnotic suggestion. Some of these folks reputedly can be hypnotized (with no other anesthesia) before surgery and feel no pain. But even if you're not in this group, chances are high that hypnosis can help you: About 60 to 79 percent of people are moderately susceptible, and the remaining 25 to 30 percent are minimally susceptible.

Children and young adults are often good candidates for hypnosis, perhaps because they're so open to suggestion and have active imaginations.

If you don't trust your therapist, or don't believe that hypnotism can work for you, it probably won't. Hypnotism can only work if you're willing for it to work and you have a clear idea about what you want it to do for you.

Possible harmful effects

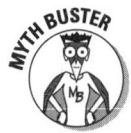

Contrary to popular belief, you cannot be hypnotized against your will and forced to do the evil deeds of a mad scientist. While you're hypnotized, you are simply in a state of focused relaxation — not a coma.

Hypnosis can be dangerous, however, if you're suffering from a serious psychiatric condition (particularly psychosis, organic psychiatric conditions, or antisocial personality disorder). These people should consult with a psychiatrist familiar with hypnosis before trying it.

Resources for finding a good hypnotist

To find a competent hypnotherapist, check with any of the organizations listed under hypnotism in this book's appendix. These groups can refer you to practitioners near you with acceptable training and certification.

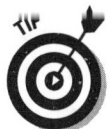

If your hypnotist also happens to be a licensed health care professional, you may be able to get reimbursement from your health insurer. Using a licensed health care practitioner is a good idea anyway. Because no states license hypnotherapists per se, this license — plus certification by the American Board of Hypnosis or the American Council of Hypnotist Examiners — is a good clue to competence.

A good therapist will

- ✔ Explain the different stages of consciousness to you
- ✔ Assure you that hypnosis won't make you do anything you don't want to do
- ✔ Review your past experience with hypnotism and answer your questions
- ✔ Often offer to do a demonstration on someone else
- ✔ Never promise to perform miracles

Methods for hypnotizing yourself

Many people believe that all hypnosis is self-hypnosis — that is, by trusting in the hypnotist you essentially brainwash yourself. So even if you go to a hypnotherapist, you can't regard her as anything more than a facilitator who helps you hypnotize yourself.

But according to a formal school of hypnosis, you can put your mind into a high state of concentration without a facilitator. Most people have found themselves in this place naturally — by daydreaming, losing themselves in a novel, or spacing out as they drive. The idea is to get yourself into an altered state during which your whole attention is focused in a single place.

Can these altered states affect your behavior in any way (besides making you miss your exit or having to pretend to know what your boss was saying)? Well, experiencing these altered states probably can't cure your stage fright or stop your smoking as effectively as formal sessions with a hypnotherapist might. But you can certainly try self-hypnosis to work toward these kinds of goals — as well as to relax and/or distract your mind from pain or cravings.

If you want to use self-hypnosis most effectively, you're best off starting with directions from a trained therapist — who will help you make sure that you're doing it right. You'll discover how to relax yourself (whether that means swinging a pendant in front of your eyes or meditating) and use your thoughts to contact your unconscious mind. When your unconscious takes over and tells your body what to do (such as lifting an arm), you're in an hypnotic state and ready to respond to suggestion.

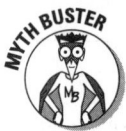

Watch out for books and audiotapes promising to target your subliminal mind to help you stop smoking, improve your personality, or whatever — especially if they promise to make these changes overnight. Effective hypnosis of any sort often needs to be tailored to your particular mind (by a teacher or yourself) and almost always requires weeks or months of practice.

Using Guided Imagery: When Wishful Thinking Works

If the idea of chocolate chip cookies baking in the oven makes your mouth water, you know what guided imagery is all about. Vivid mental images can change many bodily functions, including increasing your blood sugar, stomach secretions, and saliva flow; slowing your digestion; and heating or cooling your skin. Many people know how to control these functions naturally: for example, athletes who "psych" themselves into a better performance or dental patients who "will away" pain by imagining themselves on a tropical island while the dentist drills!

Guided imagery and cancer

Guided imagery got a lot of publicity when researchers started recommending it to cancer patients. By picturing an aggressive army of white blood cells attacking cancer cells and flushing them out of the body, patients try to get their real immune systems to do the same thing. Unfortunately, even after two decades, no one has been able to prove that this approach makes any difference in long-term survival. However, using imagery does seem to make coping with illness easier by helping relieve pain and anxiety and minimizing nausea and weight loss that can occur with radiation and chemotherapy.

When you practice guided imagery, you use these powers in a systematic way — getting your body and/or mind to do what you want by imagining it. If that sounds to you like a relaxation technique (see Chapter 17), you're right. Many people use guided imagery as one of many ways to get stress out. But, as this chapter shows, guided imagery may also help you relieve specific ailments — and even understand (and control) the emotions that sometimes accompany them.

Proof and evidence: Small, but growing

An *image* is the way you represent things inside your head. The most vivid images call on all five senses, so that you can see, hear, smell, taste, and touch the image. When you practice guided imagery (or, as it's sometimes called, *imagery*), you work to conjure up images that will produce desired effects on your body and mind.

Can imagery really work? Certainly it can relax you and distract you from pain. In fact, many healing traditions have relied on imagery as a healing tool for centuries. When you consider the solid scientific studies showing cures for specific ailments, though, the answer is hazier.

The evidence we do have comes mainly from the experience of physicians and other practitioners who have found that guided imagery has helped countless patients. These patients often used guided imagery together with other mind-body techniques — including biofeedback, hypnosis, meditation, and assorted relaxation methods. These experiences aren't enough to prove that guided imagery can heal you, but they are enough to suggest that this approach may be worth a try — especially because it's a relatively harmless (and often inexpensive) technique.

How to use your imagination

Guided imagery involves no more effort, risk, or expense than finding the time and space to play with your thoughts. If you're using this method to relax, for example, all that's necessary is to get yourself comfortable, take some slow relaxing breaths, and imagine yourself in a pretty, tranquil setting such as a beach or a mountaintop.

Try to feel this setting as though you were really there. If you're thinking of a beach, try imagining the sound of the surf, the smell of the breeze, and the taste of the salt. Take your time and enjoy each sensation.

The more "real" your image, the better it seems to convince your body that it's really happening. So get all your senses working. If you're thinking of an artillery attack, make sure that you picture the troops, smell the gunpowder, hear the exploding shells, feel the rumble of tanks, and so on.

If you don't have a "good" imagination

Don't despair. If your imagination just isn't going to conjure up a virtual image for you, focus on a single sense — perhaps a favorite flavor or tune or the feeling of a light breeze against your neck.

You can use any image you want, tailoring it to your interests. If beaches make you think of flies and sandy swim trunks, think about curling up in your favorite armchair instead. If you don't like war images, think about serving your troubles out with a tennis racket.

If worse comes to worst, join a group or class for ideas. Or invest in an imaging audiotape. Sometimes soothing suggestions from another person can shift your imagination into gear.

Good candidates for guided imagery

If you're looking for a low-risk way to beat stress, guided imagery may be worth a try. This method uses the same kind of mental persuasion that occurs during many other relaxation and meditation techniques (see Chapters 17).

Guided imagery can also be a good option if you have physical symptoms that haven't responded as well as you'd like to other therapies. Stress-related symptoms seem to respond particularly well. (By the way, at least half — and probably more — of all physical ailments originate from stress or other emotional or social problems.)

No one really knows whether guided imagery works better for certain people than others — but you increase the odds of success if you practice regularly, learn to relax, and believe that this approach can help you.

Possible harmful effects

Guided imagery is one of the most harmless healing approaches. Like any approach, though, you should never use it as a substitute for regular medical care or use it by itself to treat a serious condition.

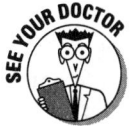

Guided imagery can lead you to overmedicate yourself. That's because — if the imagery is working — it can reduce your need for pain-relievers or other medications. You can even end up undermedicating yourself. ("Wow, I feel so much better now, I bet I can lay off this blood pressure medication.") So let your M.D. know if you're using guided imagery in case you need your dosages adjusted.

Guidance for using guided imagery

Whether you want to use guided imagery to relieve a symptom or to better understand the emotional roots of an ailment, you can get help from books, audiotapes, or a trained therapist. For more information, check out the appendix at the end of this book.

Don't forget to check courses offered by your local hospital — or to ask a trusted alternative care provider or mental health practitioner for referrals. Remember, too, that if an M.D. refers you for guided imagery training as part of therapy, you may (hope springs eternal) even get some help from your insurance company.

Applying Mind over Matter: Biofeedback

Biofeedback has been so heavily documented by scientific evidence — and so widely accepted in the health care world — that calling it alternative is difficult. But because biofeedback is based on the idea that the mind and body are linked — and the mind can control the body — fitting this approach into conventional medicine's view of the world is difficult. And you can't expect most M.D.s to recommend this technique without a lot of prompting.

Whether you're looking for a low-risk way to help treat anxiety, asthma, tension headaches, chronic pain, or many other disorders — or you just want to discover some nifty ways to control your blood pressure, pulse, and other supposedly "involuntary" functions — read on!

The mind takes control

Most people think that they can't control blood pressure, body temperature, brain waves, digestion, muscle tension, heart rate, and the like. And most of the time, they're right; these basic bodily functions are normally regulated automatically by the nervous system. Usually, you don't even notice them. But it turns out that — with biofeedback training — you can change these normally involuntary functions at will!

Talk to your blood pressure

Suppose that you're trying to control your blood pressure. A therapist hooks you up with electronic sensors to a machine (see Figure 18-1) that can measure blood pressure and then translate the reading into a picture or sound (the *feedback*). As you think different thoughts, you observe the changes in the feedback (usually a series of tones or a computerized image).

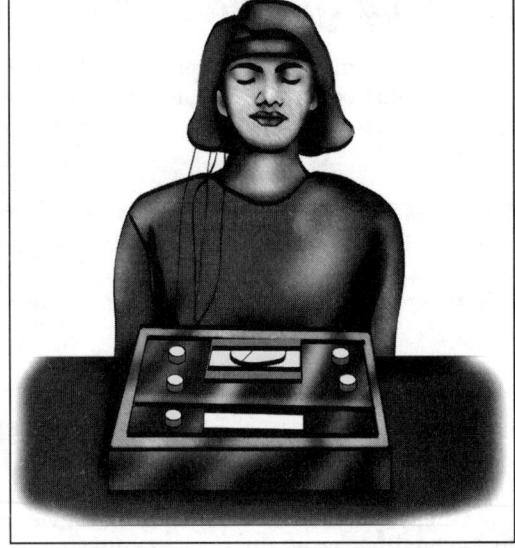

Figure 18-1:
A woman uses the feedback from a biofeedback machine to learn to control her blood pressure.

Eventually, your mind figures out what you have to do to get your blood pressure into the normal range — and how to make that happen even in the real world. Table 18-1 lays out the most common forms of biofeedback and the conditions they're used to treat.

Table 18-1		Common Types of Biofeedback	
Type	**What's Measured**	**Basic Method**	**Used for**
Brain wave	Electrical activity in the brain	Sensors placed on scalp	Alcohol and drug addiction, brain damage, epilepsy, hyperactivity, insomnia
Breathing	Breath rate, rhythm, volume, and location	Sensors around chest and abdomen or around mouth and nose	Anxiety, asthma, hyperventilation
Electrodermal response	Sweat gland activity	Sensors attached to palm or fingers to measure electrical current (the more sweating, the more current)	Anxiety, overactive sweat glands
Electromy-ography	Muscle spasms and tension	Sensors placed on the muscle group in question	Incontinence, muscle pain, physical rehabilitation, stress, teeth grinding (TMJ), tension headaches, torticollis ("wry neck")
Finger pulse	Pulse rate and amount of blood in each pulse (the higher these are, the more wired your autonomic nervous system is)	Sensor attached to a finger	Anxiety, irregular heartbeat, hypertension
Skin temper-ature (also called *thermal biofeedback*)	Blood flow changes (the more blood flows, the warmer the skin)	Temperature sensor *(thermistor)* taped to finger	Anxiety, hypertension, migraines, Raynaud's disease

Biofeedback can even help relieve problems you aren't directly trying to alleviate. If you find a way to control your skin temperature or blood pressure, for example, you may discover that other problems — especially those that stemmed from an overactive autonomic nervous system — disappear, too! Some people also find themselves feeling more in control of their health, and more hopeful about life in general.

Practice, practice, practice!

How long you'll have to wait for results of biofeedback depends on many factors, including your age, general health, ailment, and overall motivation. At the very least, biofeedback will take at least a few office sessions (each lasting 30 to 60 minutes) to help simple problems — and many ailments will require dozens of sessions. One fact is clear: The more you practice, the quicker you'll achieve desired results. Practicing at home can even reduce the number of office sessions you need. If you can, talk to other people that have used biofeedback successfully; you may lose heart on your own.

But don't try to be your own therapist by purchasing biofeedback devices on your own. Unless you have very specific instructions from a professional therapist on how to use these gizmos, you'll only waste your time and money because most of these devices are so complicated to figure out that they usually end up left in the back of the dresser drawer.

Asking your therapist to estimate the number of treatments you'll need can help keep your expectations realistic — and give you a benchmark by which to decide that it's time to put your time and money elsewhere.

Times to consider biofeedback

Just because biofeedback works for some people with your condition doesn't guarantee that it will work for you. (Actually, the same is true for any form of therapy.) You may have a form of the condition that biofeedback can't help, or you may just be one of the few people who doesn't respond well to biofeedback.

Even so, it can't hurt to ask your health care provider about biofeedback if your current therapy isn't working for you (and, while you're at it, ask to be referred to a qualified therapist!). In some cases — especially stress reduction, Raynaud's disease, and certain types of headaches and other pain — biofeedback may be the treatment of choice. If you need to control asthma, diabetes, or epilepsy; recondition muscles; or recover from stroke, biofeedback may well be a useful addition to your overall treatment plan.

Paying for biofeedback

Biofeedback can cost you — sessions can run up to about $150, and in most cases you'll need quite a few of them. The good news, though, is that private insurers will often help pay, provided that you're using the biofeedback for a reimbursable disorder.

Possible harmful effects

Unless you panic during deep relaxation or just get bugged by electronic blips and beeps, don't expect any problem from biofeedback. The instruments are safe, and the electricity rarely enters your body — except during electrodermal biofeedback (the kind that measures sweat), and the amount of current is minuscule. Just to be cautious, though; check with your M.D. if you have a serious heart condition or an implanted pacemaker (or other implanted electronic device) before using this form of biofeedback.

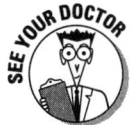

If you're taking any medications for your condition, checking with your M.D. after therapy begins is a good idea. If biofeedback works for you, you may need to reduce your dosage — only your doctor knows for sure.

Resources for finding a qualified therapist

You're the one who does the real work in making biofeedback heal you. But you will need a qualified therapist to hook you up to the equipment every time, answer your questions, monitor your progress, and offer suggestions. You can find this type of therapist in many different fields of health care — including medicine, nursing, psychology, social work, physical and occupational therapy, and so on.

Finding someone who knows what they're doing may take a little more legwork. No formal licensing is available for biofeedback therapists, but certification from the Biofeedback Certification Institute of America is a bare minimum requirement. Your best bet is to make sure that the therapists have all the standard training and licensing in their respective fields — and that they have some (successful!) experience using biofeedback on other people with your disorder.

Check out this book's appendix for organizations that can steer you to competent biofeedback therapists in your area.

Chapter 19

Thinking Positively: Optimism and Other States of Mind

In This Chapter

▶ How optimism, hope, and a sense of control may be good for you

▶ How having a sense of humor can improve your health

▶ What prayer and faith may do for you

▶ Why support from friends and family makes a difference

▶ How a pet can make you healthier

▶ How to develop a "survivor personality"

*B*y now, almost everyone has heard of the Type A personality: the driven workaholic who supposedly is at high risk for heart disease. Well, credible evidence is starting to show that being a Type A personality isn't the only risk factor. Shouldering any kind of negative emotion — especially powerlessness, hostility, anger, suspicion, and resentfulness — may not only increase your odds of heart disease but jeopardize your health in general.

No one can avoid these feelings all the time, of course. But the happiest people somehow know how to buffer them by keeping life's inevitable tragedies from spoiling the good stuff. And these folks may be the healthiest people as well. This chapter fills you in on the growing evidence that you may be able to improve your physical health just by changing the way you think and feel about your life.

Your Attitude Can Make You Sick

All the advice to "keep the sunny side up" if you want to be healthy sounds all warm and fuzzy, but almost too good to be true. Actually, though, a load of evidence shows that your attitude about life can improve your health and even speed your recovery from a serious ailment or surgery. The attitudes that seem to help the most are optimism, hope, and, above all, a feeling that you have some impact on the quality of your own life.

How optimism may affect your body

No one really understands how or why a positive attitude helps people recover faster from surgery or cope better with serious diseases — diseases as serious as cancer, heart disease, and AIDS. But mounting evidence suggests that these effects may have something to do with the mind's power over the immune system. One recent study, for example, polled healthy first-year law students at the beginning of the school year to find out how optimistic they felt about the upcoming year. By the middle of the first semester, the students who had been confident that they would do well had more and better functioning immune cells than the worried students. (See Suzanne C. Segerstrom, Ph.D., et al., "Optimism is Associated With Mood, Coping, and Immune Change in Response to Stress," *Journal of Personality and Social Psychology*, Volume 74, Number 6, June 1998.)

Some researchers think that pessimism may stress you out, too, boosting levels of destructive stress hormones in your bloodstream (see Chapter 17). Of course, it's also possible that having a positive attitude toward life makes you more likely to take better care of yourself. And you're more likely to attract people into your life (and keep them there) — which in and of itself may boost your health (see the section, "Social Support and Health").

How to keep the sunny side up

We're not saying that you should deny life's darker side or interpret every calamity as a blessing. But when calamity does strike, try not to give in to despair or fatalism. Concluding that you personally have been singled out for suffering, refusing to see any silver lining, and abandoning all hope may not only be a recipe for illness: Such attitudes are also not such great ways to go through life. Try to recognize that your grief and pain, however real and deep, are only part of a larger picture — and that this picture includes many elements of pleasure, success, and meaning.

Another approach is to try to "use your pain" for good. Many people who have suffered from life-threatening and incapacitating illnesses — including cancer, heart attack, and the like — say that they consider their illness to be "a gift." The illness taught them to value each day, appreciate the moment, and get their priorities straight. Sometimes they discover that they have the power to do things they never knew that they could.

Losing a breast to cancer, for example, has led some women to stop pouring all their energies into cultivating perfect bodies. As a result, they discover other interests and talents, such as French literature, tutoring, or race walking. Being forced to give up a high-powered job because of a disabling illness has given other people the time they always wished they had to pursue sculpting, chamber music, gardening, or other passions. We're not saying that you should wish cancer, heart disease, or AIDS upon yourself, of course; but if you keep an upbeat perspective, even life's blows can bring rewards beyond your wildest imaginings.

Remember that even if you can't change the circumstances of your life, you can change your attitude! If you need help, talk to a health professional about whether psychotherapy, support groups, or other structured approaches might help you.

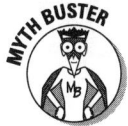

Attitude definitely seems to influence the course of illness. But some people take this link too far and make you feel that your bad attitude caused your disease or is keeping you from healing. Walk the other way if anyone makes you feel guilty for being sick or treats your physical ailments as if they were emotional or mental problems (included are physicians who banish you to a psychiatrist when you have no *obvious* signs of physical illness).

Laugh It Up

No one can prevent all tragedy and pain, but you can stop yourself from succumbing to them. And one of the best ways you can stop yourself is by laughing through the tears. Even if you're doing just fine right now, retaining a childlike capacity for joy and laughter may keep you healthier longer (and will certainly keep you happier).

Yukking it up can be a powerful antidote to stress, which has been linked to all sorts of unhealthy bodily changes. Plus, seeing the lighter side of things can help put suffering in perspective, fill you with hope and other positive emotions, take your mind off your pain, and may even do wonders for your immune system.

Still don't take humor seriously? You will if you check out a few of the dozens of therapeutic humor-related Web sites. You can get to most of these by starting with the International Center for Humor and Health (www.humorandhealth.com), a nonprofit organization that aims "to spread the healing art of laughter." Or try the American Association for Therapeutic Humor (ideanurse.com/aath/). You may find some of the humor silly or irreverent — but you may also find yourself chuckling in spite of yourself.

If you're not Web-oriented, get a copy of the Norman Cousins classic *Anatomy of an Illness As Perceived by the Patient* — Paperback Rei Edition, Bantam Doubleday Dell Publishers (August 1991). This book movingly describes how Cousins overcame a disabling and supposedly irreversible disease by routing out negative emotions — and doing a lot of laughing.

A Few Words about Prayer

Can praying make you well? Can praying for *someone else* make *them* well?

Don't laugh. Highly respected figures in the health care field are saying that it's time to take prayer and religion seriously — and many of their colleagues are listening. We're talking about people who are highly regarded even in the conventional medical world, including cardiologist Larry Dossey, M.D., and Harvard Medical School's Herbert Benson, M.D. Courses on spirituality and healing are cropping up at prestigious medical schools, and future doctors are learning how to talk to patients about religious issues. Hospitals and managed care organizations are looking for ways to restore pastoral care services that waned with recent budget cuts. Even the staid *Harvard Health Letter* recently ran a lead story about the burgeoning interest in faith and spirituality among both doctors and patients.

Faith and healing — longtime partners

Faith and healing have been linked from the beginning of human history. From day one, people assumed that they could get well by appeasing wrathful gods — who presumably made them sick as punishment for bad behavior. Pastoral care has long been a part of tending to the sick and dying, usually for purely religious reasons.

Out of the mouths of babes

A joke is currently circulating among second-graders that crystallizes a key message about prayer and faith healing. (Actually, this joke is often told in various forms by experts on alternative medicine, but we figure that by using this version we can skip the onerous permissions process):

A man was drowning, and a boat approached him. "Hop in," said the boat driver. But the drowning man replied, "No thanks. God will save me."

Soon another boat arrived. "Get in," said the driver. But again, the drowning man said, "No thanks. God will save me."

Finally a third boat came. "Get in, or you'll drown," said the driver. "No, thanks," said the drowning man. "God will save me."

Well, the man drowned and found himself face-to-face with God. "What happened?" he said to God. "I believed in you. Why didn't you save me?" "I sent you three boats," said God. "What more did you want?"

In other words, don't be surprised if the healing you pray for happens to come in the form of a drug or operation — or even a mainstream M.D.!

Researchers are finding increasing evidence that people who consider themselves religious — or who feel supported by their community — often recover faster from illness than their peers and may even have lower rates of depression, stress, illness, and death. Various studies have linked prayer and religious belief to faster recovery from surgery, substance abuse prevention and control, and a lower incidence of Alzheimer's disease, as well as a decrease in emphysema, suicide, heart disease, high blood pressure, and cirrhosis of the liver.

Remember that the "spirituality" in these studies didn't necessarily mean belonging to any particular religion or using a specific form of prayer. It usually meant having a belief system that recognized some intangible presence or power that made life feel ordered and meaningful. Generally, people classified as "religious" or "spiritual" go through life feeling peaceful and contented (even in times of suffering), and they carry a sense that the world is filled with infinite possibilities.

The reasons prayer may help

Many people believe that prayer itself — or the intervention of some higher power — explains such remarkable results. But other factors may be at work. For example, religious people probably take better care of themselves than the general population — they often eat healthier diets and avoid smoking and drinking. Just getting community support through prayer groups, church socials, bingo, or other interactions can make people feel better (see the section, "Social Support and Health"). So can the more stable marriages that can be linked to regular attendance of religious services. And in some cases, just believing that praying (or God) can heal may have made people feel better physically.

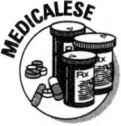

But even when investigators design their analyses to eliminate the power of suggestion and other explanations, they *still* find that faith in and of itself seems to make a difference. How? Many investigators think that the effects have to do with the *relaxation response* (see Chapter 17): the lowered pulse and other changes in body function that come from reducing stress. Prayer, and spirituality in general, may help promote certain mental states that reduce stress and elicit this response.

Nonlocality: Praying for others

Some people think that there may be more to prayer than its ability to put you in a meditative state. These folks think that praying for someone far away — maybe even someone who doesn't know they're being prayed for — can make a difference. Joan Borysenko, Ph.D., for example — a well-known clinical psychologist, bestselling author, and cofounder and former director of the Mind/Body Clinic at the New England Deaconess Hospital — believes that this long-distance healing may be possible because all minds may be interconnected as part of a single universal consciousness. "This sounds pretty hocus-pocus," she admits, "but it's certainly an idea that's been kicked around from early times. And there's definitely something to it — even if we don't understand it from a scientific perspective."

Borysenko is talking about *nonlocality:* the idea that your mind can affect *other* bodies. She tells stories about people in one room who changed the vital functions (breathing rate, pulse, blood pressure, and so on) of a person in another room — merely by thinking frightening or relaxing thoughts about them.

"That's both good news and bad news," Borysenko said at the Casa Colina Whole Health Forum in March 1998. "Because what it means is that if perhaps we're thinking loving thoughts of somebody, it may register non-locally. But it also means if we're thinking bad thoughts — saying someone is hopeless, etc. — we're kind of putting a curse on them. . . . As a psychologist, I like to think that we're just one big cosmic case of multiple personality disorder."

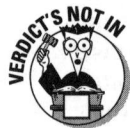

Western scientists can't explain nonlocality at all. Nor can they explain why so many people believe they have experienced extra-sensory perception (ESP), near-death experiences, or full-scale apparitions of lost loved ones.

No irrefutable evidence distinguishes these experiences from mere delusions, provoked by misfirings of certain parts of the brain (though many baffling stories can't be so easily explained away). But if Harvard's Herbert Benson, M.D., has his way, this situation may soon change — see Benson's *Timeless Healing: The Power and Biology of Belief* (Fireside: 1997). Dr. Benson, who believes that humans are "wired for God," is trying to scientifically measure the effects of praying for others.

Of course, for the truly faithful, scientific evidence is unnecessary. That's what faith's all about. And even if faith and prayer don't make people physically healthier, they undoubtedly make a lot of people live happier and more fulfilling lives.

Social Support and Health

One (of many) reasons that your attitude can affect your health is that a bad attitude can drive other people away. And interaction with other people is vital for your health. Human beings are social animals. So it's no surprise that people thrive when they have good relationships with friends, family, and people in general. More surprising, perhaps, is that these relationships can also affect physical well-being — and not just because being nasty to your doctor or shouting obscenities at her receptionist will keep you from getting optimal treatment.

The power of intense social support to help you better cope with physical illness goes above and beyond the powers of medications and other therapies. According to psychotherapist Joan Borysenko: "The [scientific] literature says clearly that although good habits are important — eating right, exercise, not smoking, etc. — none are as important as high self-esteem and the ability to give and receive love and to develop intimacy with other humans."

Borysenko talks a lot about the "Four F's" — family, faith, friends, and fun — that seem to be essential to happiness (and probably good health).

Evidence that social support may work

An ever-mounting number of large-scale studies have linked social support to specific health effects. Among the most intriguing are studies linking social support (either in the form of organized groups or one-on-one support) to longer survival time for women with breast cancer; higher levels of natural killer cells (a sign of a stronger immune system) in people with certain cancers, and increased mobility and reduced swelling of joints in people with rheumatoid arthritis.

Many studies also show lower Caesarean section rates, shorter labor, and decreased need for anesthesia in women who have a female companion experienced in labor and delivery — called a *doula* — accompany them through labor. Social support has also been shown to decrease depression after strokes; and perhaps even lower chances of developing heart problems and dying prematurely (especially in people who have a spouse or other confidant).

Despite these exciting findings, don't be fooled into thinking that tea and sympathy alone can cure a serious ailment. But a strong support network may well boost the healing powers of a broader treatment plan.

Beware of loneliness and isolation

Not only are studies showing that socializing can make you feel better — but plenty show that loneliness and isolation can be hazardous to your health (even though we all need a little "alone time" now and then). Adults with few social connections — especially those without spouses, close friends, family, church membership, or other group affiliations — have unusually high risks of dying at any given age. (On the other hand, having an unhappy marriage or getting divorced appears to threaten your health.)

Of course, social and emotional support may be helpful indirectly. If someone loves you, they're likely to take care of you — scrub the toilet bowl for you, make sure that you take your meds and go to rehab, that sort of thing. Someone who loves you may also encourage you to take care of *yourself:* eat better, exercise, stop smoking, and so on. And just having that person around may motivate you to be better to yourself.

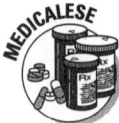

But even when investigators eliminate as many of these extraneous factors as possible, something about social ties alone seems to affect human health. Quite possibly, social ties help prompt the faith, hope, optimism, and other attitudes that may buffer you against stress. Evidence already suggests that strong social support alone is enough to reduce the output of stress hormones and boost the strength of immune cells (though no one — yet — has directly proved that these changes themselves make your health better).

Whatever the explanation, having satisfying relationships may well be just as crucial — if not more crucial — to good health as is stopping smoking, exercising regularly, or watching your fat and fiber intake.

Support groups

If you don't have a strong support network at home, you can often find one through an organized group of people suffering from the same ailment as you are. Some groups are just a bunch of patients sitting around talking. Others are led by a doctor, nurse, or other health professional. Support groups also exist for spouses and children of people suffering from many different conditions.

What a little support group can do for you

Besides the possible health benefits that may come from company, here are some other benefits you may get from joining a support group:

✔ Coping skills for frustrations that come from living with a serious illness

✔ Ideas about new therapies and funding sources

✔ Assurance that you're not alone

✔ A chance to turn off that "brave front" that you may maintain all day

✔ A chance to laugh

✔ A chance to cry

If you can't find a support group nearby, consider the many chat lines now flourishing on the Internet. You'll find the same moral support and other benefits (see the sidebar, "What a little support group can do for you") as in any face-to-face group. Chapter 4 gives you the low-down on finding a support group, both real or electronic.

Don't take the advice from any support group member as gospel. However sympathetic — or even knowledgeable about a disease — no one except your personal health care practitioner is qualified to diagnose your particular condition or dispense treatment advice. But, by all means, go ask your practitioner about any good ideas you glean from the groups.

A Warm Puppy Can Make You Better

If human support groups aren't your thing, at least consider a puppy. Evidence shows that social support can come in the form of four-legged friends as well. In fact, having a furry friend in your life can be just as good for your health — maybe even better — than a human confidant, at least if you're an animal lover (and you're not allergic, of course!).

Pet ownership has been linked to many medical benefits, including reduced blood pressure, increased mental alertness, lowered rates of depression, better survival rates from heart disease, and — for people with physical disabilities — well-being in general. Some hospitals, hospices, and nursing homes even have formal "pet therapy" programs (specially trained animals visit patients). Dogs seems to be the most healthful, but any pet will do.

Some people attribute these benefits to a pet's unconditional love — something you can't expect even from the most loving spouse. Plus, people with pets may get more exercise, and caring for a pet engenders positive emotions such as responsibility, empowerment, and love.

Feng Shui: How your surroundings may affect your health

Forget people and pets — even the lampshade in your living room may make a difference to your health. *Feng Shui*, the Chinese art of placement and design, is based on the idea that the space people live in — homes, offices, and neighborhoods — is inextricably connected to their health, vitality, and prosperity. From one perspective, this theory is just common sense. (If you spend your life in a dank, dark room, you're bound to start feeling pretty bad.) On the other hand, the precise connection between any particular mirror or crystal sold by a Feng Shui supplier and your personal recovery from disease is tenuous, to say the least.

A Sense of Control

Feeling that you have some say in your own life seems to be good for you — both emotionally and physically. People who don't believe that they have any control over their lives develop a sense of passivity and helplessness — and this sense has been linked to poor health in the same way that feeling loved and hopeful have been linked to better health.

If you have any doubt about just where your attitude stands, see whether you have the characteristics of what some people call "the survivor personality." According to Bernie Siegel, M.D., at the March 1998 Casa Colina Whole Health Forum, survivors:

- Find meaning in their work, daily activities, and personal relationships.

- Express anger appropriately. "If you don't express appropriate rage and resentment, destruction results," Dr. Siegel said. "You need to be able to say if you're not treated with respect or loved. . . . If you find you have no energy to get angry, say 'God, this is your problem.' People have been cured of incurable illness by saying this."

- Ask for help. Survivors know that they can't control everything. They can express their needs to friends, family, and health professionals — and complain when their needs aren't met.

- Say no to nonpriorities.

- Make time for play.

- Learn from their pain and depression — and then get on with living.

- Choose healthy behaviors that meet their own needs — not someone else's ideas about what's good for them.

- Don't let outside duties keep them from meeting their basic needs. Survivors remember that they are precious people first, and mothers, employees, or otherwise upstanding citizens second.

Part VI
Herbs and Other Natural Approaches

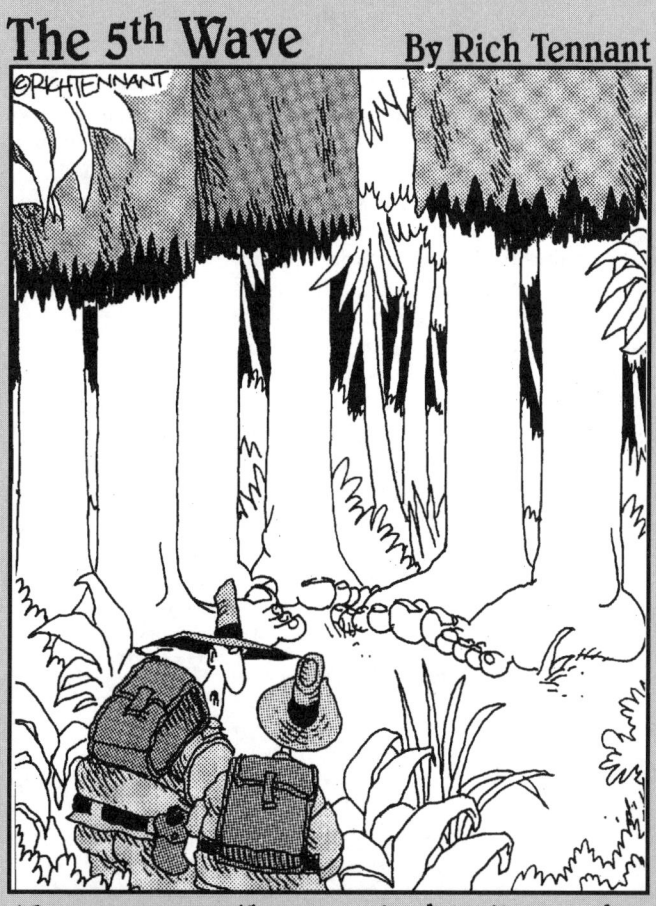

The 5th Wave   By Rich Tennant

"Legend has it there's an herb in the jungle that, when eaten, imparts great size and strength. Let's ask these natives. Perhaps they've heard something."

In this part . . .

We're not exactly sure what "natural" means — but we do know that it's a big part of what alternative medicine is supposed to be about. In some cases, natural is about cheap and easy "lifestyle" approaches to health — eating right, exercising, living clean, that sort of thing. In this part, you discover the best of these approaches, as well as find out how to avoid the more extreme versions of "natural living" that are big wastes of time and money. You can become an instant pro at navigating the wild-West world of herbal remedies, aromatherapy, and natural "dietary supplements" — so that you'll be able to side-step advertising hype and use and choose products that are safe and effective. You also discover just what "natural" energy — in the form of electricity, magnets, light, and sound — may sometimes do to heal you, plus what it probably won't do (regardless of whatever practitioners may tell you).

Chapter 20

Finding Out about Herbs and Botanicals

. . . .

In This Chapter

▶ Thinking about herbs as drugs

▶ Finding herbal remedies that work

▶ Understanding why natural doesn't necessarily mean safe

▶ Using herbal remedies safely

. . . .

*N*o drugstore or supermarket today is complete without devoting an aisle to echinacea, ginseng, aloe vera, and scores of other herbal remedies. Coupons for St. John's wort and ginkgo now appear in the same flyers as coupons for steak sauce, toilet bowl cleaner, and fruit roll-ups. With an estimated two billion dollars devoted each year to herbal supplements in the United States alone, herbal medicine is big business — no question about it.

The plus side of this herbal craze is that people are considering alternatives to the often serious side effects (and expense!) of conventional drugs — and sometimes even finding alternatives that work. The minus side is that herbal remedies are often so loosely tested and regulated that using them safely and effectively can take extra effort. But never fear. All the extra effort you'll have to make is to read this chapter!

Herbal Healing — Nothing New under the Sun

People have used (or tried using) plants and herbs to treat illness as long as they have been treating their ailments. In fact, herbal remedies remain the main and often the only form of healing in much of the world. Even many of the old stand-bys that you can find bottled up in modern medicine cabinets are based on active ingredients first found in plants.

The many modern drugs derived from plants include aspirin (originally from willow bark and later from meadowsweet), reserpine (a blood pressure medicine and tranquilizer from Indian snakeroot), and morphine (from the opium poppy). Listing all the other examples could easily fill the rest of this chapter — but you get the idea.

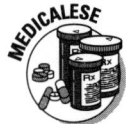

By the way, herbal medicine is essentially the same thing as *botanical medicine*, *phytomedicine*, and *phytotherapy*.

Whole Plants versus Extracts

About one-quarter of all prescription drugs are derived from herbs. But the typical Western approach is to pinpoint an "active" chemical in a plant — some little part that seems to do the work — and then extract it or synthesize it in a laboratory. For traditional Chinese and Indian healers — as well as other proponents of herbal and other medicinal plant remedies (also known as *botanicals*) — the holistic interaction of the active ingredient with all the other natural compounds in the whole plant maximizes healing. Isolating specific ingredients (and eliminating the rest of the plant) may not only reduce healing power, they argue, but also remove built-in buffers that minimize side effects.

Who's right? The question of whether whole plants or extracts are more effective — and/or safer — is a topic of heated debate. Fairly persuasive arguments can be made for both sides, and we won't bore you with them. The bottom line is that these arguments remain theoretical — with the "evidence" on both sides coming largely from folklore, tradition, logic, and sometimes even astrology. The answer will only come when herbal products are tested for safety (including long-term safety) and efficacy and then compared one by one to conventional medicines that purport to have similar actions.

The Essence of Herbs

If you're thinking about trying an herbal remedy but are overwhelmed by the number of choices, you've come to the right section. We give you the basics of what you're likely to see on the shelf — and introduce you to some of the most promising (and popular) remedies available.

Using infusions, decoctions, and tinctures

Herbal remedies can be made from flowers, leaves, fruits, or whole parts of plants. You can use the whole, fresh plant direct from the garden or produce section or buy one of various preparations. These preparations come in several different forms, each with a somewhat exotic-sounding — but easily understandable — name:

- **Teas, infusions, and decoctions.** *Teas* are made by steeping or soaking about a teaspoon of herb in a cup of water for a few minutes. "Herbal teas" have an innocuous reputation, but remember that they're only as safe as the individual herbs used to make them.

  If the steeping goes on much longer (10 to 20 minutes), the tea becomes an *infusion* — a stronger solution of the herb. And if one or more herbs are boiled rather than steeped (as often happens with barks and roots), the result is a *decoction*.

- **Tinctures.** An herb is soaked in alcohol, glycerin, or a mixture of water and alcohol and the resulting solution is strained off to form a *tincture*.

- **Extracts.** If you filter or distill out some of the alcohol from a tincture, you have an *extract* — which, ounce for ounce, is usually more potent than a tincture of the same herb. Look for *standardized extract* because it's guaranteed to contain an exact amount of the active ingredient (or what's thought to be the active ingredient) in any given dose.

- **Tablets and capsules.** As with conventional drugs, these pills are made by removing all the liquid from an extract, powdering the remaining herb, and shaping it into tablets or capsules. Many herbalists prefer tinctures and extracts because as many as 30 to 40 percent of herbal tablets and capsules contain little or none of the active ingredients of the herb listed on the label.

- **Injections.** Despite misleading claims that herbal remedies get into the bloodstream less directly than conventional meds (and therefore are slower and safer), a shot of an herb gets to work as fast as any other drug. By the way, injections are serious business and need to be done under the supervision of a qualified practitioner.

- **Oils, creams, and ointments.** Obviously, these forms are meant to be rubbed on the skin (unless it's broken or irritated; thick ointments called *salves* can be used on "weepy" lesions — that is, wounds oozing clear liquid).

No one form is necessarily better or safer than another — although obviously you're going to want a topical version (oil, cream, or ointment) if the herb can't be safely taken internally!

In Chinese and Ayurvedic medicine, herbs are often blended together (or blended with animal or mineral substances) and can augment or regulate each other's effects. But proper mixing is an art form — not something to try at home.

Finding herbs that work

No perfect way exists to determine which of the many herbal remedies work, which are safe, and which herb and dose are right for you. Packaging promises aside, data from scientifically valid experiments are still too scarce. Using the best evidence that exists right now, though, Table 20-1 lists commonly used herbs that seem relatively safe (if used correctly). Many of these herbs seem to help certain conditions (though by no means every condition their proponents claim that they help). We include a few other herbs because they've become popular even without solid proof that they work.

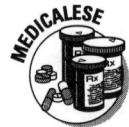

By the way, we include the scientific (Latin) names for each herb in paren-thesis. The Latin name usually contains two parts: the genus and the species of each herb. We include only the genus (one word), however, if several species of the herb are sold for similar purposes.

Table 20-1	Herbs to Know (And Maybe Love)		
Herb	**Parts Used**	**Most Likely Benefits**	**Comments**
Aloe (*Aloe vera* or *Aloe barbadensis*)	Gel and dried juice from leaves	Heals wounds and burns	Often the juice is mixed with gel and, if taken internally, can have a laxative effect.
Arnica (*Arnica*)	Flower heads	Relieves pain and reduces inflammation	Safe for external use only.
Astragalus (*Astragalus membranaceus* or huang qi)	Roots	Boosts immune system, increases stamina, promotes healing, and relieves colds and breathing problems	Evidence pretty thin for benefits in human beings, especially for treating cancer and AIDS. Avoid if you have a fever.
Black cohosh (*Cimicifuga racemosa* or black snakeroot, rattleweed, rattleroot, bugbane, bugwort, or squaw root)	Roots	May help treat rheumatoid arthritis, premenstrual syndrome, menstrual cramps, and menopausal symptoms	Evidence about safety and efficacy slim.

Herb	Parts Used	Most Likely Benefits	Comments
Bromelain (*Ananas comosus*)	Stems of pineapple plants	Relieves inflammation	
Chamomile (*Chamomilla recutita* — which is the same as *Matricaria recutita* and *Matricaria chamomilla*)	Flower heads	Relieves digestive disorders (including infant colic) and possibly inflammation (including teething pain)	Avoid if allergic to asters, chrysanthemums, ragweed, or other members of the daisy (*Asteraceae*) family.
Chili peppers (*Capsicum*)	Fruits	Reduces pain and tenderness and soothes digestive woes	The active ingredient, capsaicin, is usually used as a cream. Can be irritating both internally and externally — as anyone knows who has come into contact with a hot one! Avoid using around eyes.
Cranberries (*Vaccinium macrocarpon*)	Fruits	Prevents urinary tract infections	
Dong quai (*Angelica sinensis* or *polymorpha* — also called *Chinese Angelica*)	Roots	Relieves menstrual cramps and irregularity, plus menopausal symptoms	Evidence for efficacy mixed. May cause skin rashes and sensitivity to light.
Echinacea (*Echinacea augustifolia* or *purpurea*)	Leaves, flowers, and roots	Prevents and relieves cold symptoms, boosts immune function, and speeds wound healing	Use an extract of the fresh or recently dried whole plant — though products sold in the U.S. often aren't adequately labeled.

(continued)

Table 20-1 *(continued)*

Herb	Parts Used	Most Likely Benefits	Comments
Echinacea *(continued)*			Prolonged use may reduce effects. Avoid if allergic to plants in the daisy family. Consult M.D. if pregnant or if you have tuberculosis or autoimmune disease.
Evening primrose *(Oenothera biennis)*	Seed oil	Relieves skin rashes (allergic eczema) and possibly pain and inflammation	Evidence for benefits controversial. Watch out for adulteration with cheaper oils.
Feverfew *(Tanacetum parthenium)*	Leaves	Relieves migraines and possibly arthritis	Avoid if allergic to plants in the daisy family. Watch out for bogus products that don't contain any actual feverfew. Daily use (especially of non-capsule forms) can lead to mouth sores.
Garlic *(Allium sativum)*	Bulbs and sometimes leaves	Lowers blood pressure and thins blood, possibly even fights infection and cancer	Large amounts required for benefits (leading to flatulence, stomach distress, and maybe fewer friends, unless you're taking the "odor-free preparations!). Avoid large doses if taking aspirin or other blood-thinning drugs.
Ginger *(Zingiber officinale)*	Roots (rhizome)	Relieves motion sickness and nausea	Research on motion sickness limited. Gargantuan doses (well over the standard 4 grams a day) may produce life-threatening side effects. May cause bleeding if used with blood-thinning medications.

Herb	Parts Used	Most Likely Benefits	Comments
Ginkgo (*Ginkgo biloba*)	Leaf extract	Boosts circulation, memory, and may relieve symptoms of thinking disorders, perhaps including Alzheimer's disease, related to diminished blood supply to the brain	More data needed about efficacy, effective dosage, and long-term effects. Side effects may include gastro-intestinal distress, headaches, and allergic reactions. May be dangerous when used with blood-thinning medications, including aspirin.
Ginseng (*Panax* — comes in three varieties: American ginseng, Siberian ginseng, and Asian ginseng)	Roots	Boosts immunity or energy and stimulates "anti-stress" hormones	Many "ginseng" products contain little or none of the (rather costly) active ingre-dient (genosenides), *Panax ginsena* form may raise blood pressure. If you have diabetes or an estrogen-dependent cancer, see an M.D.
Hawthorn (*Crataegus laevigata*)	Fruits, leaves, and flowers	Lowers blood pressure and relieves some heart ailments	Use only under the supervision of a qualified professional.
Horse chestnut (*Aesculus hippocastanum*)	Seeds	Treats varicose veins, hemorrhoids, phlebitis, and other vein problems, plus numerous injuries	Never take internally or apply to broken skin.
Kava (*Piper methysticum*)	Roots, stems	Reduces stress and anxiety	No proof yet from clinical trials and can be intoxicating in large doses. Long-term use can lead to dry, scaly skin.

(continued)

Table 20-1 *(continued)*

Herb	Parts Used	Most Likely Benefits	Comments
Licorice *(Glycyrrhiza glabra)*	Rhizomes, roots	Relieves inflammation and ulcers, including mouth and throat sores and suppresses coughs — most other claims are speculative	Use only the deglycyrrhizinated form; other forms can lead to serious fluid retention, high blood pressure, and altered heart beat.
Milk thistle *(Silybum marianum)*	Fruits (seeds)	Prevents liver disease (including hepatitis and cirrhosis)	Injections and pills work better than teas (milk thistle dissolves poorly in water).
Myrtle *(Myrtus communis)*	Leaves, oil	Calms cough if diffused into a room	Used as aroma-therapy.
Onion *(Allium cepa)*	Bulbs	Thins blood, and may help prevent stomach and intestinal cancers	
St. John's wort *(Hypericum perforatum)*	Leaves, flowering tops	Treats mild and moderate depression; relieves chronic nerve pain; creams and salves relieve inflammation and promote healing	Depression should first be diagnosed by a health professional. More data needed about effective dosage, side effects, and long-term safety. Can cause sensitivity to light and dangerously interact with other drugs.
Saw palmetto *(Serenoa repens)*	Ripe fruits	Relieves benign prostate enlargement (BPH)	Large-scale and controlled studies still needed to confirm efficacy and long-term effects. Avoid tea versions because the herb dissolves poorly in water. Use only with professional supervision; may cause gastro-intestinal distress and nausea.

Herb	Parts Used	Most Likely Benefits	Comments
Stinging nettle (*Urtica dioica*)	Overground plants or roots	Relieves gout, inflammation, urinary problems, and possibly allergic symptoms	Use only if boiled or dried. Large doses may upset stomach or block elimination.
Sweet wormwood (*Artemisia annua — also called Sweet Annie*)	Entire plant	Fights parasites (especially malarial parasites)	Do not overboil.
Uva ursi (*Arctostaphylos uva-ursi;* also called bearberry)	Leaves	May relieve mild bladder and urinary tract pain	Large doses may cause ringing in the ears, vomiting, convulsions, or fainting. Prepare teas with cold water.
Valerian (*Valerian officinalis*)	Roots	Relieves anxiety and maybe insomnia	Recent controversy about whether really relieves insomnia. Taking 450 mg a day for under 2 weeks (teas or extracts) seems safe, but overdoses can lead to blurred vision, excitability, and changes in heartbeat.

If you want to know more about any specific herb, the best source is Varro E. Tyler's *The Honest Herbal* (New York: Pharmaceutical Products Press, 1993). This manual sensibly describes just what is known — and not known — about over 100 different herbs. You may also want to invest a copy of the American Herbal Products Association's *Botanical Safety Handbook,* published by CRC Press (call 800-272-7737) or contact the Council of Responsible Nutrition for its *CRN Reference on Evaluating Botanicals* (1998). And, of course, for more background on using herbs safely and effectively, get a copy of *Herbal Remedies For Dummies* by Christopher Hobbs (published by IDG Books Worldwide, Inc.) into your hands as soon as possible.

To stay up to speed on the latest research, you can subscribe to HerbalGram, a quarterly publication of the American Botanical Council and the Herb Research Foundation. Contact the American Botanical Council, P.O. Box 201660, Austin, TX 78720. Or call 512-331-8868, fax 512-331-1924, or visit the HerbalGram Web site at www.herbalgram.org/herbalgram/index.html to subscribe.

No matter where you look, you probably won't find any studies showing that a given herb doesn't work, by the way — mainly because these so-called "negative" studies rarely get published. But if no one pushing an herb on you can cite a valid scientific study (in a peer-reviewed journal such as *The New England Journal of Medicine*, *The Lancet*, or *The Journal of the American Medical Association*), assume that none exists. And although excellent evidence does suggest that certain herbal remedies work, many other herbal remedies are routinely used without any valid proof about safety or efficacy. Again, we don't mean that any given remedy *doesn't* work or *isn't* safe. We just mean that no one knows yet.

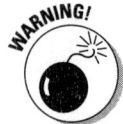

Remember that even the herbs that *may* work aren't necessarily the best way to handle your particular ailment.

The Meaning of "Natural"

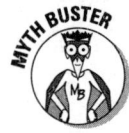

Sorry, but myths aside, "natural" has nothing to do with safety, and herbs can do plenty of harm. On the other hand, the idea that "natural" means ineffective is also a myth — as is the idea that herbs and other "natural" remedies are ineffective but also have dangerous side effects (which is the nonsensical line of many conventional docs). Many herbal remedies work and work safely — but there's nothing magical about them. You have to use them with the same care and respect that you'd use with any conventional medication.

Natural doesn't equal safe

Like any other alternative, treating yourself with herbal remedies can seriously threaten your health if it keeps you from getting professional medical help for a serious condition. Plus, in far too many cases, hyped and overpriced herbal remedies can threaten your bank account.

But there are other more specific ways that herbs can get you into trouble. The most obvious way is by poisoning you. Some herbs — such as hemlock and arsenic — are natural poisons. Others can cause damage when taken over long periods or time or in high doses, or if eaten at certain times of the year. And even the safest of herbs — such as the ones people cook with — can be toxic if taken in large enough quantities. Eating a whole nutmeg, for example, can poison you — but eating that much would be difficult.

Herbs that are safe for one person aren't necessarily safe for another — and the amount of herb that's safe for your friend can be dangerous for you. Herbs that help one ailment can aggravate another one. Echinacea, a generally safe immune-system booster, can worsen symptoms of Type I diabetes, HIV-related diseases, or rheumatoid arthritis. Even lowly garlic can cause life-threatening bleeding if used by people taking blood-thinning medications (anticoagulants) such as warfarin (Coumadin).

Yes, deaths from herbal remedies are rare, and most plant poisonings are minor. But don't be fooled into thinking that herbal remedies aren't drugs, even when they're called "natural products," "dietary supplements," or "nutriceuticals." Herbal remedies can have side effects just like any other drug, and they can interfere with the effects and safety of other herbs. Whole plants can be just as dangerous as extracts (ever eat a poison mushroom?). And because herbs are generally not as well-regulated or as thoroughly tested as conventional medicines, you take on additional risks when you use them.

Of course, given the well-known side effects of many highly-regulated conventional drugs, you may decide these are risks worth taking (especially if you take the steps we describe later in this chapter to minimize them). But to think that you're not taking risks at all just because these products are "natural" is a big mistake. Table 20-2 shows some of the more popular herbal remedies that carry substantial risks — despite glowing acclaim from many herbalists and popular books and articles.

Table 20-2	Herbs of Ill-Repute
Herb	_Why You Should Avoid It_
Borage (_Borago officinalis_)	May damage the liver.
Chapparal (_Larrea tridentata_)	Safe in teas (though it doesn't seem to do much), but tablets can damage the liver.
Comfrey (_Symphytum_)	If taken internally, can cause liver problems and even death — especially in children; external use seems safe.
Ephedra or ma huang (_Ephedra_)	Linked to nervousness, insomnia, headache, high blood pressure, irregular heart beat, heart attacks, stroke, psychosis, and is especially unsafe if you have heart disease, diabetes, or thyroid disease.
Foxglove (_Digitalis purpurea_)	Difficult to predict how much active ingredient is in any given plant — and taking a bit more than the recommended dose can be fatal.
Jin bu huan (Chinese medicine)	May cause heart and breathing problems in children and liver damage in adults.
Life root (_Senecio aureus_)	Can cause liver problems and even death — especially in children.
Lobelia (_Lobelia inflata_)	Risks far outweigh benefits; large doses can cause vomiting, coma, convulsions, and even death.

(continued)

Table 20-2 *(continued)*	
Herb	**Why You Should Avoid It**
Mistletoe (*Phoradendron lecucarpum* is American mistletoe; *Viscum album* is European mistletoe)	Can dangerously slow heartbeat, lower blood pressure, and constrict blood vessels; the European version is claimed to be less toxic than the American version and remains a popular cancer treatment in Germany.
Sassafras (*Sassafras albidum*)	May cause cancer and now banned in the U.S. as a flavoring or food additive but still sold as an herbal remedy — though no evidence exists of therapeutic value.
Yohimbe (*Pausinystalia yohimbe*)	Currently banned in the United States for over-the-counter sale; side effects include gastro-intestinal distress, tremors, anxiety, high blood pressure, rapid heart rate, weakness, paralysis, and psychosis — avoid unless under the supervision of a qualified practitioner.

Natural isn't always pure

Most of us assume that the days of snake-oil hawkers are long-gone. Today people have all these built-in government regulations to protect them from out-and-out fraud. When it comes to herbal and other "natural" medicines, however, everybody in the United States is still living in the Wild West. Unless a product claims to cure a specific disease or condition, it's regarded as a dietary supplement — not a drug. This label means that distributors don't need to prove that it works — or that it's safe (see sidebar, "The Dietary Supplement and Health Education Act — the law behind the hype").

Without good quality controls, you have little way to determine what was put into the product, or what you're about to put into yourself. Far too many herbal products claiming to be ginseng or echinacea, for example, don't contain enough of the active ingredients to do much for you. Other products contain too much active ingredient to be safe.

Ephedrine is the active ingredient in the herbal remedy ephedra (ma huang) that is used for insomnia, allergies, asthma, even weight loss. One widely publicized study led by the University of Arkansas's Bill J. Gurley, Ph.D., for example, found that the amount of ephedrine in a single brand varied more than 130 percent from one lot to the next. Only one of ten ephedrine products analyzed listed the amount of ephedrine it contained on the bottle. Plus, the amount of raw ma huang listed on the bottle did not correspond to the actual amount of the active ingredient ephedrine.

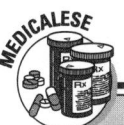

MEDICALESE

The Dietary Supplement and Health Education Act — the law behind the hype

In 1994 — for reasons that were more politically than scientifically based — the U.S. government passed the Dietary Supplement Health and Education Act (DSHEA). This act considers herbs (and vitamins) to be "dietary supplements" (and not drugs), which means that they can be marketed without proof of safety or efficacy. The only limitation is that sellers can't claim that these products diagnose, prevent, or treat specific diseases.

But that limitation is little obstacle for most marketers. Manufacturers have endless tricks to imply that their product heals or prevents a condition without making the claim directly.

Some packagers of ginkgo, for example, say that their product "promotes mental alertness" instead of "treats Alzheimer's disease." Some packagers of kava — an herb that purportedly relieves anxiety — call it a cure for the "yuppie blues" (whatever those are) without ever using the word "anxiety." Such statements are allowed, as long as promises include a disclaimer (usually in fine print) disclosing that the statements have not been evaluated by the Food and Drug Administration. (The FDA is now trying to crack down on these abuses, but they probably underestimate the wiles of the advertising industry.)

Without good quality controls, you run the risk of buying a product grown with toxic pesticides, adulterated with unlabeled ingredients, or contaminated with toxins. In past years, certain herbs have been found to be contaminated with arsenic, mercury, lead, tranquilizers, prescription painkillers, hormones, and other lovely surprises.

Natural doesn't always work

In many countries, herbal remedies are unstandardized, which means that each batch and brand can contain different amounts — even different types — of the active ingredients. Because the amount of active ingredient can vary in a growing plant (or any living thing), having a standardized extract goes a long way toward assuring yourself that you're getting what you pay for — and that you'll be using a safe and effective amount of it.

Even if an herbal medication contains the right amount of a "proven" ingredient — and even if that ingredient has the potential to help you — it may not work. Without regulated manufacturing, shipping, handling, and storage procedures, herbal remedies can easily lose whatever potency they may have had after exposure to moisture, air, or light. Such exposure is common when herbs are sold in bulk or powdered into capsules.

Tips for Safe and Effective Use

All doom-saying aside, herbs hold lots of promise for human health. It's just that in most cases people don't have enough data to know how to use them safely and effectively. But you can minimize risks by keeping a few basic tips in mind before you use any herbal product.

Most of these tips boil down to respecting the power of herbs — for both good and bad — combined with good old common sense and a healthy dose of skepticism. And if you experience any side effects at all, stop taking the remedy immediately. Call a physician if you develop a headache, rash, severe nausea, vomiting, breathing problems, or any other serious reaction.

Get expert advice

Don't dose yourself with herbs unless you know what you're doing (or, better yet, are under the supervision of a professional who does). Unless you're prepared for a strip search and physical exam in the aisles, too, don't expect the clerk in the health food store or supermarket to know what's right for your particular body either — or whether this new product will interact with some treatment you're already using.

In Europe, herbs are called phytomedicines

Europe is probably the safest place to use herbal remedies. In most countries, regulatory agencies have few, if any controls on these remedies. In the United States, this situation exists because herbal remedies aren't considered drugs, and thus escape the watchful drug arm of the FDA. In contrast, in many European countries a long and uneventful history is enough to get an herbal remedy — often called a *phytomedicine* — into the official system — as long as no formal scientific evidence proves that it isn't safe or effective.

The advantage of welcoming herbal remedies into the mainstream is that herbal remedies are better regulated and standardized. Whatever brands of ginkgo or milk thistle you buy in Germany, for example, you can feel confident

that they were manufactured according to the same standards and that they all contain a standardized dose. The other advantage of the European approach is that studying the effects of herbal remedies is a lot easier. With so many patients officially using these remedies, researchers have been able to gather decent data about their benefits and side effects. In fact, most of what is known right now about herbal remedies comes from European reports (especially German monographs).

By the way, ginkgo was the top-selling phytomedicine (from herbs and other plants) in Germany in 1996, followed by St. John's wort, horse chestnut, yeast (to treat diarrhea or acne), hawthorn flower and leaf, myrtle, saw palmetto, and stinging nettle root.

Your best bet is to see a licensed or certified healer, have a thorough exam, and mention any underlying conditions, other treatments you're currently using, and reactions to past treatments. And if you're being treated for some other condition, be sure to tell your regular M.D. about which herbal remedy you're planning to use — and how much of it.

Get the good stuff

You'll cut out a lot of risk just by keeping the following basics in mind when you shop for an herbal or natural product:

✔ Buy only from licensed or certified healers, or reputable health food stores, after consulting an experienced practitioner about which stores are reputable. Look for vendors who follow the literature about contamination and adulteration and can identify questionable brands (which they presumably don't carry). Generally avoid most chain-pharmacy herbal brands, which are rarely well-controlled for quality or standardization.

✔ Ask questions about where products came from. Usually there's no way to know from the label alone if the package contains the ingredients it says it does — or whether it's contaminated. Remember that salespeople often figure that they can say whatever they want — particularly if no one is recording their words. Get promises in writing, if possible. (See Chapters 3 and 8 for more about how to recognize credible evidence — and reputable vendors.)

✔ Don't be fooled by brand names. A lot of mainstream companies are jumping on the herbal bandwagon by slapping medical-sounding labels on herbal teas and other products. Just because a company is known for quality teas or vitamins doesn't mean that it knows anything about treating depression — or that its new herbal "health care" products undergo the same quality control procedures as its older products.

✔ Look for bottles with the word "standardized" on them. When possible, choose products that meet USP (United States Pharmacopeia) standards. A nongovernment organization, the USP develops standards for purity and potency for all prescription and over-the-counter drugs in the United States, and a few vitamins, minerals, and herbs.

Find out what you're using

Do everything you can to find out what species of herb — and what part of the plant — you're using. Also confirm that you're using the species and part known to work (refer to Table 20-1). If the saw palmetto you're taking is made of roots instead of ripe berries, it won't do you the least bit of good.

Reliable books (including this one and *Herbal Remedies For Dummies*), trusted health professionals, responsible merchants, and scientific papers are good sources of information. Labels and advertisements are usually not. Of course, you'll have to use the label to find out the contents of specific products — and if this information isn't included, leave the product on the shelf.

Start on a low dose — and stay that way

More is definitely not better when you use herbal remedies. The safest course is to start using the lowest dose and frequency recommended and increase that amount only if you don't improve (an even safer course, though often not possible, is to try changing your diet, lifestyle, or attitude to find out whether you can avoid taking any kind of drug — herbal or otherwise). Remember that many herbs work more slowly than conventional drugs — so just because you don't see immediate results doesn't mean that you should increase the dosage right away.

Whatever you do, don't go over the maximum recommended dose to get more or better effects. If you're not satisfied with the results, see a health professional about other approaches to your problem.

Vulnerable people should see a health professional before taking herbs

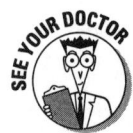

Certain people should never take herbal remedies on their own. The following groups should always seek the supervision of a health professional before using herbal remedies:

- ✔ Babies and children
- ✔ Pregnant women or women trying to get pregnant
- ✔ Anyone with a chronic or serious illness (including heart disease, cancer, diabetes, infectious diseases, autoimmune disorders, or arthritis)
- ✔ Anyone taking other medications

Use traditional herbs traditionally

If you don't use traditional medicines the way they were traditionally used, you can't expect to get the same effects — or the same safety record. Often this approach means working with an herbalist or other healer trained to use and understand herbs.

According to Dr. William Prensky, a leading authority on Chinese medicine and acupuncture, some herbs may carry an inherent ability to soften each other's negative effects. If the traditional remedies are administered according to the traditional body of knowledge, he says, they appear to be just as safe as any other medical approach.

"But that's not what's happening," Prensky — who was speaking at a conference on alternative medicine run by Oxford Health Plans — continued. "In our arrogance, we think we'll find the active ingredient and extract it . . . and put it onto the health food store shelves. . . . These [herbal] drugs should be given only by people trained in the lore in which they arose and applying those principles."

Chapter 21

Using Scents and Sensibility: Aromatherapy

In This Chapter

▶ How aromas can help your body, mind, and spirit

▶ What essential oils are all about

▶ How to use aromatherapy safely

Can what goes into your nostrils actually change the way you feel and even help you stay healthier? Actually, this theory isn't all that incredible. You know that the aroma of fresh-baked bread can make your digestive juices start flowing, right? Or the smell of varnish or chalk can conjure up your third-grade spelling bees? If nothing else, smells can make you more (or less) pleasant to be around, which could indirectly affect your health. (We'll leave the examples to your imagination.)

Aromatherapy uses the power of scent — particularly the power of fragrant oils extracted from plants — to heal. Some of its benefits have been scientifically proven; many others are wishful thinking and hearsay. This chapter separates the proven benefits from the speculative — and gives you tips on how to use aromatherapy safely and effectively.

The Power of Odor

Aromatherapy involves inhaling *essential oils* from plants, or rubbing them into your skin. Essential oils are the stuff that makes the plants smell — extracted from the plants and concentrated. You can also use the oils in a more diluted form called a *hydrosol*.

Essentials of essential oils

Aromatherapists say that essential oils do more than just make you smell good. They lift your mood and affect virtually every system in your body — circulation, hormone levels, heart rate, nervous system, digestion, elimination, you name it. Some of these effects — including the ability to alter brain waves, kill germs, lower blood pressure, or reduce inflammation — are due to the chemistry of the essential oils. Other effects are attributed to a spiritual power (which supposedly emerges when oils are artfully blended together) that helps balance body, mind, and spirit.

The power of aroma makes good sense (scents?) when you think about it. The sense of smell is one of the most primitive (just look at your dog). The first cranial nerve (olfactory) goes directly into the most fundamental, primitive regions of the brain. The ability to smell (perceive and react to foreign molecules) is the most basic sense. Even white blood cells can do it. Different smells are bound to cause change in the human nervous system.

People often confuse aromatherapy, herbal remedies, and homeopathy. While attempting to prove (or disprove!) aromatherapy, some authors of popular books even cite studies that have nothing to do with essential oils or hydrosols — any study involving a plant that smells will do. To be fair, the very limited scientific data available about real aromatherapy makes sneaking in a few irrelevant examples very tempting!

Power to fight disease — a big maybe

Other than the power to evoke memories and improve moods, the proven benefits of aromatherapy are few. Theoretically, aromas have the potential to heal. We already know that emotions can alter heart rate, pulse, blood pressure, and maybe even the way the body copes with disease — so it only stands to reason that by evoking emotions, smells can also influence the body. But there's a big difference between potential, theoretical effects and actual proof that a specific essential oil relieves a specific ailment.

So, why are so many people telling you that essential oil A can cure your toenail fungus and essential oil B can relieve your stomach cramps? Good question. The vast majority of these recommendations are based on tradition — not on actual studies that prove that any given oil produces these effects or that it is more effective (or safer) than any other treatment.

Yes, a few scattered reports show that inhaling lavender oil (see Figure 21-1) may help promote sleep and that various scents pumped into a laboratory can calm hyperactive rodents. Inhaling certain essential oils can relax or energize you or help clear your sinuses or bronchial passages. Rubbing other essential oils on your skin may help relieve burns, infections, and other skin conditions — or just make your massage more relaxing (see the section, "Scents Worth Considering" for the details). But we're talking about maybe one small study for each of these effects — not knock-you-dead proof.

True, sick people exposed to pleasant odors often *believe* that they feel better — but so far, objective tests of performance and perception of pain show no differences. Still, if you find a safe essential oil that relieves your stress, insomnia, stuffy nose, or skin condition, go for it. Expectations that aromatherapy can cure serious disease, though, are premature.

Figure 21-1:
Some reports show that inhaling lavender oil may promote sleep; other essential oils may offer different benefits.

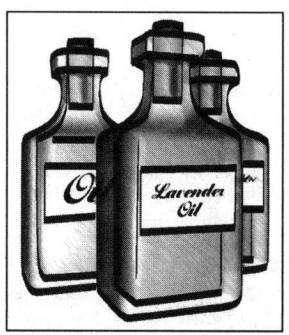

Scents Worth Considering

Table 21-1 describes some aromatic oils that have a lot of promise, even if all their powers haven't been proven. For more information about these (and many other essential oils) — including what they do, how they're made, what they can be blended with, and how to use them safely, contact any of the information resources listed under aromatherapy in the appendix.

Table 21-1	Some Popular Essential Oils	
Essential Oil	*Most Promising Applications*	*Comments*
Black pepper (Piper nigrum)	May reduce smoking withdrawal symptoms	
Clary sage (Salvia sclerea)	Relieves anxiety, burns, skin rashes	Avoid while drinking alcohol or if pregnant or have high blood pressure

(continued)

Table 21-1 *(Continued)*

Essential Oil	Most Promising Applications	Comments
Eucalyptus (*Eucalyptus radiata*)	Clears sinuses and bronchial tubes; may ease arthritis pain and help clear pimples or boils	Use through a vaporizer (diffuser) or as a chest rub; never take internally — and never use aromatherapy of any sort to treat asthma without an M.D.'s permission
Everlast (*Helichrysum italicum* — also called Everlasting)	Treats scars, bruises, wounds, and swelling	Use only highly diluted
Lavender (*Lavandula angustifolia*)	Relieves stress; small amounts can treat cuts, burns, insect bites, and other skin conditions	Use undiluted; avoid use in early stages of pregnancy
Neroli (*Citrus aurantium*)	Relieves tension, particularly relaxing as a massage oil	
Niaouli (*Melaleuca quinquenervia* or *Melaleuca viridifloral*)	Relieves acne, boils, and skin irritations; helps ease breathing problems due to allergies	For breathing problems, vaporize or use as a chest rub
Peppermint (*Mentha piperita*)	Relieves nausea, motion sickness, indigestion	Unsafe for babies and toddlers; can cause insomnia
Roman chamomile (*Anthemis nobilis*)	Relieves stress; can make massage more relaxing	Avoid during early stages of pregnancy
Rosemary (*Rosmarinus officinalis*)	May help relieve gas and other digestive disorders, boost mood, and smooth skin	Avoid if pregnant or have epilepsy or high blood pressure
Tea tree (*Malaleuca alternifolia*)	Helps heal wounds, soothes irritated skin	
Thyme (*Thymus vulgaris*)	May help fight infections, relieve joint pain, soothe coughs and sore throat	Avoid if pregnant or have high blood pressure

How to get some scents into your life

If you want to try aromatherapy, you can consult an *aromatherapist* — that is, a person who claims to be an expert in aromatherapy. Because many countries require no standard training program or licensing to practice, only you can judge the competence of a practitioner (see Chapter 6 for basics on how to make that judgment) — but contact one of the organizations listed in this book's appendix if you need help.

Try choosing an aromatherapist who knows a lot about organic chemistry and the systems of the human body and who has extensive experience blending essential oils. If you live in a country (such as Great Britain) with legal standards for aromatherapy training and certification, all the better. Another good bet is to consult someone with stellar credentials in another field of health care — Ayurvedic medicine, naturopathy, or traditional Chinese medicine, for example.

Plenty of beauty salons and spas offer aromatherapy facials and aromatherapy foot massage, alongside pedicures, reflexology foot massage, and other mysteriously named special treatments. This kind of pampering can make you feel great (at least emotionally) — but it can also cost you a bundle. Aromatherapy facials and massages can easily cost $65 or more, and the mysterious specials can run you hundreds of dollars.

Even buying essential oils — assuming that they're really pure — can be costly because the process takes a whole lot of plant to produce a tiny bit of oil. But there's no question that using aromatherapy at home is the frugal way to go. Here are some ways you can do it:

- Inhale a few drops of essential oil from a handkerchief or cotton ball.

- Pump fragrant molecules into the air with a steam inhaler or a device called a *diffusor*.

- Drop the essential oil into your bath.

- Add a few drops to a hot or cold compress (apply to aches and pains).

- Rub creams or lotions that contain essential oils into your skin.

- Take the oils internally (orally, rectally, or vaginally) — usually a bad idea. If you do start putting these substances into your body, consider them as herbal remedies and take precautions accordingly — preferably under the supervision of a knowledgeable health care practitioner (see Chapter 20).

- Freshen your air by adding a few drops to your laundry, humidifier, or old (aroma-challenged) potpourri.

If it smells good, do it? — an unsafe idea

People who assume that sniffing is a lot safer than ingesting can get themselves into big trouble. Anyone who likes the smell of gasoline — or who knows the dangers of sniffing glue — can understand the risk. Just because essential oils happen to be derived from plants and sold over-the-counter to anyone who plops down the money does not make them safe. In fact, in many countries the safeguards for essential oils and other herbal products are no more rigorous than for foods (see Chapter 20 for details) — even though some of these products, if used incorrectly, can cause serious and even life-threatening reactions.

Always keep the following safety tips in mind:

✓ Use only diluted oils — except lavender oil used for burns and insect bites.

✓ Use the oil according to directions. Don't use more than is recommended, and if the label says to dilute the oil yourself, by all means do so.

✓ Test for allergic reactions first before trying a new oil. Put a drop inside your elbow and wait 24 hours to see whether you develop a rash.

✓ Know what you're taking — in other words, find out the Latin (genus and species) name, which is the only name that differentiates one form of the oil from another. Oils called eucalyptus, for example, could be from one of several different plants.

✓ Make sure that the oils come from a reputable company. Herbs that aren't grown in the right soil and weather, harvested at just the right age and season, and distilled properly, yield essentially worthless oils.

✓ Never take oils from eucalyptus, hyssop, mugwort leaf, thuja, pennyroyal, sage, or wormwood internally and never apply oils of *any* kind to the eyes.

✓ Store essential oils in a cool place (some even require refrigeration) and discard after the expiration date (usually a couple of years).

✓ Keep essential oils away from children and avoid oils during pregnancy — except under a physician's direction. (Many diluted oils seem safe to use but you're better off with professional guidance.)

Chapter 22

Playing with Your Food: Nutrition

● ●

In This Chapter

▶ Foods that can help keep you healthy

▶ Two diets that fight hypertension and lower cholesterol

▶ The scoop on fasting, juicing, macrobiotics, elimination diets, anticancer diets, and the Ornish diet

● ●

*N*o one doubts that people's health depends on food. Without enough food or water, people wither and die. Without enough vitamins, they develop serious deficiency diseases such as scurvy, rickets, and beri-beri. Without enough protein, they can't grow, repair, and replace cells or make hormones and enzymes required for basic biochemical reactions.

Too much food or the wrong kinds of foods can be equally bad. Eating mainly high-fat, high-calorie foods will, at the very least, leave you overweight — which in turn leaves you prone to heart disease, stroke, diabetes, and other life-threatening diseases. Drinking grapefruit juice can raise blood levels of certain medications. Eating nut oils can leave a highly allergic person gasping for breath.

Isolated examples aside, nutritionists still know very little about why eating specific foods or eating foods in a specific way can promote or restore health. Plenty of "experts" will tell you what to eat and how to eat it, but most of this advice is based on inconclusive data — or on hunches, tradition, and, frankly, moralism (anything that tastes good is assumed to be bad for you, for example). That's why using food as medicine was traditionally regarded as unproven at best and downright wacky at worst.

Now, however, nutrition is quickly leaving the "alternative" ranks. Credit goes mainly to many solid studies that are starting to remind mainstream docs about the food-health connection. This chapter fills you in on some of the most exciting new discoveries. It also gives you the scoop on some popular alternative diets and how to tell the worthy ones from the bogus and downright dangerous ones.

Eating to Stay Healthy

Until quite recently, physicians learned almost nothing about nutrition in medical school. Sure, traditional healing systems from all over the world stressed the importance of nutrition in health and healing. Early versions of conventional medicine even recognized that diet and health were inextricably linked. But because few studies showed specific ways that diet could prevent or treat disease, mainstream medicine's policy of ignoring nutrition as a subject of instruction made a certain amount of sense.

Once upon a time "healthful eating" meant finding a way not to starve. But today, both doctors and nutritionists in affluent countries are focusing on finding ways to use special foods or diets to prevent, maybe even treat, disease. You can get the details in *Nutrition For Dummies* by Carol Ann Rinzler (published by IDG Books Worldwide, Inc.).

Most M.D.s will also readily tell you that the best strategy for staying healthy is to eat a lowfat, high-fiber diet, heavy on the fruits, vegetables, whole grains, and legumes.

And now even mainstream docs are convinced that diet can sometimes work as well as drugs. Physicians are raving about the following two diets:

✔ **The DASH diet for hypertension.** The Dietary Approaches to Stop Hypertension — or DASH — diet involves eating a diet low in total and saturated fat and high in fruits, vegetables, and lowfat dairy foods. For some people, this diet can prevent — and treat — hypertension as well as conventional medicines (and without the side effects). For more information, call 1-800-575-WELL or check out the DASH home page at dash.bwh.harvard.edu.

✔ **The American Heart Association Diet for mild hypertension, high cholesterol, or noninsulin dependent (Type II) diabetes.** Put together by the American Heart Association and the National Cholesterol Education Program, this two-step diet decreases the typical Western diet's levels of saturated fat and cholesterol — and so may help lower blood pressure, reduce cholesterol levels, and (in people with Type II diabetes) control blood sugar. For more information, contact the American Heart Association at 800-AHA-USA-1 or check out their Web site at www.amhrt.org.

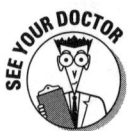

Don't throw out your medicines yet! No one who has high blood pressure or heart disease should expect these diets to substitute for medications without first consulting their physician. Plus, no one knows yet whether these diets keep working over the long run.

Maybe mom was right about those fruits and vegetables

Can an apple a day keep the doctor away? Well, maybe. Broccoli or cauliflower may work even better. Besides being chock-full of vitamins, minerals, and fiber, fruits and vegetables may also contain substances called *phytochemicals* that seem to have cancer-fighting properties. Among the most promising veggies right now are broccoli (especially the sprouts!) and other cruciferous vegetables such as cauliflower and cabbage. And, cancer-fighting aside, don't forget that filling up on fruits and vegetables will leave less room for ice cream and cheeseburgers.

Eating the Alternative Way

The DASH and AHA diets are mainstream — period. Ah, how the world has changed! But never fear. Plenty of other diets that claim to treat cancer, heart disease, and allergies with diet are still borderline alternative medicine — or way over the border.

Elimination diets

If drinking milk makes you break out in hives or eating peanut butter causes your throat to swell up, elimination diets are hardly an alternative approach — they're the *only* approach. To stay healthy you have to eliminate the offending food from your diet.

Banning certain foods from your diet to cure specific diseases — such as rheumatoid arthritis, irritable bowel syndrome, migraine headaches, and hyperactivity — is another matter. Yeah, it could work — theoretically speaking. After all, many folks are allergic or sensitive to certain foods (especially dairy products, eggs, nuts, shellfish, soybeans, and wheat), and eating too many of these foods could conceivably provoke or worsen chronic diseases and disorders. Although no one's actually proven that you can completely obliterate chronic ailments with diet alone, you can sometimes alleviate symptoms by laying off certain foods.

So, if you find that eliminating wheat or dairy products from your life makes your arthritis feel better, go for it. Just don't get your hopes up.

Fasting

Stop eating to get well? Almost every religion and healing system has recommended that you do so occasionally for the sake of your spiritual, and often your physical, health. Today, alternative healers say that going without food for days or weeks at a time can purge your body of poisons *(detoxify you)* and give your hardworking digestive system a rest.

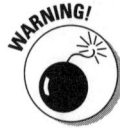

But M.D.s warn of dire consequences from fasting; we shiver just to write about them. The headaches and weakness some people develop when they skip meals are just the tip of the iceberg. Depriving yourself of nutrients for too long can lead to life-threatening changes, including fainting, anemia, gout, irregular heart beat, kidney or liver failure, and infections.

We have to agree that fasting longer than a couple of days can be downright dangerous. The popular notion that symptoms associated with fasting are just "the toxins coming out" has no science behind it whatsoever. Still, if you're basically healthy and well-nourished, you can fast for a day or two if it makes you feed good or helps you kick off a weight-loss plan.

Fasting *can* be a way to pinpoint food sensitivities: You start by eating virtually nothing and let foods back into your life one at a time as long as you stay symptom-free. Laying off food can be a good idea (and sometimes unavoidable), too, if you have the flu or some other stomach upset. Fasting may even help relieve the symptoms of some inflammatory and autoimmune diseases. But you can't fast forever, and eventually you'll have to start eating again and face the same old issues that led you to fast in the first place.

If you do decide to fast for a day or two, be sure to drink plenty of fluids. Get clearance from your M.D. if you have any serious or chronic condition.

Juicing

Juicing advocates say that consuming fruits and vegetables in liquid form is healthier than munching on them. If you've been to a juice bar lately, you may have sampled some of their recipes — carrot-beet juice, for example, or concoctions of garlic, lemon, grapefruit, and olive oil. Drinking this stuff is supposed to strengthen your immune system and clean out your insides.

Usually you have to prepare the juices yourself to make sure that you're using fresh and uncontaminated ingredients — and this process can be messy and rather expensive. You can also take dehydrated fruits and vegetables in capsule form for the same effects.

No one's denying the proven benefits of produce. Fruits and vegetables are chock-full of all kinds of vitamins, minerals, and other goodies (collectively known as *phytochemicals*) that seem to keep people healthier and probably even protect them from heart disease and cancer. Because nutritionists don't usually know which of the phytochemicals are doing the good work, most advocate eating whole fruits and vegetables — not just popping a pill containing one or two select ingredients.

Okay, so produce is good. But does it have to be pulverized? Not really. True, packing your daily dose of vitamins into a single glass of juice can be more efficient than gnawing on celery sticks all day — though more of a pain to prepare. But you still need to do some chewing (or — if you can't chew — find some other way) to get enough fiber into your diet. (Juicing cuts down fiber content, and the fiber gives you the bulk to feel sated and so keep your overall calories down.) Still, if you like the taste and don't mind the inconvenience and expense, bottom's up.

Macrobiotics

One of the most popular alternative nutritional regimens around, macrobiotics asks you to eat a lot of whole grains and cooked vegetables. And we mean a lot. Several variations exist, but you'll get about half your calories from whole grains, about 25 percent from sanctioned vegetables, and the rest from beans, sea vegetables, and soups. Sometimes fish and nuts are allowed, but you have to lay off all animal proteins (meat, dairy, and eggs), alcohol, coffee, herbal teas, many fruits and vegetables, and processed foods, as well as vitamin or mineral supplements.

As much a way of life as a way of eating, macrobiotics also asks you to balance yin (or contractive) foods with yang (expansive) foods. (If this kind of talk sounds like gobbledegook, see Chapter 9.)

Supposedly, eating this lowfat, high-fiber way can help prevent heart disease — and maybe it can. But whether it can prevent — or treat — cancer, as advocates claim, is more uncertain, as is the overall safety of this diet. Here's what you have to know about macrobiotics:

- ✔ You have to be psyched to follow this regimen. If everyone in your household is going along with you — especially those involved in cooking and shopping — it can be done, but eating in restaurants can be a challenge.

- ✔ Sticking to the macrobiotic regimen can cheat you out of essential amino acids, vitamins, and minerals — and endanger your health.

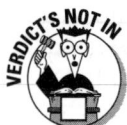

✔ Anecdotes and testimonials aside, no one has ever proven that this diet can prevent or cure cancer. Dropping your anticancer treatment to try a macrobiotic diet could be the last decision you ever make. (Macrobiotic purists say that their diet and cancer drugs don't mix — you have to choose one or the other.)

✔ Babies, children, pregnant women, and people with cancer or other serious illnesses should use this diet only under the supervision of an M.D. If you really want to pursue this route, try to find a solid conventional physician who also has extensive experience and training in macrobiotics.

If you're healthy and insist on trying macrobiotics anyway, at least do it safely. Make sure that you're taking multivitamin supplements (even if they're not "officially" permitted) and consider talking to a qualified nutritionist to make sure that you're getting all the nutrients you need. (See the appendix for resources that can help you find one.)

Anticancer diets

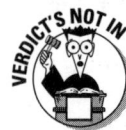

The Gerson Diet, Hoxsey Treatment, wheatgrass diet, megadose vitamin C diet, Livingstone-Wheeler Treatment — if you're suffering from cancer, chances are someone will mention these (or other) anticancer diets to you. Almost all of them involve rigorous and dramatic changes in the way you cook and eat — emphasizing fresh fruits and vegetables and whole grains — and promise that they can reverse even advanced cancer.

Mainstream doctors beg to differ. Sure, most of them suspect that certain eating patterns and foods can increase your lifetime risk of developing some cancers — but most will give you the thumbs down if you suggest using a special diet to cure a cancer that has already developed (especially if it has already spread). They'll tell you that the alternative options play on your desperation by promising to cure the uncurable without all the nasty side effects and expense of surgery, chemotherapy, radiation, and other mainstream cancer therapies. We agree that your first line of attack for many cancers is mainstream medicine — because, if the cancer is caught early enough, these therapies often have a real chance of working.

But, obviously, mainstream cancer therapy doesn't have the greatest track record in the world. So, if you've tried standard therapy to no avail, aren't anticancer diets and other lifestyle changes worth a try? Maybe. No diet has ever been proved to cure or reverse cancer. Period. But many of the diets at least have to potential to give you a sense of control — which, in turn, can have a positive impact on your health (see Chapter 19).

Again, don't try any dietary approach to cancer unless you've tried the more standard approaches first — and told your regular M.D. what you're up to. One thing we know for sure is that inadequate nutrition will hasten a cancer demise — and efforts to prevent malnutrition can prolong life. So keep away from any diet that doesn't meet basic nutritional needs.

The Ornish approach

Dr. Dean Ornish is a conventionally trained M.D. who says that he knows how to prevent — even reverse — heart disease using only diet, meditation, and love (yes, love). Dr. Ornish claims that this approach is cheaper — and longer lasting — than drugs or surgery. And more and more experts — including mainstream docs and insurance companies — think that he's right.

The Ornish Plan involves an extremely lowfat, vegetarian diet — based on fruits, vegetables, legumes, and whole grains — together with a regular program of mind-body approaches, including progressive relaxation exercises, yoga, guided imagery, and even support groups to help get some emotional intimacy into your life. (That's where the "love" comes in.) See Chapters 17, 18, and 19 for more details on these mind-body approaches.

If you want the details of Dr. Ornish's diet and program specifically, your best source is the horse's mouth: *Dr. Dean Ornish's Program for Reversing Heart Disease: The Only System Scientifically Proven to Reverse Heart Disease Without Drugs or Surgery* (Ivy Books/Mass Market Paperback Reprint Edition: February 1996), in either book or audiotape format (Random House Audio: December 1991).

The downside of the Ornish plan — assuming that it works — is that it's hard to follow. You have to radically change your eating habits and your lifestyle as well. But many people are willing to make these sacrifices when they're fighting for their lives. Plus, now that Dr. Ornish (with ConAgra) is packaging his own prepared foods, sticking to the diet may be a little easier.

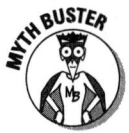

Viewing the Ornish plan as a cookie cutter approach to reversing heart disease is a big mistake. Just because this plan may *potentially* reverse heart disease in some people doesn't mean that it necessarily will for you. If you have coronary artery disease or atherosclerosis, discuss this approach with your physician, but realize that in some cases conventional approaches (including bypass surgery or angioplasty) may be necessary.

Chapter 23

Taking Vitamins, Minerals, and Other Supplements

In This Chapter
▶ Understanding the role vitamins, minerals, and trace elements play in your body
▶ Determining the amount of vitamins and minerals you need
▶ Choosing the best way to get nutrients — from foods or supplements
▶ Sorting through supplements that may help you and those that probably won't

*N*obody questions the importance of vitamins and minerals. Technically vitamins and minerals are called *micronutrients*. *Nutrients* are chemicals used by the body to conduct basic operations of life; *micronutrients* are simply nutrients that the body only needs in small amounts. Many nutrients are called *essential* because humans can't live without them. Because the body can't make these essential nutrients itself, you have to get them from outside sources — usually either foods or dietary supplements (anything other than food that provides nutrients).

Nothing alternative there. But many people stray from the beaten path by consuming vitamins, minerals, and other "natural" nutrients in doses higher than mainstream doctors and nutritionists recommend. Why would anyone want to do this? Well, many people (including, unfortunately, people trying to sell you the stuff) believe that supplementing your diet with high doses of these substances has amazing powers not only to keep you healthy but even to treat some diseases usually considered incurable.

Frankly, the whole area of dietary supplements is fraught with controversy. Everyone has an opinion — and most of these opinions are based on inconclusive evidence at best. The plus side of all this controversy is that the conventional medical world is waking up and starting to reexamine some dusty old doctrines. The minus side is that a lot of the advice you get is not only misguided, but hazardous to your health.

This chapter gives you the background you need to separate the helpful from the harmful advice and make reasonable choices given today's limited state of knowledge in the realm of vitamins, minerals, and other dietary supplements.

ABCs of Dietary Supplements

If you want to know everything worth knowing about dietary supplements, we recommend checking out *Nutrition For Dummies* by Carol Ann Rinzler (IDG Books Worldwide, Inc.). Otherwise, just stick with this section for a bare-bones overview of the topic — just enough information for you to navigate the supplement aisles and advertisements with your wits about you.

All you need to know about vitamins

Vitamins are organic chemicals (containing carbon, hydrogen, and oxygen) that promote healing, prevent deficiency diseases, and regulate various body functions — including building bones, skin, nerves, and blood.

You can't get along without at least minuscule amounts of 11 specific vitamins: vitamin A, vitamin D, vitamin E, vitamin K, vitamin C, and the B vitamins: thiamin (vitamin B1), riboflavin (vitamin B2), niacin (vitamin B3), pyridoxine (vitamin B6), folate (the synthetic form is folic acid), and cobalamin (vitamin B12). Most nutritionists now say you also need biotin (vitamin B7) and pantothenic acid (vitamin B5), two other B vitamins.

These (and nonessential) vitamins are divided into two groups: fat-soluble (A, D, E, and K) and water-soluble (all the rest). As you'd expect, the fat-soluble vitamins dissolve in body fat, meaning that they stick around in your body if you take more of them than you need and may lead to toxic effects. Conversely, surplus water-soluble vitamins are just carried off in the urine.

All you need to know about minerals and trace elements

Essential minerals are chemical elements found in nonliving things that get incorporated into plants and animals and are necessary for life. They come in two forms: *major minerals* (stuff you need a fair amount of to survive) and *trace elements* (stuff you need in only minuscule proportions).

The major minerals include calcium, chloride, magnesium, phosphorus, potassium, sodium, and sulfur. Trace elements include chromium, copper, fluoride, iodine, iron, manganese, molybdenum, selenium, and zinc.

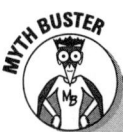

One last thing you need to know — life is complex

Everywhere you look, you can find a chart or a person making claims about what a vitamin, mineral, or other supplement will do for you. Although many of these claims are basically true, they tend to oversimplify the way the body works.

Most nutrients work in concert with each other. For example, if you don't have enough vitamin E, vitamin A can be destroyed in your gut. Without enough vitamin D, your body can't absorb calcium and phosphorus. And without niacin, pantothenic acid, and magnesium, vitamin B1 can't do much for your digestion.

So just because a study shows that a single nutrient may help prevent a certain condition doesn't necessarily mean that popping a few pills of that nutrient will help you. No matter how much calcium you take to prevent osteoporosis, for example, it won't do you the least bit of good if you're not getting enough vitamin D. That's one of the reasons why most nutritionists recommend getting nutrients from your diet whenever possible. (Another reason is that many foods contain phytochemicals, natural substances that may have anticancer and other disease-fighting properties.)

If you're a healthy adult, eating a balanced diet gives you an effective and ample mix of vitamins and minerals — no thinking or calculations necessary. That's the best news we've heard all day.

All you need to know about other dietary supplements

A *dietary supplement* is just something you add to your diet — presumably to make up for nutrients you're not getting in your food. Alongside the shelves of vitamin and mineral supplements, you may also find some other supplements, often called "natural" because they're usually made out of hormones, amino acids, enzymes, or herbs. These aren't really foods, but, at least in the United States, they are called dietary supplements anyway, as long as their manufacturers don't directly claim that taking them will treat or prevent a disease (in which case, they would be considered "drugs").

As with vitamins and minerals, these natural supplements are sold on the premise (even if it's not stated explicitly) that your body can't naturally get — or make — enough of this stuff to keep you healthy or cure what ails you.

The Scoop on RDAs and DRIs

How many vitamins and minerals do you need? The answer depends on who you are, who you talk to, and what you hope to accomplish.

The conventional line is that most people need a set intake of these substances every day. These set intakes come in two forms: DRIs or RDAs.

✔ DRIs, or *dietary reference intakes,* used to be called RDAs, which stood for "recommended dietary allowance." But it's a good thing they got renamed because everyone was always confusing them with the kind of RDAs that still exist (recommended *daily* allowances). In any case, DRIs are standards developed by the National Research Council's Food and Nutrition Board. They come in the form of a range of values that differ depending on your age, reproductive status, and so on.

✔ RDAs, or *recommended daily allowances* (sometimes called U.S. RDAs), are the recommendations that often appear on food-package labels indicating how much of each nutrient you need to prevent deficiency diseases — and, as of recently, sometimes the amount needed to provide actual health benefits. RDAs offer a single number no matter who you are, usually the highest number you'd find on the DRI charts (except for pregnant and breast-feeding women) — so the amount listed may well be more than you need.

As new research comes in, these charts are modified accordingly. No matter how up-to-date, though, both the RDAs or DRIs can sometimes recommend less of a nutrient than you personally need. If you're suffering from a chronic disease, for example, or if you're taking certain medications, you may need extra vitamins and minerals. The same is true for smokers, vegetarians, dieters, pregnant or nursing women, children, adolescents, and elderly people.

Because everyone is different, use the RDAs and DRIs as general guidelines. But talk to a professional health care provider to determine the amount that's right for you.

Orthomolecular medicine

Orthomolecular medicine is a controversial therapy during which people use high doses of vitamins, minerals, and amino acids to prevent and treat disease. The term *orthomolecular,* coined by Nobel Prize-winner Linus Pauling, Ph.D., means "balanced molecules." In fact, the goal of this therapy is to get all these nutrients into perfect levels of balance in the body, a process that may require megadoses of supplements. Some early studies show that some forms of orthomolecular medicine may help in the treatment of AIDS, asthma, cancer, depression, heart disease, lymphedema, schizophrenia, and stroke — but much more research needs to be done before anyone should consider this a miracle therapy.

Can You Get Enough Vitamins and Minerals from Food Alone?

The conventional line is that you should basically stick to the DRIs or RDAs, getting as many vitamins and minerals as you can from your foods. But many alternative providers say that these official recommendations are way too low — and if people ate enough food to give them the vitamins and minerals they needed, everyone would weigh over 600 pounds.

The answer, supposedly, is super-high doses of vitamin and mineral supplements — popularly known as *megadoses*. No one really knows when a reasonable dose becomes a megadose or what exactly the word means. For some people, a megadose means enough vitamins and minerals to do damage. For other people, it means enough vitamins and minerals to do you some actual good. In this book, we just use the term to mean more than the conventionally recommended dosages.

Megadoses may help — possibly

On the plus side of the megadose controversy, increasing evidence suggests that at least some of the recommended allowances may be too low and that higher doses may help prevent the onset of chronic diseases. Studies show that higher-than-recommended levels of certain nutrients — especially calcium, magnesium, folate, niacin, beta-carotene, and vitamins C, D, and E — may help prevent certain serious diseases, including osteoporosis, heart disease, and certain forms of cancer.

Even so, most of the claims made for megadoses — including the late Nobel Prize-winner Linus Pauling's infamous contention that massive amounts of vitamin C can cure cancer (not to mention the common cold) — are mainly big talk and quite often can get you into real trouble.

Hazards of megadoses

In most cases, the risks you take loading yourself up with super-high doses of nutrients outweighs the (still uncertain) benefits. How can natural stuff like this hurt you? Easy. Table 23-1 shows some of the awful consequences of swallowing too many vitamins; the sidebar "Mineral madness" shows why taking too many minerals is a bad move, too.

Table 23-1	Vitamin Overdoses: How Much Is Too Much for Healthy People?
Vitamin	**Overdose**
Vitamin A	15,000 to 25,000 IU retinoids a day for adults (2,000 IU or more for children) may lead to liver damage, headache, vomiting, abnormal vision, constipation, loss of hair, loss of appetite, a low-grade fever, joint pain, sleep disorders, dry skin, and dry mucous membranes. A pregnant woman who takes more than 10,000 IU a day doubles her risk of giving birth to a child with birth defects.
Vitamin D	2,000 IU a day can cause irreversible damage to kidneys and heart. Smaller doses may cause muscle weakness, headache, nausea, vomiting, high blood pressure, retarded physical growth and mental retardation in children, and fetal abnormalities.
Vitamin E	Large amounts (more than 400 to 800 IU a day) may cause upset stomach, dizziness, or increased blood pressure.
Niacin	Doses higher than the RDA raise the production of liver enzymes and blood levels of sugar and uric acid, leading to liver damage and an increased risk of diabetes and gout.
Vitamin B6	50 mg a day may (temporarily) damage nerves in arms and legs, and hands and feet.
Vitamin C	High doses of vitamin C (particularly by intravenous infusion) can push iron levels in the bloodstream to toxic levels before the vitamin itself leaves the body.

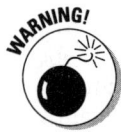

One result of megadosing that neither chart shows — but that we can't emphasize enough — is that even too many of the water-soluble vitamins can do serious damage. Many people acknowledge the risks of excess fat-soluble vitamins (because excess amounts stick around in body fat); but they also believe that excess "water-soluble" vitamins are harmless because they get "washed out" in the urine. (See the "All you need to know about vitamins" section for more on fat- and water-soluble vitamins.) But this idea is not necessarily true.

Where you get nutrients may make a difference

Assuming that you do decide to supplement your diet, is using a "natural product" — that is, something pulled out of a real-life plant or animal — any better than using a substance made in a laboratory?

Mineral madness

Omigosh. Here's another reason not to gulp down megadoses: Taking too much of one mineral can affect your elimination of, or make it hard (maybe even impossible) for your body to use, one or more other minerals.

This list shows which mineral megadoses can affect your ability to absorb and use other minerals and trace elements.

If You Get Too Much of This Mineral	Your Body May Not Be Able to Absorb or Use This One
Calcium	Magnesium, iron, zinc
Copper	Zinc
Iron	Phosphorus, zinc
Magnanese	Iron
Molybdenum	Zinc, copper
Phosphorus	Calcium
Sulfur (protein)	Molybdenum
Zinc	Copper

Most experts say no way. Nobody with even rudimentary knowledge of chemistry (or its history) can claim that a grain of difference exists between vitamin C made in a lab or that pulled out of a rose hip. Chemically, they are usually identical substances (though the "natural" one often costs a lot more).

Buying organic doesn't mean a whole lot either, at least in terms of how well the product will work. Yes, a certified organic supplement may protect you from exposure to pesticides. But the plant that was grown under these pristine conditions has no way of knowing whether the nutrients it grew in were organic or not.

However, in spite of these theoretical arguments, a few studies *do* suggest that natural forms of vitamins and minerals sometimes seem to work better. Recently, for example, a study showed that natural vitamin E gets delivered to a growing fetus more efficiently than a synthetic supplement; this study is consistent with previous research showing that natural vitamin E is retained better and is more biologically active than synthetic vitamin E. The natural and synthetic vitamins are chemically identical — except that their molecules are arranged in such a way that the natural E is a kind of mirror-image of the synthetic E. So, conceivably, they could work slightly differently in the body. But because one of the sponsors of these studies was the

Natural Source Vitamin E Association, we'd like to see similar results from other researchers. For more information, see *The American Journal of Clinical Nutrition* 67 (1998): 459–464, 669–684.

If you want to make sure that you're getting natural vitamin E, look for "d-alpha-tocopherol" in the list of ingredients. The synthetic version begins with "dl," rather than just "d."

Stay tuned. All we can say right now is that, when it comes to harnessing the protective effects of vitamins and minerals, the best sources seem to be whole foods. If you want to maximize the protection against heart disease and certain cancers associated with specific vitamins and minerals, for example, your best bet is to get your nutrients from fresh fruits and vegetables. Popping a nutrient-packed pill — even when the nutrients were derived from natural sources — gives you less protection (see the sidebar, "If you don't like broccoli, can you pop a pill?").

Supplements That May Help

Proper diet is still the best way to get the vitamins and minerals you need. But get real; not everyone eats a perfect diet. So, sometimes, a supplement or a multivitamin pill makes sense.

Boosting certain nutrients above recommended levels may even help stave off certain chronic diseases — even though, in most cases, nobody's proven that *supplements* are the best (or even an effective) way to boost them.

If you don't like broccoli, can you pop a pill?

Nutrition is a field fraught with controversy, but just about everyone in it has only nice things to say about fruits and vegetables. One reason is that study after study links diets rich in produce with lower rates of heart disease, certain cancers, and other serious conditions.

The result has been the burgeoning field of *nutriceuticals* — or broccoli in a pill. The reasoning goes that these foods must contain something that's good for us, so why not just package this goodie into pill form and get it quickly down the gullet? Well, several reasons — and we're not just talking about the temptation to pop the pill and then spend the rest of the day gorging on empty calories. Not only do you have to worry about getting the right dosage (and an uncontaminated product), but, frankly, no one really knows what the "goodie" is. Who's to say that the vitamins and minerals should get the credit? Other still-unknown substances lurking in the food could be the real heroes.

So until someone does a study linking dietary supplements (other than the ones already known to prevent deficiency diseases) to lower rates of disease, keep chewing.

Beta-carotene

The saga of beta-carotene is a good example of how primitive nutritional knowledge remains. The essential lesson is to roll with the punches, trying not to change your life every time a new study comes in and totally contradicts the study you read the month before.

Beta-carotene is a pigment (coloring agent) found in dark green, dark yellow, and orange fruits and vegetables (see Figure 23-1). It belongs to a family of chemicals called *carotenoids,* all of which can be transformed into vitamin A by the body (though there's currently some debate about whether they all end up as vitamin A). Because carotenoids also all have the potential (at least in a test tube) to neutralize cellular wear-and-tear, they get people really excited (see the sidebar "Antioxidants — keeping those free radicals in control").

If the term beta-carotene rings a bell, that's because it has had researchers more excited than any other carotenoid. In fact, for a while, investigators speculated that beta-carotene might help prevent heart disease and certain cancers, especially lung and throat cancers in heavy smokers. But, alas, the best studies showed that, if anything, people who took beta-carotene supplements actually increased their risk of lung cancer and heart disease! Researchers then decided that beta-carotene was still a good thing, but only if you got it through your diet — probably because fruits and vegetables contain many different carotenoids besides beta-carotene, plus other nutrients.

Figure 23-1:
Dark green, dark yellow, and orange fruits and vegetables contain beta-carotene.

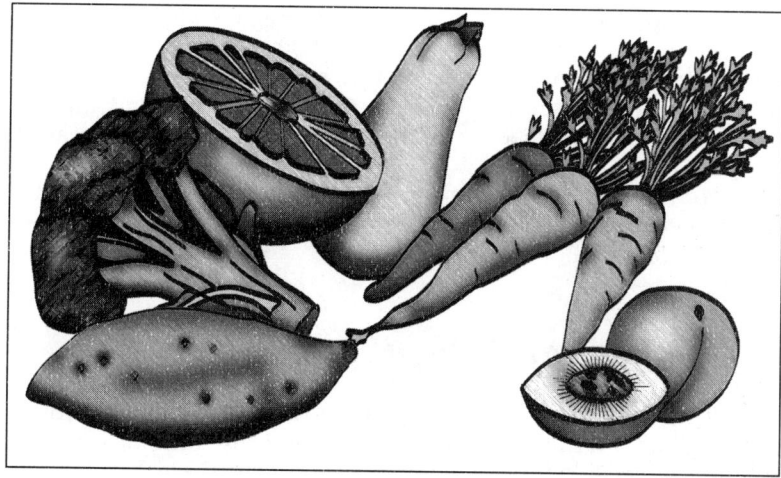

Buyer beware

Remember that — however potentially beneficial — no "dietary supplement" is guaranteed to be safe or effective. Quality control for these products is a real problem, especially in the United States, where a federal act permits manufacturers to sell largely unregulated herbal remedies, vitamins, minerals, amino acids, and hormones as long as they label them as "dietary supplements" and make no specific health claims for them. (See Chapter 20 for more about this act, called the 1994 Dietary Supplement and Health Education Act.)

Anyone who remembers the L-tryptophan horror will be wary of buying these unregulated

substances (see Chapter 8 for more on safe shopping). Back in 1989, over 1,500 people in the United States developed a chronic and debilitating disease (and 38 people died) after taking contaminated supplements of this amino acid (an over-the-counter insomnia treatment) supplied by a foreign manufacturer.

We're not saying that conventional medications don't carry their own set of risks — and, sometimes, quite substantial ones. But assuming the safety and purity of everything "natural" or "over the counter" is an equally big mistake.

But now the debate has reopened, with even newer evidence that beta-carotene supplements may be useful, after all. New data from the Physicians' Health Study — an ongoing study of 22,000 male doctors — showed that taking 50 milligrams of beta-carotene supplement every other day significantly reduced the rate of prostate cancer, at least in those doctors who had low levels of beta-carotene to begin with (probably because they ate fewer fruits and vegetables). But take note: Eating plenty of beta-carotene–rich fruits and vegetables seemed to be just as effective as taking the supplements. (Dr. Meir Stampfer reported the study findings at the May 1998 annual meeting of the American Society of Clinical Oncology.)

If you decide to go the eating route, remember to be good to your produce. Carotenoid levels plummet when produce is left in open containers, exposed to fluorescent lights, or cooked.

Calcium and vitamin D

Calcium — together with sufficient vitamin D — can play a role in preventing osteoporosis, the excessive bone loss and susceptibility to fractures that often afflicts older people, especially women. Theoretically, you can get sufficient calcium from diet alone, but the reality is that most women don't.

Antioxidants — keeping those free radicals in control

You may know that when nutritionists talk about *free radicals,* they're not talking politics. No, free radicals are nasty molecules that run amuck in your body, adding oxygen molecules willy-nilly to other perfectly nice molecules — and destroying cells in the process. This oxygen-adding process (technically known as *oxidation*) ultimately destroys cells and contributes to certain degenerative diseases, maybe even to aging itself.

So it's no wonder that antioxidants are all the rage. Supposedly, supplementing your diet with these substances — which include carotenoids (forms of vitamin A) and vitamins C and E — may help reduce the risk of cancer and heart disease. But, right now, no one can say for sure whether these supplements can

really slow or reverse disease or whether some people may have inborn defenses against free radicals that work fine without supplements, thank you very much. On the plus side, researchers are at last developing techniques that can measure just how antioxidants affect the disease process, so expect some answers soon.

Meanwhile, mixing several antioxidants together on your own probably isn't such a hot idea. Solid knowledge about how antioxidants interact with each other is just too limited right now to say whether mixing and matching can help — or hurt. If you're determined to create antioxidant cocktails, remember that you're being your own guinea pig.

Now evidence suggests that using supplements to get calcium intake up to recommended levels (which are 1,200 milligrams a day for women ages 51 to 70) may not only help prevent osteoporosis but can also make hormone replacement therapy work better — see *The American Journal of Clinical Nutrition* 67,1 (January 1998): 18–24. Calcium supplements (along with regular exercise and sufficient vitamin D) may also help women at risk of osteoporosis minimize bone loss. Some nutritionists say that intake should be as high as 1,500 milligrams a day. Because most women get about 600 milligrams a day through diet alone, supplements are something to think about.

Remember, though, that your body cannot absorb calcium without enough vitamin D. Many older people, or people who just don't get out much (sunlight is a primary source of vitamin D), are short on vitamin D and may need vitamin D supplements (about 400 IUs — international units — per day), as well. And don't forget that regular exercise can help prevent osteoporosis, too.

Fiber

Can eating soluble fiber (such as psyllium) lower your cholesterol levels? Maybe. Eating soluble fiber supplements does seem to keep the intestine from absorbing cholesterol, but you have to force 10 or so grams of it a day down your gullet to nudge your cholesterol levels even a bit lower. Most people find it easier (and more pleasant) just to bulk up their diets with fiber-rich foods: grains, apples, citrus fruits, potatoes, kidney beans, and so on. Because eating fiber-rich foods may reduce your risk of hypertension, certain cancers, and heart disease, you get double the benefit by getting your fiber from foods rather than supplements.

Folate and vitamin B6

Folate — a B vitamin abundant in citrus fruits and green, leafy vegetables (see Figure 23-2) — made headlines in the United States when the Food and Drug Administration (FDA) doubled the recommended daily allowance for folic acid (the synthetic form of folate) and began requiring manufacturers to start fortifying every 100 grams of bread, pasta, cereal, flour, and other grain products with 140 micrograms (mcg) of folic acid.

Why all the hoopla? Besides mounting evidence that folic acid may help prevent heart disease and stroke, overwhelming evidence already shows that women who don't get enough folic acid in the early months of pregnancy have a higher risk of having a baby with certain serious birth defects (such as spina bifida). So to make sure that everyone gets enough folic acid, the FDA wants it baked into the bread people eat rather than relying on people to take supplements.

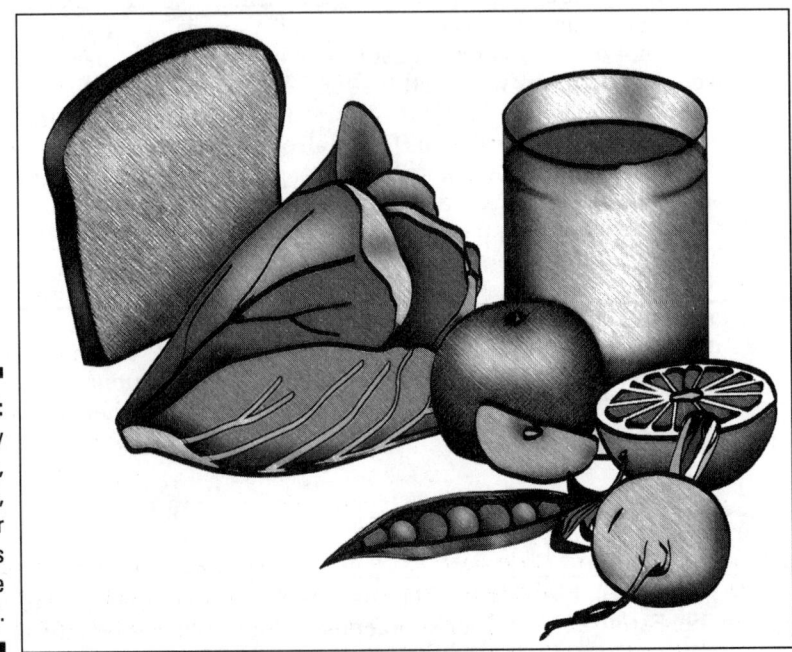

Figure 23-2:
Green, leafy vegetables, citrus fruits, and other foods provide folate.

But to get to levels of folic acid necessary to help prevent disease, you'll probably want to supplement your diet, unless you have an appetite like Dagwood Bumstead's. Taking a little extra B6 along with your folic acid may also be a good idea — especially if you're at risk for heart disease. Several studies have linked low folate and B6 intake to increased risk of heart attacks in men.

And, more recently, data from the Nurse's Health Study — which has assessed more than 80,000 nurses for 14 years — showed that high intakes of folic acid and B6 can reduce the risk of heart disease in women by 45 percent. Women at lowest risk took an average of nearly 800 micrograms (mcg) of folic acid and almost 6 milligrams (mg) of B6 a day — levels much higher than the current recommended daily allowances. To get 800 micrograms per day of folic acid from foods alone would require drinking 6 cups of orange juice, eating 11 cups of romaine lettuce, 33 eggs, or 7 cups of broccoli. To get 6 milligrams per day of B6 would require eating 11 pounds of lean beef, 5 pounds of potatoes, 9 bananas, 36 ounces of chicken breast, or drinking 57 cups of milk! — according to *The Journal of the American Medical Association* and *The Council for Responsible Nutrition* 279,5 (February 4, 1998): 359–64.

Even these studies don't prove conclusively that shoring up on folate or B6 will necessarily cut your risk of heart disease. (Other reasons could account for the fact that people with high intakes of these vitamins were healthier.) Real answers won't come until someone does an experiment requiring one group to take supplements and another group to take placebos; then researchers wait to see whether the people in the first group have lower rates of heart disease.

For now, you probably can't go wrong taking a multivitamin with folate and vitamin B6 every day. But don't skimp on the best dietary sources of these vitamins either: avocados, bananas, broccoli, chicken, cold cereal, eggs, fish, hamburger, milk, orange juice, potatoes, romaine lettuce, spinach, and whole wheat bread.

If you do take multivitamins or other supplements, check with your doctor to make sure that you're absorbing vitamin B12 properly.

Iron

Remember those old commercials for "iron-poor blood?" They suggested that if you felt fatigued or run-down, the reason was an iron deficiency, and the answer was boosting your blood with iron pills.

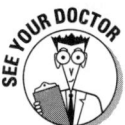

Some people really do need extra iron — especially children, teenagers, women in their childbearing years, and people with ulcers or certain intestinal diseases. But if you're a man — or a woman past menopause — your fatigue probably isn't due to an iron deficiency. In any case, the best way to find out is just to have some blood taken from your fingertip and analyzed by an M.D. Whatever you do, don't decide on your own that you're iron-deficient and treat yourself with iron supplements (which can be dangerous if you suffer from certain genetic disorders).

Magnesium

Magnesium is important for nerves, heart, and fat metabolism, and many people have abnormally low levels of this essential mineral (which often works in conjunction with calcium). Some complementary and alternative medicine gurus want to treat everything with intravenous injections of magnesium — without a whole lot of evidence backing them up. But magnesium supplements (in pill form) may indeed be useful in treating insomnia, asthma, migraine, hypertension, and PMS — and in helping people live longer after heart attacks.

Magnesium can be fatal in high doses, but, fortunately, you would need to take vast quantities of magnesium supplements to overdose. (Diarrhea is usually the first sign that you're overdoing it.) Intravenous magnesium injections, sometimes used to treat abnormal heart rhythms, are another matter; we suggest avoiding them unless you're under the care of a highly skilled M.D.

To be safe, never take more than 350 milligrams per day as supplements, though most people without kidney disease can go as high as 500 milligrams. And because magnesium often works in conjunction with calcium, make sure that you're getting enough calcium every day, too (see the earlier section "Calcium and vitamin D"). Magnesium is abundant in bananas and many other plant foods, including dark green fruits and vegetables, beans, grains, nuts, and whole seeds.

Omega-3 fatty acids

Omega-3 fatty acids — often called "fish oils" because (surprise!) they abound in many fish — are naturally occurring fats that seem to help reduce the risk of heart disease by keeping arterial walls clear and preventing blood clots from lodging in them. If eating two or more servings a week of salmon, mackerel, sardines, bluefish, or other omega-3 rich fish isn't your thing, you can get the same benefits by taking daily supplements of 1,000 milligrams of fish oil per day.

Another way to get your omega-3 is to substitute canola or olive oil for all other oils in your diet whenever possible. You can also learn to love flax-seeds or flaxseed oil, which are both chock-full of omega-3 fatty acids.

Vitamin C

Moderate doses of vitamin C may reduce the risk of certain cancers and heart disease, plus help you resist viral infections and maybe even relieve your sniffles and sneezes — but not *cure* your cold (or your cancer). The doses we're talking about — around 250 milligrams per day — are higher than currently recommended, although recommended levels may be increased any day now.

Don't bother taking more than about 250 milligrams of vitamin C per day. Not only is ingesting more than this amount pointless, but if you take above 500 milligrams, the excess water-soluble vitamin is just excreted in the urine. Plus, when you get over about 500 milligrams, vitamin C starts generating *free radicals,* substances that damage your genes. Oddly, at lower doses, vitamin C protects you against free-radical damage (that is, it acts as an *antioxidant*).

Do you need to supplement your diet with extra vitamin C? Probably not. Eating the recommended five servings a day of fruits and vegetables gives you plenty (though, for many people, this task is more difficult than it sounds).

Vitamin E

For years, vitamin E has intrigued scientists as a possible means to slow the advance of disease, and maybe even stop the aging process. Because vitamin E has antioxidant properties (see the sidebar, "Antioxidants — keeping those free radicals in control"), researchers thought that it may be able to halt the rampant destruction that leads to degenerative disease and cell death.

Most of the studies about vitamin E's powers — and there have been plenty of them over the years — have been disappointing. But some researchers now say that high doses of vitamin E may slow the progression of Alzheimer's disease and Parkinson's disease and reduce the risk of prostate cancer. The most convincing evidence of all suggests that vitamin E supplements may help protect against heart disease and prevent heart attacks.

If you suffer from heart disease — or are at high risk of having a heart attack — talk to your M.D. about the possibility of vitamin E supplements. Just remember that taking more than about 400 IUs a day can raise your blood pressure or make you feel pretty sick.

By the way, if vitamin E sounds like a great excuse to start smoking, stop exercising, or start chowing down donuts every day, forget it. No matter how much vitamin E you take, your risk of heart disease will be just as high if you don't keep the other controllable risk factors for heart disease (including weight, cholesterol levels, and smoking habits) in check.

Supplements You Probably Don't Need

Regardless of what you hear on TV or read in bestsellers, many "hot" supplements are more hype than hope. We're not saying that the substances in this section don't work. Some have great potential. But, right now, the data is so thin that potential risks (to your wallet and/or your health) outweigh potential benefits.

Chromium

Ever hear those mysterious commercials for chromium picolinate? The implication is that this miracle drug — which only the in-crowd knows about — can help burn fat, reduce cholesterol, stabilize blood, and even prevent heart disease, diabetes, and osteoporosis, to boot.

What's the truth? Well, the trace element chromium does seem to have something do with the way the body handles blood sugar, and it *may* help treat diabetes (if you have diabetes, talk to your M.D. about this supplement). And because chromium picolinate is an easily absorbed form of chromium, it *may* theoretically have effects on blood sugar too. But when it comes to helping people lose weight, chromium has yet to prove itself. That's why diet and exercise are still much better proven (and cheaper) ways for most people to get and stay healthy and fit.

By the way, your body only needs very small amounts of chromium to survive, and no one knows too much about the best ways to get it into your diet. For now, count on American cheese, broccoli, calves' liver, wheat germ, and yeast as top chromium-containing foods.

Coenzyme Q-10

You've probably heard the ads for Coenzyme Q-10, at least subliminally. Supposedly, this wonder supplement — also known as CoQ-10, ubiquinone, or vitamin Q — treats cancer, heart disease, obesity, and nerve and muscle problems. Some ads claim that it can make you a better athlete, or even stop you from aging.

Here's the reality: In the test tube, this fat-soluble nutrient acts as an antioxidant, so it has considerable promise as a tissue protector. But proof that it can lower LDL cholesterol, protect heart tissue from damage, shrink tumors, or do much of anything else in *real, live human beings* doesn't exist — at least not yet.

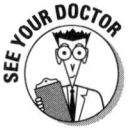

So, for right now, though CoQ-10 appears to be safe, it probably isn't something you need — unless you have congestive heart failure. Some clinical experience, especially in Japan, suggests that CoQ-10 can help real people with congestive heart failure. That's why — even though CoQ-10 is no substitute for conventional treatment — you may want to talk to your M.D. about the possibility of supplementing your regular therapy with a little CoQ-10.

DHEA

According to the latest hype, taking one dose a day of a miracle supplement called DHEA can take 20 years off your age and increase your lifespan — not to mention boost your immunity, blast your fatigue, jumpstart your sex drive, lift your mood, build your bones, reverse your Alzheimer's, melt your fat, and prevent just about every disease known to humankind (including osteoporosis, diabetes, heart disease, and cancer). Hey, why not? DHEA is a miracle drug — isn't it?

Did you really think that we'd say yes? Being sold as a fountain of youth, this supplement is actually a naturally-occurring hormone called dehydroepiandrosterone that declines in the bloodstream as people age. Some DHEA promoters conclude that taking supplements of DHEA should therefore prevent the aging process. Others say that declining levels in older people might just mean that you need less DHEA as you get older.

What's the truth? Right now the risks of DHEA outweigh the known benefits. Frankly, no matter what the packages say, no one really knows how (or if) this stuff works. Some limited research suggests that DHEA may help improve memory, fight depression, and boost levels of natural killer cells. In single studies, DHEA supplements helped elderly patients endure flu shots and relieved symptoms of lupus. But, so far, no outstanding evidence shows that taking DHEA supplements is the best (or even a safe) way to help these or any other conditions. Plus, always think twice before ingesting substances that you're body already makes — DHEA included — or your body may forget how to make these products on its own.

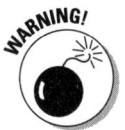

Long-term effects of taking DHEA remain a mystery. Some studies indicate that DHEA can damage the liver, masculinize women and increase their risk of heart attack, and stimulate the growth of certain cancers. So, unless you're participating in a research study, are under close medical supervision, and are using less than 50 milligrams a day, stay away from this one for now. (If you insist on taking it, at least make sure that you have frequent checkups to measure liver function, cholesterol levels, and testosterone levels.) No doubt about it — you are manipulating critical hormones with DHEA. This is something you don't want to do out of a vitamin store.

Glucosamine and chondroitin

Glucosamine is a naturally occurring compound that, when taken as a supplement, is supposed to build and strengthen cartilage. Because cartilage protects the bones from grinding together at the joints, it helps relieve the symptoms of osteoarthritis, a condition that occurs when cartilage breaks down. *Chondroitin* is another natural compound that stops production of enzymes that break down cartilage — so, at least in theory, it may also help keep the new cartilage intact.

Studies on real people who are using these compounds remain limited. Several small clinical trials do suggest that glucosamine and chondroitin can ease pain and improve mobility at least as well as standard treatments for osteoarthritis (such as anti-inflammatory drugs). But until longer and larger studies are done, no one can assess the risks or the long-term benefits of taking these supplements. And so far no one has shown that taking these compounds can actually cure or reverse the degenerative process.

If you're willing to live with these unknowns, you may want to try these compounds, especially if you're fed up with the expense and side effects of standard treatments. Talk to your M.D. first, though, particularly if you have diabetes. Also, remember that these supplements can be just as pricey as standard treatments. Plus, like all unregulated "dietary supplements," it's buyer beware when it comes to knowing just what's in the bottle.

Melatonin

Melatonin is a hormone produced by a tiny gland in the brain. It seems to affect many bodily processes, particularly the body's *circadian rhythm:* the biological events (including sleeping and waking) that recur every 24 hours or so. So it makes a certain amount of sense that melatonin could potentially help relieve insomnia or stave off jet lag.

Can it? Well, taking melatonin supplements (1 to 2 milligrams) a couple of hours before bedtime may help you fall asleep, but it won't help you sleep any longer or better. As for jet lag, some studies show that taking small doses of melatonin at various intervals on the day you travel can help reset your bedtime. Other studies show that this approach doesn't do a thing — or can even make jet lag worse.

Even so, if your best friend's testimonial has you sold on melatonin (and many people swear by this hormone despite the lack of conclusive evidence), remember this: Like all so-called "dietary supplements," melatonin is loosely regulated in many parts of the world, so you may not be getting pure melatonin. Even if you are, you're subjecting your body to a potent hormone that could cause still unknown dangers. (One study has already shown that taking melatonin can leave eyes prone to damage from bright light.) So you're safest waiting until better data come in.

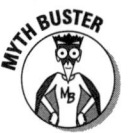

Can melatonin also prevent cancer and degenerative diseases — as is so often claimed? Sorry, but so far the evidence just doesn't exist.

Shark cartilage

Someday (over the rainbow) researchers may discover that taking supplements made from finely powdered connective tissue (cartilage) of the shark can help block cancer from spreading or relieve the symptoms of arthritis. Someday. The stuff has some really cool properties in a test tube — such as blocking the growth of new blood vessels, the kind that tumors bank on as they spread. But sharks have a long way to go to prove that they have something to offer human beings — besides terror.

Sure, with your M.D.s okay you can try shark cartilage together with more conventional treatments for cancer and arthritis. So far, no one thinks that ingesting shark cartilage can hurt you — as long as you make sure that you get it from a reputable manufacturer. (If it's not white, it's not pure.) And never take these supplements if you're pregnant, have heart disease, or recently had surgery.

Zinc

Can taking zinc supplements relieve your cold and boost your immune response? Major studies several years back suggested that they could, and a lot of people (including supplement manufacturers) got really excited. Now you can get zinc lozenges in the candy rack at the supermarket — and, if you've ever stood there with your head stuffed and nose running, you may have thought about picking up a pack.

Before you jump on the zinc bandwagon, remember that the final word won't be in for a while. Yes, some studies do suggest that zinc gluconate lozenges can take a few days off your cold. Even more studies suggest that they can't. You find the same kinds of contradictions when you look at the effects of zinc on immunity. Why these studies contradict each other may have something to do with the exact type of zinc pill involved — some people think that certain flavoring agents such as sorbitol or citric acid may deactivate the zinc.

In the meantime, will trying zinc to relieve your runny nose and watery eyes hurt you? Only if you take too much — in large quantities (more than 2,000 milligrams or so), zinc can produce nausea, vomiting, stomach pain, and diarrhea. Taking even moderate amounts of zinc for too long can also leach copper out of your body, so be sure to add copper supplements if you're taking zinc for more than a month or so.

Chapter 24

Playing with Physics: Energy Medicine

In This Chapter

▶ Finding out about electromagnetism and what it has to do with humans

▶ Using electricity to heal (including electroacupuncture)

▶ Evaluating the healing potential of magnets, light, color, and sound

*E*nergy medicine is one of those annoying terms that everyone uses differently. Some people use the term to mean healing approaches that aim to balance or unblock an invisible "vital energy." This particular form of energy medicine is sometimes called *balancing*. (It's also sometimes called *energy therapy* or *biofield therapeutics,* just to add to the confusion.) You can find out more about this kind of energy medicine — which includes polarity therapy, *Qi Gong*, Reiki, or therapeutic touch — in Chapter 16.

Other people use the term "energy medicine" to describe methods in which the sufferer (or the healer) hooks up with a universal spirit power — perhaps by praying or by going into a trancelike or meditative state. (See Chapter 17 on meditation and Chapter 19 on attitude.)

But wait! There's more. We use the term "energy medicine" in this chapter to describe a form of healing in which practitioners manipulate not some vague vital energy or spirit, but energy of the Western kind: electromagnetic energy, in the form of electricity, magnetism, light, or sound waves.

Human Lightbulbs and Magnets

You may think that electromagnetic energy belongs in physics class, but it's a natural part of biology, too. (Electric eels are a prime example.) In fact, the human body emits its own electrical and magnetic fields, just like everything else in the universe — and mainstream doctors use these fields all the time, whether they're doing MRIs (magnetic resonance imaging) to image body parts or electrocardiograms (EKGs) to measure heart rhythms. And everyone's heard of electric shock therapy to treat certain mental disorders.

Electromagnetic energy has been put to a dizzying number of medical uses over the years, many of them quite effective. Applying this energy to the body can speed wound and fracture healing, repair tissue, strengthen bones, and even encourage the incorporation of bone grafts. Investigators are looking at all sorts of potential uses of electromagnetism, including the treatment of nerve damage, diabetes, heart attack, stroke, and cancer.

But the evidence for these more ambitious applications isn't in yet. So it's no surprise that mainstream doctors look somewhat askance at some of the ways alternative healers are using electricity and magnetism right now. And this skepticism is understandable, especially given the famous quacks who have promoted electric and magnetic devices as cure-alls over the years.

The Body Electric

This section describes some of the more popular alternative uses of electricity in health care. But note that in some countries many of these techniques have already been accepted as mainstream.

Electroacupuncture biofeedback

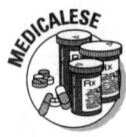

Acupuncturists say that the body is made up of invisible energy channels (*meridians*), each associated with different organs in the body. Along these meridians are hot spots, called acupuncture points, where the energy can be measured and manipulated (see Chapter 15 for details). During electroacupuncture biofeedback (which is also called *electroacupuncture according to Voll — or EAV*), practitioners measure the energy emitted at these points with special instruments. They measure this energy in terms of *electrical conductivity* — that is, how easily electrons flow at any given point.

Advocates of this approach say that — if you're normal and healthy — electrical conductivity is lower at acupuncture points than elsewhere in the body. Abnormally high or low readings mean that the corresponding organ isn't working right, maybe due to disease, infection, toxins, or food allergies.

Ideally, this kind of screening can help nip serious illnesses in the bud and maybe cut health care costs in the process. No one knows for sure whether it really can — yet. Even so, this technique is already widely practiced in Europe and Japan and is used experimentally in the United States.

More MORA, please

This "natural" therapy holds that healthy people emit smooth electromagnetic waves. If you get sick, the waves get out of kilter. The MORA is a machine that not only analyzes the smoothness of these waves but corrects wayward ones and returns them to the body — presumably to correct the problem.

Some alternative doctors use the MORA to treat muscle pain, skin disease, headaches, and circulation problems. Others use the MORA to alter and then transmit colored light into body tissues, which is a kind of color therapy (see the section, "Color therapy"). Still other practitioners have patients try promising homeopathic remedies (see Chapter 12) until the MORA starts to emit smooth, healthy waves.

Whether this approach works is an open question. But as far as anyone knows right now, it's probably not dangerous, except perhaps by delaying better understood treatments and shrinking your bank account.

Pain relief and TENS

Buzz away your pain with a little electric current? Believe it or not, this approach can really work — and work so well that even mainstream doctors now use it regularly to treat chronic pain! And most insurance companies will help pay for it!

We're talking about *transcutaneous electrical nerve stimulation* — which, fortunately, everyone calls TENS for short. By applying an electric current to certain nerves, you stop them from conducting pain messages to the brain, and maybe stimulate the body to produce natural painkillers to boot. A less electricity-intensive device called an *electro-acuscope* can also zap pain, probably by stimulating tissue repair. Ah, relief!

The Attraction of Magnets

Using magnets to heal the body is yesterday's news. Anton Mesmer, an Austrian physician, gave these things a try back in the late 18th century, claiming that he could manipulate "animal magnetism" in the body by waving magnets or his hands over people or putting them into giant magnetized tubs. Later, his theories inspired countless charlatans and "magnetic healers" to hawk their cures at various medicine shows, promising that they could restore "magnetic fluid" to proper balance and so cure asthma, nervous disorders, and just about anything that ailed folks.

Today, alternative healers are still making claims for magnets. They tell stories of magnets relieving chest pain overnight, melting away kidney stones, dislodging plaque from arteries, calming stress, and curing infections and insomnia — plus curing all sorts of mental and psychological disorders.

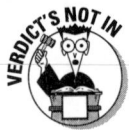

So far little solid evidence supports these claims — nor the specific benefits of applying small magnets to key points, subjecting yourself to magnetic fields generated by giant machines, or sleeping in magnetic beds covered with magnetic blankets. Therapy with powerful electro-magnets (not the little stationary ones you can put in your shoes) does seem to help broken bones heal faster. One small study suggests that low-intensity magnets may relieve post-polio pain (though no one knows how well or how long). Another study suggests that magnets may relieve diabetes-related nerve pain, and quality research on other painful conditions is starting to happen.

Meanwhile, many people swear that placing small (stationary) magnets on key points relieves otherwise intractable pain — and it might. But until better data come in, we can't say whether these effects are due to the placebo effect or the magnets themselves. But, hey, if a magnet can make your pain go away, who cares why? (Just don't place a magnet directly over a pacemaker or other implanted electronic device.)

Let There Be Light

Light, or lack thereof, can control what goes on in your body. When you get hungry, when you sleep, and when you wake all depend on the pattern of light and darkness you experience. If you've ever gone to sleep in a totally dark environment (such as a basement apartment with no windows) and found yourself waking up at 2 in the afternoon, you know what we mean.

Light therapy uses light — natural or artificial, white or colored — to relieve stress, boost mood, and treat various medical problems. Some of this therapy isn't the least bit alternative. Putting newborn babies under intense light is a routinely prescribed way to treat jaundice. Exposing people to carefully timed bright lights can reset the biological clock, helping people overcome jet lag or cope with the stresses of shift work. And sitting under fluorescent light for about 15 minutes a day can help people overcome seasonal affective disorder (SAD, a condition in which people become depressed during dreary, gray days of winter but bounce back to their usual contented selves as soon as spring sunlight returns. See the section "Bright light therapy").

Today, even conventional doctors by and large accept these and other therapeutic uses of light therapy (also known as *phototherapy*). But data proving many other grandiose claims have not yet seen the light.

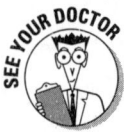

Consulting a health care professional — usually an M.D. — can be a good move before trying light therapy. For one thing, you'll get a diagnosis of your ailment. (You don't want to get treatment for SAD, for example, if your real problem is clinical depression.) Plus, you may get some help from your insurance company if an M.D. prescribes light therapy.

Full-spectrum light therapy

Full-spectrum light therapy calls on all the wavelengths of light contained in sunlight — including all the colors of the rainbow (the visible spectrum), ultraviolet, and infrared light. Sometimes it calls on the sun itself, and sometimes full-spectrum light generated artificially.

Some alternative healers say that full-spectrum light therapy can relieve numerous ailments — including depression, hypertension, insomnia, migraines, premenstrual syndrome, rashes, and various metabolic imbalances. Some healers even say that it can help prevent colds and sore throats — and even certain forms of cancer. Proof, however, remains elusive.

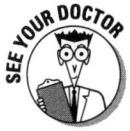

If you have serious eye problems — such as cataracts or glaucoma — get clearance from an eye doctor before trying light therapy of any sort.

Bright light therapy

The light used in bright light therapy is less intense than full-spectrum sunlight and doesn't contain any ultraviolet rays — but it's still plenty bright. Some alternative healers say that steeping yourself in bright white light in the intensity of 2,000 to 50,000 lux can not only keep you alert and productive but also treat various eating, sleep, and menstrual cycle disorders. The research proving these claims is marginal at best. What we do know is that some people using bright light therapy experience temporary headaches and blurred vision.

Using bright light to treat SAD is not alternative. What is alternative is the notion that you have to use special therapeutic light boxes (sold at health food stores and by mail-order catalogs) or full-spectrum lamps to get any benefits. Any old incandescent lamp will do, provided you sit under it for at least 15 minutes a day during the hazy days of winter.

Ultraviolet light therapy

Usually, you hear about the dangers of ultraviolet light. You have to protect yourself from these rays if you want to avoid sunburn and snow blindness and — down the line — premature wrinkling, skin cancer, and cataracts and other eye damage. But most destruction comes from a specific wavelength of UV light known as UV-B light. At least part of other wavelengths of UV light, especially UV-A, may actually do some good.

In a fairly mainstream technique called *PUVA light therapy*, patients take a light-sensitive drug. The UV-A rays chemically activate the drug to help clear up vitiligo, psoriasis, and other skin conditions. (Never use this therapy if your rash may be due to an infectious disease.) Some researchers are also trying to treat the autoimmune disease, *lupus erythematosus,* with UV-A light — but the jury is still out on effectiveness.

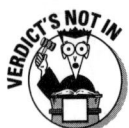

More controversial are attempts to manage cancer, AIDS, asthma, rheumatoid arthritis, and serious infections by removing a pint or so of blood, irradiating it with UV light, and reinjecting it. Supposedly, this procedure restores chemical balance and blasts out disease-causing microorganisms.

Cold laser therapy

Laser beams can do all sorts of neat healing tricks — and mainstream doctors use many of them. Among the best known laser beam feats are clearing up skin conditions, resculpting corneas, and performing "bloodless" surgery.

Alternative healers claim that *cold laser therapy* (also called *soft* or *low-level laser therapy*) can also control pain and clear up infections. Some acupuncturists use low-level laser beams in lieu of needles to stimulate acupuncture points *(laser acupuncture),* and many healers combine laser treatments with other alternative treatments such as herbs, dietary supplements, and homeopathic medicines. Although lasers work no better than the old-fashioned acupuncture needles, they're probably safe.

Color therapy

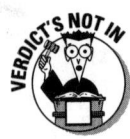

If you're susceptible to the powers of a gorgeous sunset or you know how crummy dark gray walls can make you feel, you can understand the basis of color therapy. Different colors may not only alter moods but may even alter chemical balance in the bloodstream. Color therapy uses this power of color to help heal and keep you healthy. The problem is that the evidence for specific effects — concrete data proving that red light relieves skin rashes, for example, or that flashing white lights ease pain — is slim at best.

We're not saying that color therapy doesn't work — just that most of the stories about the way specific approaches can heal are based on individual studies or just plain individuals. But many forms of color therapy — many tried in one form or another since antiquity — are easy, cheap, and generally safe. And, who knows? They may actually help you.

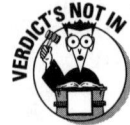

Whatever the health effects, here are some ways (some more sensible than others) to get a little color in your life:

✔ **Look at a red rose or bright yellow buttercup, repaint walls or decorate a room with objects in your personal "healing color," or focus colored lights with "health-enhancing energies" through a prism, crystals, or colored floodlights onto the skin.**

✔ **Ingest dyes that absorb specific colors of light and then become chemically activated to kill cancer cells** *(photodynamic therapy).*

✔ **Eat ground or powdered gems of various colors.** Because most gemstones are pretty much chemically inert — like rocks — this idea doesn't make a whole lot of sense.

✔ **Visit a color therapy practitioner to get your** *auric field* **diagnosed.** Also called *rainbow body,* the auric field is a layer of eight colors that supposedly surrounds human bodies. The colors are bright and clear in healthy people, faded in sick ones.

✔ **Think of specific colors as you inhale and exhale** *(color breathing).* Advocates of this largely data-free approach say that breathing in "turquoise" (whatever that means) and breathing out "red" can boost your immune system. Supposedly, breathing in "yellow" and breathing out "violet" can boost your mental powers. Hey, if you understand how to breathe in yellow, you're pretty smart as far as we're concerned.

The Soundness (Sometimes) of Sound Therapy

Music soothes the savage breast — and the civilized one, too. Sound therapy uses sound waves — sometimes in the form of music, sometimes not — to promote physical, mental, and emotional health. It's a pretty sound idea, so to speak, though many of the specific health claims made by sound therapists haven't yet been supported by scientific data.

Sound healing

Sound healing involves one of many methods — some of them dating back to ancient Tibetan, Ayurvedic, or Chinese healing traditions — that use sound waves to balance the body's natural vibrations. Whether the sound waves come from a tuning fork, computer, or the patient's own voice, they are directed at the patient — sometimes at the problem area, sometimes at acupuncture points — to melt away pain and tension. Some practitioners even claim that specific frequencies of sound delivered at certain intervals can destroy disease-causing microorganisms, relax muscles, alleviate depression, improve blood flow, speed healing, and reduce swelling — plus maybe even promote recovery from spinal cord injuries.

Despite the popularity of various forms in Asia and certain European and South and Central American countries, sound healing is still considered experimental at best by U.S. health authorities.

Music therapy

Sure, maybe some smooth jazz can calm you down or a Strauss waltz can help you navigate a ski slope, but can music really make you better physically? In many cases, yes.

You can do music therapy on your own — and you probably already do. Just playing a favorite song or piece of music can lift your spirits or just plain relax you. Listening, playing, and even moving to music can lower your blood pressure, reduce stress, and maybe even make you smarter and healthier. (A colleague of ours just completed a doctoral study showing that senior citizens who play musical instruments cope better with the trials and tribulations of aging — and may even suffer less from physical disabilities, or at least notice them less.)

For people suffering from serious learning disabilities, autism, Alzheimer's disease, speech disorders, stroke, behavioral or social problems, or visual and hearing impairments, a music therapist can be the way to go. Some music therapists even specialize in using music to ease symptoms of multiple sclerosis, rheumatoid arthritis, and — though research isn't quite as strong here — other forms of chronic pain. Depending on your situation or preferences, you can work with a therapist one-on-one or in a group, as well as combine music therapy with other psychological therapies or psychiatric medications.

Skeptics argue that some of music's "effects" may really result from a little uninterrupted rest (because white noise often works the same wonders as music). But other studies show that specific kinds of music — usually classical — work best, even for people who say that they despise classical music. Another form of music, or even a steady drumbeat, may work for you, though, especially if it's your thing.

Maybe that's why conductors are one of the longest-lived professions (unlike doctors).

Part VII
Specific Conditions

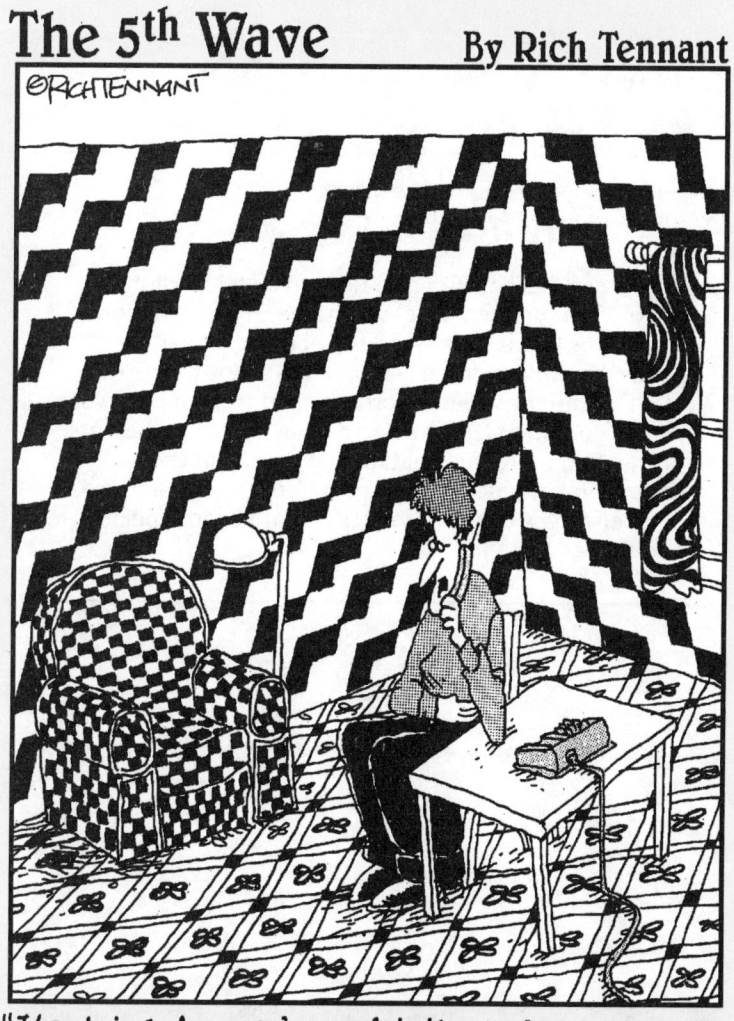

"I've tried Ayurveda, meditation, and aromatherapy, but nothing seems to work. I'm still feeling nauseous and disoriented all day."

In this part . . .

*1*f you suffer from allergies, fibromyalgia, prostate problems, premenstrual syndrome, sinus infections, arthritis, or headaches — or any of numerous other specific health conditions — this part is for you. We fill you in on the "best bet" alternatives to treat and prevent specific conditions, plus let you know where in the book you can find more information about each of them. Equally vital, we alert you to commonly recommended, but often bogus or dangerous, alternatives for specific conditions.

Best-Bet Alternatives
for Specific Conditions

• •

*W*e'll 'fess up: To us, the most important single recommendation that we can make for alternative treatment involves the mind-body approach. Why? Because mind-body medicine is the "heart and soul" of alternative medicine. Whenever you are sick, you are upset, by definition. This emotional distress adds "stress" to the healing process. And pre-existing "stress" may have had a role in the development of the illness.

Even most mainstream doctors concede the profound connection between the mind and physical illness. Mind-body techniques may benefit the underlying ability of the body to heal. And even if these approaches don't really change the underlying course of your illness, they often help you *suffer less* in the process.

Mind-body medicine probably gives you the greatest "bang for your buck" in all of alternative medicine. Discovering how to do relaxation routines, yoga, or visualizations — or even to just sit in a quiet place, breathe rhythmically, and let your mind get quiet — is cheap and easy to learn, very low-risk, and applicable to all sorts of problems.

And so, though we may mention mind-body techniques for some of the conditions below, you can assume that we recommend addressing the "stress" of any illness with the mind-body approach of your choice. Exploring one of these techniques is a fruitful voyage of discovery and a foundation of alternative medicine.

Allergies and asthma

Runny nose, itchy red eyes, wheezing, coughing, sneezing, stiff swollen joints, upset stomach, and hives — allergic reactions are no fun, whether caused by pollen, mold, animal dander, drugs, insect venom, chemicals, or food. Conventional remedies may provide some relief, but often only after costing a pretty penny or causing heavy-duty side effects. So it's no wonder that many people turn to alternative options. But don't forget that — although not always possible — the best way to beat an allergy is to avoid whatever is causing the symptoms.

Asthma sufferers should never substitute herbal remedies for conventional ones without clearance from an M.D. Treating asthma with herbal remedies can land a person in the hospital (or worse) — either because the remedies are dangerous or because using them delays effective treatment. Serious asthma is nothing to play around with.

Certain alternative approaches may help relieve allergic symptoms:

- **Aromatherapy:** If you're all clogged up, massaging fragrant oils around the nostrils or inhaling them from a cloth can clear you out fast. Favorite oils include lavender *(Lavandula angustifolia)*, niaouli *(Melaleuca viridiflora)*, eucalyptus *(Eucalyptus globulus)*, and peppermint *(Mentha piperita)*. (See Chapter 21.)

- **Ayurveda:** Ayurvedic doctors attribute allergies to digestive problems — whatever conventional allergy tests show. So expect to make dietary changes if you want to get with the program — a program that may also include herbal and cleansing *(detoxification)* routines. (See Chapter 10.)

- **Chiropractic or osteopathic:** Manipulation of the upper- and mid-back may reduce asthma symptoms. Just how long the effects last remains a mystery. (See Chapter 13.)

- **Herbal remedies:** Taking a whiff of horseradish can clear out your sinuses — at least temporarily. So can squirting a little salt water up your nostrils. Inhaling the vapors of ginger tea can soothe inflamed sinuses, and smoothing evening primrose oil on your skin may relieve allergic rashes. Dozens of other herbs are used to prevent or relieve allergy symptoms, too — including cayenne pepper, chamomile, garlic, onion, echinacea, elder flower, ginkgo, goldenrod, stinging nettles, and yarrow. Any of these can be worth a try if used appropriately. (See Chapters 20 and 25.)

  You can be allergic to the herbs you use to treat your allergies! Stinging nettles, in particular, cause many people grief. And never use ephedra, bee pollen, or royal jelly unless you're under the supervision of a qualified physician. (The latter two probably won't do much, anyway.)

- **Homeopathy:** These remedies are tailored to symptoms. That's why you may take one remedy for hives, another for itchy eyes, and still another for upset stomach mixed with runny nose. Usually these remedies involve minuscule amounts of the stuff that provokes the symptoms (not all that different from conventional allergy shots, except that the amount of active substance in a homeopathic remedy is so tiny that no instrument on earth can measure it). The idea is to goad your body into healing itself. (See Chapter 12.)

- **Massage:** Some techniques have been shown to improve breathing in asthmatic children. (See Chapter 16.)

- **Nutrition:** If you're allergic to a particular food, changing your diet can be essential. Even if conventional allergy testing (skin tests) don't show the source of your troubles, you may want to eliminate suspected foods from your diet to find out whether symptoms let up — or try eating one food at a time and gradually adding new foods to see which, if any, provoke your symptoms. You may also find that avoiding dairy products or wheat can put the brakes on mucus production and that spicy foods can open up your nasal passages. As for other "anti-allergy" diets, evidence is scanty, and expert recommendations conflict. But, hey, if cutting caffeine, white sugar, or whatever from your diet makes you feel better, go for it. (See Chapter 22.)

- **Traditional Chinese medicine:** Besides offering special herbal concoctions (including ginseng tea) to relieve runny noses, these healers may try changing your immune response with various acupressure and acupuncture techniques. Acupuncture in particular has been shown to help relieve asthma symptoms in children — and the evidence is strong enough that even many conventional doctors are starting to notice. (See Chapters 9, 15, and 16.)

- **Vitamins and supplements:** Evidence that these can prevent or relieve allergic symptoms is thin. Yes, vitamin B12 or magnesium supplements may help prevent asthma, and some studies suggest that vitamin C is a "natural antihistamine" and a natural cure for asthma and allergies — but no one knows for sure. And, sorry, but the same is true for vitamin A or B-complex vitamins, bioflavenoids (stuff found in the white part of citrus fruits), and zinc lozenges. (See Chapter 23.)

Athletic performance and sports injuries

Can natural remedies make you a better runner or boost your athletic power? Maybe. One thing is for sure, though: If you hurt yourself on the field, certain alternative remedies can come in handy.

Sports injuries. If conventional approaches aren't easing the pain from strains, pulls, and tears, one or more of these alternative approaches may help:

- **Bodywork:** These methods can improve muscle function, expand range of motion, and increase balance and coordination after a physical injury. (See Chapter 16.)

- **Chiropractic:** Chiropractors — especially those who specialize in sports — often have much to offer injured joints and muscles. (See Chapter 13.)

- **Herbal remedies:** Arnica (at extremely diluted — *homeopathic* — strength) and bromelain are herbal remedies that may be taken to reduce inflammation and relieve pain. Use arnica externally; don't ingest it. (See Chapter 20.)

- **Homeopathy:** Several homeopathic remedies reputedly speed the healing of tendons and ligaments or relieve various forms of pain. These medicines probably won't hurt you — but use them in conjunction with more time-tested methods. (See Chapter 12.)

D-6 Best-Bet Alternatives for Specific Conditions _____

- **Massage:** These techniques can be just the thing to relieve aches and speed healing in overused or injured muscles. They can also help prep muscles for a strenuous workout. (See Chapter 16.)

- **Traditional Chinese medicine:** These healers can whip up some soothing linaments for aches and pains. And acupuncture can sometimes relieve pain and help speed healing from many types of sports injuries, especially when it is performed soon after the injury occurs. (See Chapters 9 and 15.)

Warming up with stretching exercises, using the right equipment and protective gear, drinking plenty of fluids, wearing proper footwear, and stopping when you're pooped are all commonsense ways to stop injuries from happening in the first place. Getting a physical exam before you take up a new sport or exercise is also wise, especially if you're over 40.

Performance enhancement. We're not saying that you can turn yourself into Michael Jordan or Bonnie Blair, but the following approaches can often help improve your game:

- **Bodywork:** Knowing where your body is in relation to its surroundings is an important part of athletic success — and many bodywork techniques can help improve this ability *(proprioception)*. Bodywork methods including the Alexander technique, Aston Patterning, Hellerwork, and Pilates/Physicalmind Method can help improve muscle function, expand range of motion, and increase balance. *Tai Chi,* a blend of physical and mental exercises with roots in ancient Chinese medicine, can help develop effective movement for all sports and may even help boost your cardiovascular capacity. (See Chapter 16.)

- **Guided imagery and meditation:** Visualizing yourself winning a point or a race can help make it happen. Picturing what's going to occur next also keeps you ready for action but still calm and in control. Mentally rehearsing a dive or sprint can even engrave some patterns in your brain that improve the real performance. And meditation of any kind can help train your mind to focus — vital if you're going to overcome the stress of competition and put your energies into your performance. (See Chapters 17 and 18.)

- **Nutrition:** Eating right can help improve both energy and stamina. Once upon a time, athletes were told to eat steaks and chops, ostensibly to supply energy and build up muscles. Now the advice leans more toward high-carbohydrate, low-fat meals *(carbo-loading),* ostensibly to do the same thing. This approach seems to work for a lot of people. (See Chapter 22.)

- **Stress reduction techniques:** Using relaxation and stress management skills can make a difference. When the heat is on, good athletes use the heat to their advantage — harnessing stress hormones and neurotransmitters to boost speed and power instead of collapsing in terror. (See Chapter 17.)

- **Thinking positively:** Having a "can do" attitude makes a difference for many athletes — as does believing that you have the power to control your own body. Having a supportive network of friends, family, and coaches can help, too. And, though it's a cliché, just having the drive to win can empower you. Of course, understanding that no one can win all the time — and calmly accepting that everyone eventually loses — can help keep you balanced long after the competition. (See Chapter 19.)

- **Vitamins and supplements:** You'll probably hear that taking supplements of vitamins B and E, as well as zinc, calcium, potassium, and magnesium, can help guard against muscle damage, maintain muscle flexibility, and lower susceptibility to injuries. But these claims just aren't backed by solid research. Athletes are best off eating a healthy diet (which includes plenty of magnesium, potassium, and calcium) and taking a good multivitamin to cover these vitamin and mineral bases.

Plenty of products promise to enhance athletic performance or restore muscle tone after serious injury or illness. We hate to be party poopers, but there's not enough evidence to convince us that you should throw your money at most of the following "miracle" products:

- **Performance-enhancement drugs (doping):** Any drug you take to build muscle, boost endurance, mask pain, or improve athletic performance — prescription or non-prescription, legal or illegal — is bad news (unless you need it for health reasons). We're talking about anabolic steroids, growth hormone, amphetamines, cocaine, clenbuterol, ephedrine, and even caffeine and alcohol. These substances can produce serious side effects and interact with other drugs you're taking. Plus, if you get caught using them, your athletic career is down the tubes.

- **Vitamins, nutriceuticals, and herbal "power-boosters":** Maybe you've seen some of the sports and "body fuel" products claiming to supply energy fuel, enhance anabolic activity, boost endurance, stabilize blood sugar levels, encourage fat reduction, aid in tissue repair, increase lean muscle mass, and raise growth hormone release to fight aging — often all at the same time? Or perhaps you've been tempted to try "scientifically formulated" concoctions of vitamins, minerals, essential amino acids, protein-sparing carbohydrates, natural performance enhancers, and exclusive "premium" or "supreme" blends of "energy-boosting" herbs. These products sound too good to be true. They are. (See Chapter 23.)

Autoimmune and related disorders

Conventional approaches leave much to be desired in the treatment of autoimmune disorders — conditions that arise when your immune system starts battling your own body. Drugs that keep the immune system in check *(immunosuppressive drugs)* can control a serious flare-up of symptoms but over the long haul can wreak havoc with healthy organs. No wonder that many people are looking for gentler, safer alternatives!

Many alternative approaches may help autoimmune disease — which can include chronic fatigue syndrome, some forms of diabetes, fibromyalgia, inflammatory bowel disorders (ulcerative colitis and Crohn's disease), lupus, multiple sclerosis, rheumatoid arthritis, scleroderma, and thyroid disorders. Most of these approaches haven't been proven by standards of Western science but may still be worth at try:

- **Aromatherapy:** Inhaling certain essential oils may help relieve pain. (See Chapter 21.)

D-8 Best-Bet Alternatives for Specific Conditions

- **Biofeedback:** This method can help lower stress hormones in people suffering from just about any autoimmune condition and so help control symptoms. (See Chapter 18.)

- **Bodywork and massage:** These approaches can help relieve pain, relax stiff muscles, and reduce swelling. (See Chapters 16.)

- **Cranialsacral therapy:** This approach (often performed by osteopaths, chiropractors, and massage therapists) involves a special manipulation of the skull bones to relieve pain and improve muscle function. (See Chapters 13, 14, and 16.)

- **Hypnotherapy, guided imagery, meditation, and progressive relaxation:** Just about any other relaxation technique can help suppress symptoms of many autoimmune disorders. (See Chapters 17 and 18.)

- **Nutrition:** Consulting with a good nutritionist or a nutritionally oriented physician may be your best option. Reduction of animal fats in the diet, coupled with a regimen rich in vegetables, fruits and whole grains has been shown in solid research to decrease inflammation that occurs in many autoimmune disorders. Eating deep-water fish instead of hamburger, hydrogenated fats, and cheese may make your joints less achy. Supplementation of Omega-3 fish oils, as well as gamma linolenic acid, quercetin, and evening primrose oil, may also help.

- **Thinking positively:** Feeling good about yourself and having a supportive network of friends and family may reduce symptoms of just about any autoimmune disorder. (See Chapter 19.)

- **Yoga:** The postures can help relieve stiff and painful body parts by increasing flexibility. And don't forget that regular exercise (alternative or not) can help prevent diabetes and a whole host of nonautoimmune disorders, including heart attack, stroke, depression, aging-related disability, incontinence, and possibly even certain forms of cancer. (See Chapter 17.)

Until better data come in, you're best off avoiding the following methods to treat various autoimmune disorders. We think that these methods require too much investment (of time, effort, and money) for too little reward and/or are just plain dangerous:

- **Apitherapy (bee venom therapy):** This process involves repeatedly irritating an already inflamed area with bee venom (week after week) and supposedly goads natural anti-inflammatory responses into action. But apitherapy can be painful — and even fatal in people with severe allergies — so check first with your M.D.

- **Cell therapy:** See Chapter 4.

- **Chelation therapy:** See Chapter 4.

- **Detoxification programs:** See Chapter 10.

- **Enzyme therapy:** See Chapter 4.

- **Hydrogen peroxide therapy:** See Chapter 4.

- **Hyperbaric oxygen therapy:** See Chapter 4.

- **Juice therapy:** See Chapter 22.

- **Light therapy:** See Chapter 24.

- **Magnetic field therapy:** See Chapter 24.

- **Orthomolecular medicine:** See Chapter 23.

- **Oxygen therapy:** See Chapter 4.

_____ **Best-Bet Alternatives for Specific Conditions** **D-9**

Chronic fatigue syndrome (CFS). This still little-understood illness used to be called chronic Epstein-Barr virus, and today is sometimes called chronic fatigue immune dysfunction syndrome (CFIDS) or myalgic encephalomyelitis (ME). Whatever the name, the syndrome involves longstanding fatigue that's debilitating enough to interfere with daily activities and doesn't let up even during rest, often together with symptoms such as recurrent sore throat, lack of concentration, muscle soreness, joint pain, sleep disorders, malaise, swollen lymph nodes, headaches, and persistent low fever. Although no cure exists, the following therapies may be helpful in treating symptoms:

- **Acupuncture:** This treatment may help alleviate muscle pain. (See Chapter 15.)

- **Herbal remedies:** St. John's wort may relieve depression, but don't treat depression on your own without a diagnosis from a qualified mental health professional. Echinacea may help relieve sore throat. Ginger, deglycyrrhizinated licorice, or ginseng may help, too. (See Chapters 20 and 25.)

- **Massage:** These techniques may relieve muscle pain and depression. (See Chapter 16.)

- **Meditation:** This practice may help alleviate stress and improve concentration. (See Chapter 17.)

Fibromyalgia. Also called fibrositis, fibromyositis, or chronic muscle pain syndrome, this condition is often misunderstood and misdiagnosed because its wide-ranging symptoms can occur in many other diseases. Besides having various aches and pains in the neck, shoulders, low-back, and thighs, people with this condition have specific *tender points* — areas that hurt when pressed. Other symptoms may include sleep disturbances, numbness,

headaches, and depression. No cure is known, but the following therapies may relieve symptoms:

- **Acupuncture or acupressure:** These procedures may help relieve pain. (See Chapters 15 and 16.)

- **Bodywork:** Non-Asian forms — and exercise in general — may help keep the body limber and slow the onslaught of the disease. (See Chapter 16.)

- **Herbal remedies:** Herbs may help relieve specific symptoms. Topical creams made out of chili peppers may relieve pain. (See Chapter 20.)

- **Homeopathy:** Remedies such as Rhus Tox 30X may help, but consult a good homeopath before trying any on your own.

Inflammatory bowel disorders. These disorders — which include ulcerative colitis and Crohn's disease — involve inflammation and, sometimes, sores of the digestive tract. Symptoms include chronic (sometimes bloody) diarrhea, low-grade fever, lack of appetite, malaise, weight loss, gas, and abdominal tenderness. Ulcerative colitis is usually limited to the small intestine, and Crohn's disease (also called regional enteritis or ileitis) can wreak havoc in the mouth, esophagus, and stomach, too. Some people with Crohn's disease develop joint pains and skin rashes as well.

Some inflammatory bowel disorders may be due to autoimmune problems; others may be due to food allergies. Whatever the cause, the following alternative remedies may provide some relief:

- **Ayurveda:** Some Ayurvedic healers can whip up a diet plan, combined with relaxation techniques and certain herbal remedies, that may quell symptoms. (See Chapter 10.)

D-10 Best-Bet Alternatives for Specific Conditions _____

- **Herbal remedies:** Herbalists offer various concoctions (such as marshmallow root and slippery elm bark) to reduce inflammation or calm an overactive immune system. Hard-core proof is lacking, but — assuming that the herbs are safe and are used safely — they may be worth a try. (See Chapter 20.)

- **Massage:** Combining massage with deep-breathing exercises may help control pain and improve sleep, though evidence is limited. (See Chapter 16.)

- **Nutrition:** Elimination diets can be the treatment of choice for these disorders and are often a good place to start before resorting to conventional drugs or surgery. Basically, you fast briefly and then add one food group at a time back into your diet, trying to determine which food group brings back your symptoms. If symptoms are related to food allergies, changing your diet can help enormously. High-fiber diets may help prevent both Crohn's and colitis, but often aggravate the digestive tract once disease has set in. (See Chapter 22.)

- **Vitamin and mineral supplements:** At least in theory, these may help because some evidence links deficiencies of certain vitamins and minerals (including copper, vitamins E and K, and niacin) to Crohn's disease. But so far no one has proved that taking these supplements alleviates symptoms. Taking fish oil — or just eating fish — does seem to help relieve the symptoms of ulcerative colitis. (See Chapter 23.)

Lupus. Short for systemic lupus erythematosus (SLE), this chronic autoimmune disease involves inflammation of the connective tissue (collagen) in joints, heart, lungs, brain, kidneys, blood vessels, and other parts of the body. Symptoms, which often come and go, may include joint pain, facial sores, swollen lymph nodes, light sensitivity, rashes, hair loss, headaches, fatigue, memory problems, and a characteristic butterfly-like rash across the nose and cheeks. Depending on where the inflammation is, kidney, lung, and blood problems may occur as well.

Many of the dietary and stress-management approaches we describe in the first part of this section can help relieve some of these symptoms, in conjunction with mainstream therapies. The following approaches may help, too:

- Getting regular exercise may help reduce fatigue.

- Keeping out of the sun and away from ultraviolet light may help minimize the butterfly rash.

- Taking the hormone DHEA (dehydroepiandrosterone) may help control various symptoms, according to one small study, but more data are needed to say for sure.

Multiple sclerosis. Also known as MS, this central nervous system disorder causes the nerves in the brain and spinal cord to lose their protective coating. Scar tissue and hardened (sclerotic) plaques replace this coating. Because nervous signals can't be transmitted efficiently, various movement and coordination problems result. Common symptoms — which often occur as attacks — include loss of muscle control, lack of coordination, impaired eyesight, fatigue, numbness or paralysis in the arms and legs, slurred speech, and incontinence.

Although multiple sclerosis remains incurable, these approaches may relieve symptoms:

- **Acupuncture or acupressure:** These procedures may help reduce fatigue and relax stiff limbs and muscles. (See Chapters 15 and 16.)

- **Bodywork:** Certain non-Asian forms — especially the Feldenkrais method and Tragerwork — may be useful in preserving coordination. Bonnie Prudden Myotherapy may relieve numerous symptoms. (See Chapter 16.)

- **Nutrition:** Special diets and supplements are often claimed to relieve suffering, but so far evidence remains unconvincing. One preliminary study did suggest that a lowfat diet can slow deterioration — but it's too soon to say anything definitive. (See Chapter 22.)

Rheumatoid arthritis (RA). This disease (also called RA, rheumatism, or synovitis) occurs when the membranes lining the joints become inflamed. Besides causing severe joint pain and swelling, RA can seriously deform limbs and may damage the heart, lungs, eyes, nerves, and muscles as well. That's why sufferers often resort to powerful drugs and other therapies — including many alternative approaches. Although none of these approaches offers a cure, some (in addition to the dietary approaches we mention at the beginning of this section) may help relieve pain and suffering to some extent:

- **Acupuncture and acupressure:** These treatments may help relieve pain in some (but probably not most) sufferers. (See Chapters 15 and 16.)

- **Chiropractic:** Having a chiropractor manipulate the spine and other arthritic joints can relieve pain and broaden range of motion. But avoid forceful manipulation of the upper neck because RA may loosen the ligaments in that area. Sometimes chiropractors may prescribe exercises and nutritional interventions as well to relieve arthritis symptoms. (See Chapter 13.)

- **Herbal remedies:** Evening primrose oil, or supplements of gammalinolenic acid (an essential fatty acid contained in evening primrose oil) holds some promise for RA sufferers. But reviews are mixed for just about any other herbal remedy — including the flower therapy "Rescue Remedy" and borage seed oil — as balms for pain and inflammation. Topical creams made out of chili peppers can relieve pain due to osteoarthritis (which is not an autoimmune disorder) but don't help rheumatoid arthritis pain at all. (See Chapter 20.)

- **Massage:** Gentle stretching in therapy can keep range of motion intact. (See Chapter 16.)

- **Nutrition and dietary supplements:** Some very limited (and flawed) studies show that fasting or elimination diets can help some patients, especially if food sensitivities aggravate symptoms in the first place. But eating fatty fish (such as salmon) or taking fish oil supplements may really help. Less likely to help are antioxidants (such as beta-carotene, vitamin C, and vitamin E), shark cartilage, zinc, or glucosamine and chondroitin, but any of these supplements may be worth a try with your M.D.'s okay. (See Chapters 22 and 23.)

Cancer

Cancer is not one disease but several different diseases caused by out-of-control cell growth. If you have — or think you may have — any form of cancer, your first line of attack is to see a conventional doctor — no ifs, ands, or buts about it. You also need to tell your doctor that you're considering alternative therapies to make sure that they don't interfere with your overall treatment plan.

D-12 Best-Bet Alternatives for Specific Conditions _____

Right now, no guaranteed cure for cancer exists, mainstream or alternative. The good news is that many alternative techniques can improve quality of life, relieve side effects from conventional therapies, and give seriously ill people a sense of hope. The following alternatives may help — and probably won't hurt — cancer patients:

- **Acupuncture:** Although no cure for cancer, acupuncture treatments can help beat the nausea and vomiting often associated with radiation and chemotherapy treatments. Electro-acupuncture treatments may relieve cancer-related pain. (See Chapter 15.)

- **Bodywork and exercise:** Dismiss anyone who says that *Qi Gong*, reflexology, or any other form of bodywork can cure cancer. But by all means consider using bodywork (or just plain physical exercise) to help feel more relaxed and comfortable and perhaps even relieve cancer-(or cancer treatment-) related pain and nausea. (See Chapter 16.)

- **Guided imagery, hypnosis, and meditation:** So far, no one has proven that you can think away cancer cells — and not for lack of trying. But these mind-body approaches can help you ease the side effects of cancer treatments and just plain feel better about life. (See Chapters 17 and 18.)

- **Herbal remedies:** Many herbs (including astragalus, dong quai, echinacea, and Asian ginseng) supposedly "boost" the immune system and so — theoretically — shore up the body against future or existing cancer. But the emphasis is on "theoretical." Extremely small studies suggest that shiitake or maitake mushrooms, mistletoe, extracts of the Venus flytrap, and various botanical therapies used in traditional Chinese medicine may help treat certain forms of cancer — but until better evidence is in, don't get your hopes up. Ginger, and maybe some other herbs, may help relieve nausea that often accompanies conventional cancer therapies. (See Chapter 20.)

- **Homeopathy:** Some of these remedies may relieve nausea that can result from conventional cancer therapy. (See Chapter 12.)

- **Nutrition and dietary supplements:** Over the years, many different diets, fasts, purges, and vitamin therapies have been tried to treat cancer, but so far none has managed to prove itself to the satisfaction of Western scientists — and that includes the often-hyped supplements such as beta-carotene, vitamins C and E, folic acid, selenium, vitamin B6, magnesium, zinc, and Coenzyme Q10. Stay tuned. Shark cartilage can — in a test tube — boost the immune system and block the growth of new blood vessels that tumors need to spread. But actual evidence that shark cartilage can cure cancer is nil. (See Chapters 22 and 23.)

- **Positive thinking and social support:** No one's ready to say that supportive friends and family — or a special support group — can *cure* cancer. But this kind of support (as well as keeping depression and hopelessness in check) may make coping with your symptoms easier and, in some cases, even help keep your disease in remission. (See Chapter 19.)

- **Stress reduction techniques:** Maybe stress predisposes people to cancer. Maybe it doesn't. In any case, getting negative stress out of your life is often a good idea for other health reasons. (See Chapter 17.)

- **Yoga:** It won't cure your cancer but it can relieve the stress that often comes with cancer — and probably aggravates it. Plus, some people say that yoga can help strengthen your immune system. (See Chapter 17.)

We recommend that most cancer patients avoid these approaches:

- **Massage therapy:** Though it may help some people, this therapy can be dangerous for cancer patients unless performed under the supervision of a highly skilled M.D. (See Chapter 16.)

- **Oxygen therapy:** This warning includes hydrogen peroxide and ozone therapies — because risks far outweigh the dubious benefits. (See Chapter 4.)

A diet rich in fresh fruits, vegetables, and whole grains and low in fat may well be the most effective alternative approach of all because it may help prevent certain cancers. Avoiding cigarettes is a good bet, too — and not even alternative — as is keeping consumption of alcoholic beverages, and salt-cured and charcoal-broiled foods to moderate levels, getting regular exercise, and minimizing exposure to air pollution, ultraviolet radiation (including sunlight), and industrial chemicals. Gorging on soy products (such as tofu) is looking like a better and better idea. And getting screened regularly for various cancers is a way to catch any cancer at an early and often treatable stage.

Children's ailments

Maybe you like the idea of raising a "holistic" child. Maybe you like the idea of using a practitioner who treats the "whole child" — one who asks about diet, sleep, emotions, friends, and school instead of just taking aim at a throbbing ear or wheezing chest. Maybe you'd just

like to avoid using the heavy-duty (and sometimes oddly ineffective) conventional guns to combat minor teething pain, earaches, diarrhea, and other everyday aches and pains without which no childhood would be complete.

If any of these are your concerns, you may want to consider various alternative methods to treat and prevent illness in your children. We describe useful methods for some of the most common childhood conditions in this section. If your child has a condition we don't cover here, you're almost sure to find some useful home and alternative remedies in Winifred Conkling's *Natural Healing for Children: An Essential Handbook for Parents* (St. Martin's Paperbacks,1996).

If your child doesn't respond to alternative treatments promptly or appears seriously ill, contact a qualified physician immediately. Signs of serious conditions in children include difficult or rapid breathing, coughs that last more than a week, excessive drooling, gaping cuts, high fever, lethargy, pale color, severe vomiting or abdominal pain, head injury, stiff neck — or any sudden, unfamiliar, or persistent changes in behavior or health.

One more thing: Some people think that raising a child "holistically" means shunning immunizations for classic childhood illnesses, but — despite some thought-provoking new theories linking immunizations to the rise in childhood allergies and asthma — you and your child are still better off going with the recommended immunizations right now. The risks are minuscule compared to the enormous potential benefits to both society and your child.

Asthma. This condition, often triggered by an allergen or by exercise, occurs when the bronchial tubes narrow and fill with mucus, making breathing difficult. Symptoms include coughing, wheezing, and rapid, shallow breathing. Asthma is a

D-14 Best-Bet Alternatives for Specific Conditions

potentially life-threatening condition and needs to be treated with respect and monitored by an M.D. But certain alternative approaches may sometimes reduce the need for potent prescription medications:

- **Acupuncture:** These treatments may reduce the number and severity of attacks. (See Chapter 15.)

- **Homeopathy:** Remedies are available for asthma, but don't rely on them to treat a serious attack. The same advice goes for herbal remedies and dietary supplements. (See Chapters 12, 20, and 23.)

- **Massage:** This therapy may reduce the severity of an attack and perhaps prevent future ones — though it's no substitute for conventional therapy. (See Chapter 16.)

- **Nutrition:** If a child has food allergies, avoiding them may help prevent asthma attacks. (See Chapter 22.) And if you suspect symptoms stem from low-grade food sensitivities, start with eliminating sugar, dairy, and/or processed foods, and then rotate the diet around watching for symptoms.

Keeping the child away from whatever provokes asthma attacks if possible is a good, if not foolproof, idea. Breastfeeding newborns for at least six weeks may help prevent allergies in the first place (though it is by no means a sure-fire way of preventing problems). Another smart move (besides keeping conventional medicines on hand for an emergency) is to use a device called a *peak flow meter* (available by prescription) on a regular basis to measure how much air is getting into the lungs; when air flow is sub-normal, you can adjust treatment accordingly.

Attention-deficit hyperactivity disorder (ADHD). Also called hyperactivity, attention deficit disorder (ADD), or sometimes mislabeled altogether, this condition is characterized by distractibility, impulsiveness, irritability, and, sometimes, learning disabilities. Some people think that the condition may be related to food sensitivities or allergies, although proof remains elusive.

The following methods are often used to treat ADHD, some with more success than others:

- **Biofeedback:** This technique can often work to reduce stress and help kids with ADHD learn to calm themselves. (See Chapter 23.)

- **Cranialsacral therapy:** Used by some osteopaths, chiropractors, and massage therapists, this method may relieve symptoms, though perhaps not any more than any other kind of soothing touch and attention. (See Chapters 13, 14, and 16.)

- **Herbal remedies:** Certain herbs are often advocated to calm children, but none have been proven to work — or to be safe for kids. And note that some purists say that kids should never take herbal remedies internally. But if you're determined to try the herbal approach, you're best off using an herbalist or other practitioner highly knowledgeable about herbs and how they work in children. (See Chapter 20.)

- **Massage:** A little hands-on can reduce symptoms considerably. (See Chapter 16.)

- **Nutrition:** Cutting out sugar or caffeine, avoiding certain foods or food additives, supplementing zinc, and so on have so far failed to prove their worth to mainstream nutritionists. If certain dietary changes seem to help your child, however, they may be worth trying. But avoid unscrupulous doctors who claim that they can cure your child by running mysterious blood tests to look for sensitivities and deficiencies and then selling you expensive vials of dietary supplements. (See Chapters 4, 22, and 23.)

Bed-wetting. Kids who wet their beds after about the age of 5 or 6 can cause their parents — and themselves — a lot of distress. Most kids outgrow this problem naturally, given enough time, but a few tricks can help push the process forward. Note, though, that you and your child may have to experiment a little to see which solution works for you.

Many parents find that getting the child (especially older, motivated children) actively involved in the solution — asking him or her to change the sheets, working out an action plan together, and so on — works. So does limiting drink and caffeine intake in the evening, having the child go to the bathroom just before bed, or waking the child in the middle of the night to use the toilet. Some kids respond when they're wired up to special alarms that go off and (eventually) awake the groggiest of children at the first sign of wetness; this approach often works because many children who wet their beds are sound sleepers who sleep right through the urge to urinate. This approach sounds drastic but can work surprising well — especially if the child is forced to get up, clean up, and go to the bathroom when the alarm buzzes and then rewarded with stickers or other treats for dry nights.

Whatever method you choose, remember that laying low is your best approach. Shaming or threatening a child about this problem rarely works — and often makes matters worse. And although some children respond to a reward system (stickers for every dry night or a coveted

toy after 30 dry nights), some children feel pressured by these tactics, which therefore backfire. Ultimately you and your child will have to experiment with various approaches. If nothing is working, though, see a physician to make sure that the child doesn't have an underlying physical or emotional disorder.

The following alternative approaches may be worth trying as well:

- **Acupressure or shiatsu:** These treatments may help some kids. (See Chapter 16.)

- **Acupuncture:** Although evidence leaves something to be desired, some acupuncturists say that they can help a child overcome bed-wetting problems. (See Chapter 15.)

- **Chiropractic:** One report suggests that chiropractic manipulation may help, but the strength of the data is marginal.

- **Homeopathy:** Some remedies purport to help control bed-wetting. Maybe they do, and they're probably harmless enough to try if nothing else is working. (See Chapter 12.)

Croup and colds. Everyone knows what a cold is, and some kids seem to have one just about all the time. Croup is a sometimes serious condition that affects mainly babies and toddlers, usually in the middle of the night. It happens when the airways narrow and clog with mucus, giving the child a harsh, barking cough that sounds something like a seal. Although most cases of croup aren't life-threatening, listening to your child gasp for breath can be petrifying.

Colds and croup are often amenable to classic home remedies. Running a vaporizer or humidifier in a coughing, sneezing kid's room to thin mucus secretions is one of the oldest parenting tricks in the book, and so is standing in a steamed up bathroom with a croupy baby or toddler (taking the kid out into the cool night air works well, too). And don't forget to try saltwater nose drops or gargles to clear a stuffy nose, at least temporarily. Drinking hot liquids and chicken soup makes sense, too.

Below are some alternatives that can often alleviate symptoms of these problems, sometimes so well that no medical attention is required. But keep in mind that it's easy to confuse simple croup and cough with much more serious, life-threatening disorders. That's why it's vital to call an M.D. if your baby or child has a high fever, labored breathing, excessive drooling, pale skin, or a stiff neck. And don't be embarrassed to call for help if you're unsure: It's better to be safe than sorry, right?

- **Aromatherapy:** Rubbing certain herbal remedies or essential oils on the skin — such as rubbing eucalyptus oil on a child's chest may help clear stuffy sinuses and bronchial passages. Adding a little eucalyptus oil to a vaporizer may also help. (See Chapter 21.)

- **Homeopathy:** These remedies may help — and most are so diluted that they're probably safe to try. But if you really buy into homeopathy, it doesn't make sense to use over-the-counter homeopathic remedies for anything but the most minor ailments (such as runny noses); more serious illnesses require the diagnostic skills of a trained homeopath. (See Chapter 12.)

Constipation and diarrhea. These conditions afflict kids more often than most parents would like to admit. The term constipation is a poorly defined term that is usually used to mean moving your bowels less often than desired. Note that many people (kids included) think that they're constipated when they're not: Despite what Grandma may have told you, many folks are perfectly healthy and happy without moving their bowels every day. But for kids who have obvious pain, bloating, or bleeding, constipation is a big problem. Call an M.D. if your child goes more than 3 or 4 days without moving his bowels. Though many perfectly normal toddlers go this long during the arduous power-struggle called toilet training, some children may have an intestinal blockage.

Diarrhea is just the opposite problem. Children often develop frequent, loose, or watery stools, sometimes accompanied by abdominal cramps. Unchecked, diarrhea can quickly cause serious dehydration in kids — so call an M.D. if it lasts for more than 24 hours or so.

The following alternative treatments and home remedies can often help control both constipation and diarrhea:

- **Acupuncture and acupressure:** Treatments are big maybes but could be worth a try if nothing else is helping your child's gas, nausea, or constipation problems. (See Chapters 15 and 16.)

- **Enzyme therapy:** In the form of lactase supplements, this therapy may be helpful if the child is lactose-intolerant (lactase-deficient). (See Chapter 4.)

- **Herbal remedies:** Some herbs may soothe intestinal distress but usually aren't good ideas for children, especially when so many other better-understood approaches work just as well or better. Use psyllium, a so-called natural laxative, only under the direction of a qualified practitioner. (See Chapters 20 and 23.)

- **Homeopathy:** These remedies may be worth a try but probably won't work if other, better proven methods haven't worked. (See Chapter 12.)

Best-Bet Alternatives for Specific Conditions *D-17*

- **Massage:** This therapy can often work surprisingly well. (See Chapter 16.)

- **Nutrition:** Cutting out certain foods is often the way to go to treat minor diarrhea, constipation, or other tummy troubles. Eating a high-fiber, balanced diet and avoiding irritating foods can help prevent these disorders, too — and promote good health in general. So can drinking plenty of fluids and getting regular exercise. And everyone and his grandmother knows that eating prunes or drinking fruit juice can get your bowels moving. (See Chapter 22.)

For diarrhea, offer your child the "BRAT" diet — bananas, rice, applesauce, and (dry) toast. Often a day or so of these foods will clear the problem right up. And make sure that the child drinks plenty of fluids to stave off dehydration. Avoiding fruits and fruit juices is a must.

Earaches and ear infections. Kids get a lot of earaches, many of them due to ear infections or fluid accumulation in the middle ear (the area where sound waves travel through three tiny bones toward the ear drum). Perhaps because the tube that connects the middle ear to the throat (the eustachian tube) is smaller in little kids, their ears are particularly susceptible to infection and inflammation. A child complaining of ear pain, pulling on an earlobe repeatedly, or just acting cranky or out-of-sorts may be showing signs of an ear infection.

Conventional M.D.s have been catching flak lately for treating every ear infection they see with antibiotics. Not only does this kneejerk approach promote the development of drug-resistant bacteria, say critics, but it doesn't do a thing for the many earaches and infections caused by viruses or fluid accumulation and not susceptible to antibiotics. Plus, antibiotics can have nasty side effects and burn holes in parents' wallets, even though most childhood earaches and infections clear up on their own. Overuse of antibiotics may even leave kids more susceptible to allergies and asthma later in childhood, though this claim is controversial.

Of course, a serious ear infection left untreated may occasionally lead to serious, even life-threatening complications (including deafness and meningitis). So be sure to call an M.D. if the child has a fever or severe pain. Sometimes the eardrum ruptures — which is actually part of the natural healing process — leaving a yellow discharge in its wake. It will eventually heal, but at this point it's worth consulting an M.D. about antibiotics.

Here are some alternative treatments that may help your child:

- **Acupuncture:** Treatments may help relieve pain, at least temporarily. (See Chapter 15.)

- **Chiropractic:** Some chiropractors and osteopaths say that certain head and spine manipulations can drain clogged eustachian tubes and so help relieve ear infections. Maybe — but most ear infections go away on their own, so it's difficult to know what's really happening. If you want to try this approach, see a practitioner with special training and experience in this area. (See Chapters 13 and 14.)

- **Herbal remedies:** Echinacea or garlic may boost the immune system in general and reduce the risk of ear infection — but never use these in children except under the supervision of a highly knowledgeable herbalist or other practitioner. (See Chapters 20 and 25.)

D-18 Best-Bet Alternatives for Specific Conditions

- **Homeopathy:** These remedies may help soothe the pain — and, even if they don't, they're usually safe enough to try if pain isn't too severe. (See Chapter 12.)

- **Nutrition:** Food allergies may underlie certain ear infections, although no one knows for sure. If your child is allergic to dairy products, in particular, you may find that cutting these out of the diet reduces the number of ear problems (you should be cutting these foods out anyway). Breastfeeding may reduce your child's chances of ear infections but is hardly a foolproof method. (See Chapter 22.)

Skin problems. From diaper rash to poison ivy to impetigo to insect bites, the various types of skin rashes and disorders that plague kids are far too many to mention and deserve individualized treatment. But certain alternatives can help soothe red or itchy skin, whatever the source:

- **Acupressure or shiatsu:** These treatments may help relieve pain and itching associated with skin disorders. (See Chapter 16.)

- **Herbal remedies and aroma-therapy:** Certain remedies may help prevent infection or heal rashes, including goldenseal, tea tree oil, arnica, and calendula. Jewelweed and milkweed can help heal poison ivy, and aloe vera provides welcome relief for itchiness and irritation. (See Chapters 20, 21, and 25.)

- **Homeopathy:** Some remedies may help soothe a rash and probably won't hurt to try. (See Chapter 12.)

- **Vitamins:** Vitamin E or C ointment may help bites and stings heal faster and reduce inflammation, though evidence is thin. (See Chapter 23.)

Keeping skin cool, clean, and dry is often a good way to prevent many skin rashes. And remember to call an M.D. at the first sign of fever, blistering, discharge, or appetite change.

Teething pain: When those little teeth start poking through the gums, little tykes can suffer royally. Perfectly charming babies suddenly turn into drooling, fussy beasts, and parents want to stop the suffering — and fast. Besides the old standards — cold wet rags for gumming, frozen bagels to chomp on, and over-the-counter gum-numbing drugs and pain-relievers (never aspirin for children, though), the following alternative approaches may help:

- **Acupressure:** Pressing on certain key points may provide immediate — if temporary — relief. (See Chapter 16.)

- **Acupuncture:** Treatments may relieve dental and facial pain — but taking a teething infant to the acupuncturist seems a little extreme to us. (See Chapter 15).

- **Aromatherapy:** Diluted clove or tea tree oil applied to a cloth may help, though maybe not better than any kind of wet cloth. Putting olive oil on a cloth may work well, too. But check with your child's doctor first. (See Chapter 21.)

- **Homeopathy:** Some remedies aim to cure fever associated with teething. But remember that fever (as well as vomiting and diarrhea) are not "symptoms" of teething — just symptoms of other conditions that often afflict young children, too. You may want to try a homeopathic remedy for teething *pain,* but it probably won't work any better than standard home remedies. (See Chapter 12.)

Colds and flu

Runny, achy, stuffy, wheezy, chilly, burning — there's got to be a better way to deal with colds and flu besides over-the-counter remedies that often don't work and leave you groggy or wired when they do. Surely alternative healers have a better way to deal with the common cold or flu? Well, probably not, at least as far as cures go. But some methods we describe in this section may relieve your symptoms better than conventional remedies — and often without the same nasty side effects.

Colds are common, contagious diseases caused by one of about 200 different viruses that irritate the nose and throat. Usually symptoms — which can include head and chest congestion, runny nose, sore throat, sneezing, dry cough, aches, chills, burning eyes, and headache — can be treated at home. But contact a physician if you have difficulty breathing, a temperature of 103°F or higher, a sore throat together with a fever of over 101°F (signs of more serious conditions), or you think that your symptoms may be due to an allergy. And even the most minor cold symptoms in babies two months of age or younger warrant a prompt call to the doctor.

Flu, which is short for influenza, is another common viral disease with symptoms similar to colds, plus aching muscles, general fatigue, and a fever that may alternate with chills. When flu strikes, call an M.D. if you already have a weakened immune system (from cancer, AIDS, diabetes, and so on) or another serious condition. Call, too, if your fever lasts more than 3 days or if you have trouble breathing or experience chest pain — possible signs of pneumonia.

Otherwise, the following alternative remedies may provide welcome relief for many cold or flu symptoms, though you may have to experiment a little to find what works for you:

- **Acupuncture and acupressure:** Putting finger pressure on certain key points on the head may help relieve headaches, sore eyes, and nasal congestion. Acupuncture may be something to try when colds lead to major pain — say from a sinus infection (sinusitis). (See Chapters 15 and 16.)

- **Aromatherapy:** Inhaling steam fragranced with oil from the *Eucalyptus globulus* plant — or rubbing some diluted oil on your chest — can relieve congestion. Some people prefer peppermint *(Mentha piperita)* or tea tree *(Melaleuca alternifolia)* oils. Diffusing myrtle *(Myrtus communis)* into a room can calm a cough. If you have asthma, be particularly careful, though; herbalized vapors can sometimes spark an asthma attack. (See Chapter 21.)

- **Herbal remedies:** Leading the list of herbal cold balms is the daisy-like echinacea flower, certain parts of which may help rev up the immune system and keep cold symptoms at bay. But beware. If you want results, you must use the right species — and the right parts of that species. Far too often, labels on commercial products make it hard for you to determine which part or species you're using. What you want are extracts of the fresh or recently dried whole plant, either *Echinacea augustofolia* or *Echinacea purpurea,* or roots of the *Echinacea pallida.* Don't take this herb continuously because it may stop working after a couple of weeks.

Teas, capsules, and tinctures made from other herbs — including astragalus, boneset, elecampagne, eyebright, elderflower, garlic, ginseng, goldenseal, peppermint, and yarrow — are also popular cold and flu treatments, as are certain Chinese herbal formulas, but until better evidence comes in you'll have to see for yourself whether they seem to help. Just make sure to follow our tips for safely using herbal remedies! (See Chapter 20.)

- **Homeopathy:** Many folks swear by various homeopathic remedies to prevent or treat cold and flu symptoms. We don't think that the evidence is strong enough to recommend any of these in particular, but most are probably safe enough to try. (See Chapter 12.)

- **Nutrition and dietary supplements:** If only popping a few vitamins and minerals could keep colds and flu away! But right now the only dietary supplement with any real evidence behind it is vitamin C — which, in moderate doses, may work to prevent colds and quicken recovery. You're better off sticking to a well-balanced diet rich in fruits and vegetables and all the vitamins and minerals they contain. When colds and flu do get you, avoiding dairy products *can* help thin mucus, and hot, spicy foods can clear out your sinuses — at least temporarily. Drinking eight or so glasses of water and juices every day to replace lost fluids and reduce congestion can help, too. A glass of dry red wine can help dry out your sinuses. And don't knock the power of chicken soup — even recent scientific investigations confirm that there's something in it, besides Mama's love, that relieves congestion and other cold symptoms.

Even though some studies suggest that zinc can cut down days of suffering, just as many studies say that it doesn't do diddly. Sure, right now no one says that there's any harm in trying, as long as you stick with recommended dosages. And you do need to get enough zinc in your diet if you want to stave off colds and flus. But because scientists still don't know whether supplementary zinc really helps — and know even less about long-term effects — buyer beware. (See Chapter 23.)

- **Reflexology:** Pressing or massaging the area just under the ball of your foot may help relieve coughs and wheezing. And even if it doesn't, it certainly can't hurt to try! (See Chapter 16.)

Don't forget that one of the best ways of dealing with colds and flu is preventing them. To keep your immune system ready for combat, don't bother with the "immune boosting" herbs. These may work, but the evidence is still too sparse to justify the expense. Instead, concentrate on living a healthy lifestyle: Eat a balanced diet rich in fruits and vegetables, get enough rest, exercise regularly, avoid smoking, drink plenty of fluids, take a good basic multivitamin, and keep negative stress out of your life. Avoiding people who already have colds and flu is also a good idea, as is washing hands well and not smoking.

Diabetes

Diabetes *(diabetes mellitus)* is a term that includes several different disorders, all of which involve high levels of sugar (glucose) in the blood. The two most common forms of this disease are called Type I (formerly called juvenile) diabetes and Type II (formerly called adult-onset) diabetes. Type I occurs when the body can't produce enough insulin (a hormone that removes excess glucose from the blood), which means that people with this disorder need to take regular injections of insulin. Type II occurs when the body can't efficiently use the insulin it produces. Women sometimes develop a third kind of diabetes, *gestational diabetes,* during pregnancy. The condition usually disappears after childbirth and can often be treated with diet but may leave women at risk for developing chronic diabetes later in life.

Signs of possible diabetes include excessive thirst and urination, increased appetite, weight loss, fatigue, nausea, blurred vision, frequent yeast infections, impotence in men, and frequent urinary tract infections in women. Poorly controlled diabetes may not only result in fainting, coma, and weakness but ups the risk of serious and sometimes life-threatening complications, including heart and kidney disease, circulatory problems, and eye and nerve disorders. People with diabetes should be under the care of a qualified M.D. — and people with signs of diabetes should contact a physician for an accurate diagnosis.

For just about any type of alternative therapy you can name, someone will tell you that it can help treat certain symptoms of diabetes — if not cure the disease outright. But the evidence suggests that the following alternatives may be your best bets, if used together with more conventional therapy:

- **Acupuncture:** These treatments may help relieve pain due to diabetes-related nerve problems, though it's premature to expect acupuncture or Traditional Chinese herbal medicine to prevent diabetes or reduce insulin needs. (See Chapters 9 and 15.)

- **Ayurveda:** Certain dietary changes recommended by Ayurvedic doctors may help control blood sugar levels. (See Chapter 10.)

- **Biofeedback:** This practice can help improve blood flow to hands and feet and so help prevent serious complications of the disease. It can also lower stress hormones, which in turn may help control blood sugar levels. (See Chapter 18.)

- **Exercise:** Regular exercise may help blood sugar and reduce the need for insulin shots (and it can reduce chances of getting diabetes in the first place). But people with Type I (insulin-dependent) diabetes need to shore up on carbohydrates before exercising — and keep food and drink on hand — in case blood sugar drops to dangerous levels. And anyone with diabetes should check with an M.D. before embarking on a strenuous exercise program.

- **Herbal remedies:** Certain herbs (including burdock, garlic, ginkgo, hawthorn, onion, and ginseng) may help control the symptoms of diabetes but should never be used without consent of the M.D. treating the diabetes. Adding a little garlic or onion to your diet probably can't hurt, though. Topical creams made with cayenne *(Capsicum annuum)* may help relieve diabetes-related pain in the hands and feet. And quercetin, a biologically active chemical (bioflavenoid or flavenoid) from citrus fruits, may help minimize nerve damage. (See Chapters 20 and 25.)

- **Magnetic field therapy:** These treatments may help relieve nerve pain *(neuropathies)*. (See Chapter 24.)

- **Nutrition:** The right diet can make a huge difference in controlling blood sugar levels. Although debate exists about which diet works best, no one disputes that minimizing sugar intake is essential. Filling up on complex carbohydrates and fiber is also usually a good bet. Certain foods such as okra, peas, and cinnamon may play roles in lowering the need for insulin, but your best bet is to work with a qualified health care professional to find the nature, amount, and timing of various foods that work best for you. (See Chapter 22.)

- **Relaxation, meditation, guided imagery, and hypnotherapy:** These approaches may lower stress and help keep blood sugar in check. (See Chapters 17 and 18.)

- **Vitamins and supplements:** Chromium may help regulate blood sugar levels in some people with diabetes. Many other dietary supplements appear to have something to do with the way the body uses insulin, but right now claims that consuming more than recommended doses of any given vitamin or mineral can control blood sugar or reduce need for insulin shots remain largely speculative. (See Chapter 23.)

- **Yoga:** The postures may help regulate blood sugar and keep the need for insulin shots in check, though no convincing proof exists. (See Chapter 17.)

Some forms of diabetes may be preventable by keeping your weight within normal limits, exercising regularly, and eating a balanced diet. Quitting smoking — or never starting — is a good move if you already have diabetes (and even if you don't) because it reduces your risk of heart disease.

We recommend avoiding the following treatments, all of which are too risky and/or unpleasant to justify their very speculative benefits:

- **Chelation therapy:** See Chapter 4.

- **Detoxification treatments and colon therapy (enemas):** See Chapter 10.

- **Ozone and hydrogen peroxide therapies:** See Chapter 4.

Heart disease

Chest pain, shortness of breath, dizziness, palpitations (fluttering sensations in the chest), and fluid retention can all be signs of conditions other than heart disease. But if you have any of these symptoms — or if you're overweight, sedentary, over 45, have a family history of early heart disease, smoke, or have high blood pressure, high cholesterol levels, or diabetes, you should (at the very least) have a complete physical examination by an M.D. to check the state of your heart.

If you have been diagnosed as having some kind of heart condition, no alternative can substitute for conventional medical care. But many alternative approaches can be useful additions to your overall therapy.

Arrhythmias. This term means any kind of abnormality in the heart's rhythm — too slow, too fast, irregular, skipped beats, and the like. Some people are born with arrhythmias; others develop them as a result of coronary heart disease. You can have arrhythmias without noticing them, but many people sense their hearts racing, thumping, or fluttering. Some arrhythmias are harmless, but an M.D. should check any that occur fairly often.

A few alternatives show promise in treating arrhythmias, as long as they're used in conjunction with conventional medical care:

- **Biofeedback:** This practice can help certain kinds of heart beat irregularities. (See Chapter 18.)

- **Guided imagery:** This approach can help decrease arrhythmias, especially those that don't stem from a physical abnormality in the heart. (See Chapter 18.)

- **Herbal remedies:** Hawthorn may help relieve arrhythmias and other forms of heart disease — if used under the supervision of a trained herbalist working with an M.D. (See Chapter 20.)

- **Vitamins and supplements:** Intravenous injections of magnesium seem to reduce risk of various arrhythmias. But, obviously, these injections aren't something you should try at home, and no one has ever shown that popping magnesium can make any difference. You don't want to fool around with any minerals, really, because too much or too little of many minerals can cause serious heart rhythm problems. (See Chapter 23.)

Coronary heart disease. This term encompasses many different but related conditions that involve progressive blockage of oxygen supply to the heart. In coronary artery disease, or CAD — the blood vessels *(arteries)* supplying oxygen to the heart get blocked or narrowed, usually because of the build-up of plaque over the years (a process known as *atherosclerosis*). Because the heart doesn't get as much oxygen as it needs, chest pain *(angina)* can result after and/or during exercise or stress.

If the oxygen supply becomes severely blocked — either because of narrowed arteries themselves or because a blood clot lodges in narrowed arteries — a heart attack *(myocardial infarction)* occurs. Heart attacks can be fatal, severely damage the heart muscle, or leave relatively minor damage, depending on the location and extent of the blockage. Symptoms of a heart attack include a tight, squeezing feeling in the chest (not short, stabbing pains); pain anywhere in the chest, neck, shoulders, or arms; indigestion; nausea; dizziness, fainting, and/or shortness of breath. Any of these symptoms can signal a much less serious problem, but if you're at all uncertain, remember that it's better to be safe than sorry.

Sometimes after a heart attack (or instead of one) the heart becomes so oxygen-starved that it can no longer pump sufficient oxygen-rich blood to body tissues — a condition known as *congestive heart failure*. Symptoms of congestive heart failure include bloating (in the ankles, legs, abdomen, heart, and lungs) and shortness of breath.

The following approaches may help lower the risk of serious coronary heart disease and/or relieve some of its symptoms:

- **Exercise:** Although strenuous exercise can provoke a heart attack, getting regular exercise is also one of the best ways to prevent heart disease from happening. But get an M.D.'s approval before embarking on any new exercise plan, particularly if you're over 40 or have other risk factors for heart disease. Keeping your weight within normal limits, avoiding foods high in saturated and polyunsaturated fats, and quitting smoking can make a difference, too.

- **Herbal remedies:** Hawthorn can help in the treatment of both congestive heart failure and angina because it helps the heart pump blood more efficiently and increases blood flow to the heart muscle. But it's a powerful drug (even if it's called an herb) and should be used only under the supervision of a qualified M.D. (See Chapter 20.)

- **Nutrition and vitamins:** Foods rich in natural antioxidants such as beta-carotene, vitamin E, and flavonoids (abundant in produce, tea, and wine) may help lower the risk of heart attack (but some research indicates that supplements of beta-carotene may actually increase your risk!). (See Chapters 22 and 23.)

D-24 Best-Bet Alternatives for Specific Conditions _____

Eating salmon, mackerel, sardines, bluefish, or other "fatty" fish several times a week — or just taking supplements of "fish oils" — may lower your risk of heart disease by preventing plaque build-up in your arteries. So may using canola and olive oil as your primary dietary oils or sprinkling flaxseeds or flaxseed oil (available at health food stores) on your food. (See Chapter 23.).

Phytoestrogens which are natural compounds in soy-based foods (especially in tofu and some soy drinks), may work just as well as hormone replacement therapy at keeping arteries clear and lowering risk of heart disease in women past menopause. Soy phytoestrogens may also help prevent plaque from accumulating in the main artery going to the brain and so perhaps help prevent strokes (events sometimes called *brain attacks* because they occur when oxygen supply is cut off to brain tissue rather than heart tissue). So far, though, the best evidence for these phytoestrogen effects come from studies in monkeys. (See Chapter 22.)

The amino acid derivative L-carnitine — taken as a pill or as an intravenous injection — may help the heart pump more efficiently and possibly lower the risk of angina and death. But this powerful substance should be used only under the supervision of a qualified M.D. Coenzyme Q-10 (CoQ-10) probably can't live up to all its advertised claims but may be useful in patients with congestive heart failure. And supplements of magnesium may help some people live longer after heart attacks.(See Chapter 23.)

- **Stress reduction techniques:** Any relaxation technique that relieves negative stress may cut your risk of suffering a heart attack. Whether that's bodywork, guided imagery, meditation, biofeedback, yoga, or just getting some regular exercise or vacation time doesn't make a whit of difference. (See Chapters 17, 18, and 19.)

- **Thinking positively:** Although the evidence is far from conclusive, praying, regular religious attendance, or even having someone pray for you may reduce your chances of heart disease and improve your chances and rate of recovery. Working to rid yourself of hostile and angry feelings may actually cut your risk of heart attack, too. Leaving a high-stress job or changing work conditions can also make a difference, though not possible for everyone, of course. (See Chapter 19.)

- **Traditional Chinese medicine:** These healing methods supposedly strengthen the heart with various massage, acupuncture, herbal, and dietary tactics. Talk to your regular M.D. before trying these approaches, though, to ensure that they are compatible with your overall therapy. (See Chapter 9.)

High cholesterol (hypercholesteremia). Cholesterol is a chemical manufactured in the liver of all animals — including humans — that is used to make cell walls, hormones, and other essential substances in the body. Having cholesterol circulating through your bloodstream is vital. But high levels of this stuff — particularly high levels of a form called low-density lipoprotein (LDL) cholesterol — have been linked to a high risk of coronary heart disease because LDL cholesterol promotes the build-up of artery-clogging plaque. Doctors hope that lowering LDL cholesterol (and perhaps raising high-density lipoprotein, or HDL, cholesterol) will lower this risk, and many prescribe powerful anti-cholesterol drugs to patients who can't get their cholesterol under control by changing diet and exercise habits alone.

Some of the following alternatives promise to help get cholesterol levels down without the side effects of these potent medications:

- **Herbal remedies:** Garlic has been getting a lot of press lately as a "safe, natural" way to cut cholesterol levels — and it may really help. Just remember that spiking everything with garlic or swallowing garlic pills probably won't make you the most popular person in town. Some health food stores sell coated garlic pills that promise to leave your breath more socially acceptable. (See Chapters 20 and 25.)

- **Nutrition:** Chowing down on soy-based foods may help reduce total cholesterol and LDL cholesterol, and maybe triglyceride levels, too (substances that may also be linked to an increased risk of heart attack). What you want are soy-based foods that contain natural compounds called isoflavones (also called phytoestrogens), according to recent research reported at the American Heart Association's 38th Annual Conference of Cardiovascular Disease, Epidemiology, and Prevention by John R. Crouse III, M.D., a professor at Wake Forest University Baptist Medical Center. Tofu and certain soy drinks are your best bets — but soy sauce doesn't have enough of this stuff to do much for you. (See Chapter 22.)

  Making major lifestyle changes — including going on an extremely lowfat diet and incorporating relaxation techniques into your life — may help clear clogged arteries and lower your risk of heart disease.

- **Vitamins and supplements:** Cholestin, a substance extracted from Chinese Red Yeast, can lower cholesterol levels even better than garlic in healthy adults with moderately elevated cholesterol levels. Chinese Red Yeast has been used for thousands of years in Asia as a base for red wine, as well as a food preservative, spice, and medicine. But whether the standardized extract from it is a "natural dietary supplement" or an unapproved conventional "drug" is a topic of hot debate in the United States. And no one knows yet whether it has any fewer long-term side effects than conventional cholesterol-lowering drugs. Stay tuned. (See Chapter 23.)

We recommend that you avoid the following approaches for treating any kind of heart disease, at least until better evidence comes in:

- **Chelation therapy:** This treatment probably doesn't do anything and may be dangerous. When results from a massive study at Stanford Univeristy come in (maybe next year), we should know more. (See Chapter 4.)

- **Chiropractic:** Although often perfectly fine as a therapy for other conditions in heart patients, this therapy can do little, if anything, for heart disease itself. (See Chapter 13.)

- **DHEA (dehydroepiandrosterone):** This steroid hormone packaged as a dietary supplement may actually increase risk of heart disease! (See Chapter 23.)

- **Lecithin and shark cartilage:** These dietary supplements are basically wastes of money, given the dearth of evidence showing that they work in treating or preventing heart disease. (See Chapter 23.)

- **Ozone therapy:** This approach is way too risky to fool around with if you have heart disease. (See Chapter 4.)

HIV infection and AIDS

AIDS *(acquired immunodeficiency syndrome)* is a condition caused by infection with the HIV virus. By weakening the immune system, the HIV virus eventually leaves people vulnerable to life-threatening infections and cancers *(opportunistic infections)* that people with normal immune systems usually resist.

Right or wrong, many people still regard AIDS — or even infection with HIV — as a death sentence. Promising developments in the past few years may have raised hopes somewhat, but for most victims AIDS remains an ultimately incurable condition. Some alternative healers pooh-pooh this doom-and-gloom attitude, though none of them can pull out convincing evidence that they can cure AIDS or remove every last trace of HIV from the body. What some of their methods may do, however, is relieve some of the symptoms of AIDS and maybe even reduce susceptibility to opportunistic infections.

Right now, no remedy — conventional or alternative — can wipe out AIDS completely (at least as far as we know). But many alternative therapies offer genuine hope to people infected with HIV or living with AIDS:

- **Acupuncture:** These treatments may help relieve AIDS-related nausea, fatigue, or other symptoms. (See Chapter 15.)

- **Bodywork and exercise:** These approaches are hardly cures, but they often help improve overall health and make people with AIDS just plain feel better. (See Chapter 16.)

- **Guided imagery, hypnosis, and meditation:** These mind-body approaches probably can't help you will away HIV, but you can use any of them to make living with your condition easier, and maybe even reduce susceptibility to AIDS-related infections. (See Chapters 17 and 18.)

- **Herbal remedies:** No known herbal remedy has been shown to cure AIDS or even reduce chances of AIDS-related infections. Still, some herbs can be worth trying if you use them safely and in consultation with a qualified practitioner who not only understands herbs but has experience treating AIDS and HIV infection. Taking immunity-boosting herbs (such as astragalus, echinacea, and ginkgo) may help revive an ailing immune system — and certain herbs (such as garlic) may help battle bacteria and viruses. Deglycyrrhizinated licorice can soothe the mouth and throat ulcers that often accompany full-blown AIDS. Just remember that even if these herbs have these powers, no one yet understands just how they work in helping AIDS or whether using them really makes a difference in the course of the disease. (See Chapters 10 and 25.)

- **Hyperbaric oxygen therapy:** Inhaling pure, pressurized oxygen won't drive HIV out of the body, but it may alleviate bothersome symptoms of AIDS — including numbness in the arms and legs and fatigue. It may even help stave off certain "opportunistic infections." The downside is that hyperbaric oxygen therapy costs a bundle and isn't widely available. (See Chapter 4.)

- **Stress reduction techniques:** Getting the stress out of your life may help you resist certain infections — and, in any case, will make it easier to handle any adversity that may come from living with HIV or AIDS. (See Chapter 17.)

- **Thinking positively:** Talking to other people infected with HIV can improve quality of life immensely — not to mention introduce you to new ideas about managing the condition. Social support may even help you resist infection and other AIDS-related debilities. And although keeping the sunny side up won't cure you, it may well play a crucial role in keeping you healthy. (See Chapter 19.)

- **Vitamins and supplements:** Vitamin A supplements may — and the emphasis here is on may — reduce the chances that an HIV-infected mother will pass the AIDS virus on to her unborn child. But substituting vitamins for con-ventional AIDS medications (which are pretty effective in this area) is a big mistake. (See Chapter 23).

- **Yoga:** These positions ostensibly help strengthen immunity. Maybe they do. In any case, yoga can help you relax — an important part of resisting infection and just plain feeling good. (See Chapter 17.)

Right now, you're best off avoiding the following "cures" for AIDS and HIV-infection:

- **DHEA (dehydroepiandrosterone):** Taking these hormone supplements has no proven benefits in treating AIDS and some serious potential dangers. (See Chapter 23.)

- **Ozone therapy:** Bubbling ozone though the blood is supposed to relieve AIDS-related pain and reduce susceptibility to oppor-tunistic infections. And, yes, ozone may indeed blast bacteria and viruses in a test tube. But that result doesn't mean that it will obliterate the HIV virus from a living human body. (See Chapter 4.)

New and bizarre "treatments" for HIV disease crop up daily. The vast majority of them turn out to be useless or dangerous. A very few may end up as useful adjuncts to mainstream therapy. The bottom line is that there is still no proven cure for AIDS. The conventional three- and four-drug cocktails are keeping many people alive who otherwise might not be, even though new resistance is always a problem. The alternatives may provide some degree of relief but probably do not significantly alter the course of the disease — at least so far. Healthy lifestyle measures and a positive attitude probably do as much as anything.

Hypertension

Hypertension is a condition in which blood pressure is consistently high, subjecting blood vessels to considerable stress. Blood pressure readings come as a pair of numbers (such as $^{120}/_{60}$ or $^{110}/_{80}$). The first number, called the *systolic blood pressure,* reflects the pressure on the blood vessels when the heart contracts. The second number, called the *diastolic blood pressure,* reflects the pressure when the heart relaxes. Usually a diastolic blood pressure of 90 or more is considered to be a problem, although different doctors and health organizations disagree over exactly what levels define mild, moderate, and severe hypertension.

Because high blood pressure is the only symptom of hypertension, many people with this condition who feel well stop taking their medication. In doing so, they put themselves at risk for stroke, heart attack, and kidney failure.

The following alternative methods may help control hypertension and in some cases serve as substitutes for conventional blood pressure medications and their often nasty side effects. But remember: How you control your blood pressure doesn't matter. The important

D-28 Best-Bet Alternatives for Specific Conditions

thing is that you get it down and keep it down. Assuming that your "pressure is fixed" is dangerous. This problem requires regular follow-up and monitoring.

- **Ayurveda:** Some parts of Ayurvedic medicine (including meditation techniques, dietary changes, and music therapy) may help reduce blood pressure. (See Chapter 10.)

- **Biofeedback:** This practice can help some (but not all) people with mild hypertension. It's not much help for more moderate to severe hypertension, the type that normally requires drug therapy. (See Chapter 18.)

- **Herbal remedies:** Getting more garlic and onion into your life may help thin blood and/or lower blood pressure (and may even spice up your menus), though right now evidence is mixed and limited. Taking valerian root now and then to relax may indirectly help lower blood pressure, too. Even stronger evidence suggests that hawthorn, including tea made from the hawthorn plant, can lower blood pressure — but it should be used with the guidance of a knowledgeable herbalist who is working together with your M.D. (See Chapters 20 and 25.)

- **Massage:** This therapy can significantly lower both systolic and diastolic blood pressure, plus help knock out feelings of hostility and anxiety that can contribute to high blood pressure. (See Chapter 16.)

- **Music:** Formal music therapy can reduce blood pressure (or raise it, depending on the type of music you choose). (See Chapter 24.)

- **Nutrition:** Making dietary changes alone can help get blood pressure down — or help keep it from climbing in the first place. Both conventional and alternative

practitioners alike advocate adopting a high-fiber, lowfat diet rich in fruits and vegetables, commonly known as the DASH diet. (See Chapter 22.)

New guidelines from the National Heart, Lung, and Blood Institute for the prevention and treatment of hypertension include following the DASH diet. And, though this institute is about as mainstream as you can get, none of their other recommendations will alienate people in the alternative camp. They recommend limiting salt and alcohol intake, eating lots of potassium-rich foods (such as orange juice, prunes, bananas, potatoes, and yogurt), maintaining a healthy weight, avoiding cigarettes, and doing 30 to 45 minutes of aerobic exercise most days.

- **Spirituality:** Prayer and distance healing may make a difference and certainly can't hurt. (See Chapter 19.)

- **Stress reduction techniques:** Any kind of relaxation technique — meditation, yoga, guided imagery, and bodywork included — can help relieve stress and indirectly help keep blood pressure in check. (See Chapters 17, 18 and 19.)

- **Vitamins and supplements:** Magnesium supplements may lower blood pressure a bit, probably by relaxing blood vessels, but long-term effects and safety remain unknown. Potassium and calcium supplements may help, too, at least in some people — but don't fool around with potassium supplements on your own because they can cause potentially fatal changes in heart rhythm. (See Chapter 23.)

Eating oily fish (such as salmon, mackerel, bluefish, or sardines) or taking fish oil supplements regularly may help control high blood pressure. (See Chapter 23.)

If you have hypertension, make sure that you understand the possible signs of heart attack or stroke and get emergency medical care if they occur. You should also contact a doctor if you are pregnant, develop signs of troubling side effects from antihypertensive medications, have a diastolic blood pressure reading of 130 or higher, or experience nausea, hazy vision, headaches, or confusion.

We recommend avoiding the following approaches for treating hypertension:

- **Detoxification:** These regimens to clear out your "system" are too onerous and unproven to be worth the effort. (See Chapter 10.)

- **Electrotherapy and magnetic field therapy:** These treatments haven't been proven to help. If you want to try them anyway, make sure that you're under the care of a qualified practitioner. (See Chapter 24.)

Men's health

Alternative therapies offer help for several conditions that afflict only men.

Prostate problems (noncancerous). The prostate is a small gland that encircles the neck of the bladder and urethra (the tube that transports urine from the bladder through the penis) and secretes part of the sperm-carrying seminal fluid produced during ejaculation. In many men, especially as they age, the prostate becomes abnormally enlarged, resulting in a condition called *benign prostatic hypertrophy,* or *BPH.* Symptoms include painful, weak, incomplete, and/or frequent urination and incontinence.

Another condition, called *prostatitis,* occurs when the prostate gland becomes inflamed or infected. Symptoms include pain or burning during urination, painful ejaculation, bloody semen, general fatigue, frequent urination, pelvic or low-back pain, fever or chills, and impotence.

A man with symptoms of either BPH or prostatitis should contact a physician before trying alternatives. Untreated, prostate problems can result in wide-spread infection, bladder stones, or kidney damage.

The following alternative approaches may provide some relief:

- **Ayurveda:** This medicine offers herbal remedies that may relieve congestion in the prostate. Some yoga postures derived from Ayurvedic medicine may also relieve pain. (See Chapters 10 and 17.)

- **Herbal remedies:** Saw palmetto berries may help shrink an enlarged prostate and help relieve the symptoms of both BPH and prostatitis. (See Chapters 20 and 25.)

  Extract from the stinging nettle root may help urinary retention in men with BPH. Another herbal remedy, uva ursi, may help relieve bladder pain as well. (See Chapter 20.)

- **Homeopathy:** Various remedies claim to relieve prostate problems and probably are harmless enough to try. (See Chapter 12.)

- **Nutrition:** Eating foods rich in zinc and vitamins C and E may help keep the prostate healthy, although evidence is limited. Right now, there's no particular reason to supplement a balanced diet with these vitamins and minerals, or to invest in supplements of specific amino acids, essential fatty acids, or other products promoted as balms for prostate problems. (See Chapter 22.)

- **Traditional Chinese medicine:** This system may help relieve symptoms of either prostatitis and urethritis (an inflamed or irritated urethra) with certain herbal remedies and acupuncture treatments. (See Chapters 9 and 15.)

D-30 Best-Bet Alternatives for Specific Conditions _____

Men are best off avoiding the following alternatives, mainly because the evidence that they work is too slim to justify the expense, pain, or effort involved:

- **Detoxification or colon therapy (enemas):** See Chapter 10.
- **Juice Therapy:** See Chapter 22.
- **Magnetic field therapy:** See Chapter 24.

Prostate cancer. This condition is the second most common cancer affecting men in the United States and is prevalent throughout the world. It occurs when cancerous cells develop in the prostate gland and, often, spread to many other parts of the body. Symptoms of prostate cancer can be quite similar to those of noncancerous prostate problems. They include bloody urine or semen, difficulty in controlling urine stream, burning or painful urination, and painful ejaculation.

Any man who suspects prostate cancer should see a conventional physician. All men over 50 should also be screened for prostate cancer on a yearly basis.

The alternatives that help relieve symptoms of BPH, prostatitis, and other noncancerous prostate problems may also relieve some symptoms of prostate cancer (see preceding section). Plus, eating cooked tomatoes or tomato sauce two or three times a week probably couldn't hurt because these foods contain lycopene, a substance thought to help reduce the risk of prostate cancer. But neither this approach or any alternative should be regarded as a cure or a substitute for conventional therapy.

Impotence. This term is used to describe a condition in which a man cannot achieve or maintain an erection required for a satisfactory sexual experience.

Before you turn to expensive, risky drugs (even the ones getting so much publicity right now), you may consider trying the following alternatives:

- **Acupuncture:** These treatments may help some men. (See Chapter 15.)
- **Aromatherapy:** One sort or another can increase blood flow to the penis. Men may have to experiment, though, to see which particular odor works for them. (See Chapter 21.)
- **Exercise:** Men whose impotence is due to leaking veins may find that Kegel exercises (alternately squeezing and releasing the muscles that control urine flow) can help restore normal function.
- **Herbal remedies:** Ginkgo can increase blood flow, and so — in theory — may help promote erections. But credible studies proving that this herb can actually help impotence don't exist. Evidence is even scantier for ginseng and most other herbal "sexual performance" products riding the coattails of the hot prescription impotence medications. (See Chapter 20.)

We recommend that you avoid the following for treating impotence:

- **Cell therapy and chelation therapy:** These therapies remain too risky and unproven to justify the expense and effort involved. (See Chapter 4.)
- **Magnetic field therapy:** No evidence shows that this therapy works, and it often involves sinking big money into unproven products. (See Chapter 24.)
- **Yohimbe:** Though it may increase sex drive and relieve impotence, this herb can produce serious side effects and is currently banned in the United States as a nonprescription product. If you live elsewhere and still want to try it, make sure that you're under the supervision of a highly skilled practitioner who knows a lot about this herb. (See Chapter 20.)

Mental and emotional well-being

Mental and emotional disorders include any problems that involve disturbances in behavior, feelings, or thinking — even if these problems have their origins in physical or biochemical problems. Conventional therapy often involves psychotherapy, combined with various prescription medications notorious for unpleasant side effects. As a result, many people with mental and emotional disorders are looking to milder, alternative approaches for controlling their symptoms. But if you suspect that you may have a mental or emotional disorder — or suspect one in someone you care for — get an accurate diagnosis from an M.D. and/or psychologist before attempting any treatments on your own.

Alzheimer's disease and memory loss. The term "Alzheimer's disease" includes several disorders characterized by progressively degenerating memory, thinking, and behavior. Afflicting approximately 15 million (usually older) people worldwide, Alzheimer's involves gradual memory loss, apathy, disorientation, communication problems, irritability, and, eventually, degeneration to an infantile state in which sufferers cannot communicate or care for themselves.

Right now no one knows how to cure or reverse this common and tragic condition that can be as devastating for caretakers as for the person with the disease. But some alternatives may be worth trying to help boost memory in people with or without Alzheimer's disease:

- **Bodywork:** *Qi Gong* exercises probably can't hurt to try. (See Chapter 16.)

- **Guided imagery:** This approach may help improve mental functioning and is probably harmless in any case. (See Chapter 18.)

- **Herbal remedies:** *Ginkgo biloba,* an herb that increases blood flow to the brain without increasing blood pressure, has been getting a lot of press lately as a possible memory booster and a way to slow the progression of Alzheimer's. And numerous studies suggest that large, concentrated doses of standardized extract from this herb really can boost memory, concentration, and even social functioning — though not that they can prevent or reverse serious Alzheimer's disease. Ginkgo only seems to help memory problems related to reduced blood flow to the brain. Keep in mind that ginkgo can reduce the ability of blood to clot and can be dangerous if mixed with other anti-clotting drugs, including aspirin. (See Chapter 20.)

  Other herbal remedies — including ginseng — haven't been proven to work but may be worth trying if used prudently. (See Chapter 20.)

- **Vitamins and supplements:** Vitamin E in large doses may slow the progression of Alzheimer's disease to some extent, though effects on the memory of healthy adults remain unknown. And this approach should only be tried with professional guidance, because taking more than 400 IU of vitamin E per day can lead to internal bleeding. (See Chapter 23.)

  The supplement inositol is intriguing but does not yet have enough good data to prove its efficacy yet. Use it only with physician supervision. (See Chapter 26.)

Don't bother trying the following approaches, unless better evidence for their efficacy ever appears:

D-32 Best-Bet Alternatives for Specific Conditions

• **Detoxification:** Removing mercury-based dental fillings or engaging in internal cleansing programs has never been shown to make the least bit of difference in anything but anecdotal reports. Eventually researchers may discover that certain chemical toxins or pollutants may promote Alzheimer's, but right now no one knows enough to claim that avoiding these substances is worth the effort (or even possible).

• **Hyperbaric oxygen therapy:** This therapy can be costly and dangerous and doesn't seem to work in treating Alzheimer's anyway. (See Chapter 4.)

• **Lecithin:** This dietary supplement made from soybean oil, has never been shown to do anything for Alzheimer's in any double-blind, placebo-controlled study. (See Chapter 26.)

• **Nutrition and dietary supplements:** Making dietary changes or taking vitamin or mineral supplements — which, in theory, may help prevent or reverse Alzheimer's — have never been shown to help real live people.

Anxiety disorders. Just getting worried now and then (everyday anxiety) is not a medical disorder. But when it becomes frequent or severe enough to interfere with daily activities, it becomes an official health problem. Psychiatrists usually classify anxiety disorders into different categories, including *phobias* (persistent, irrational fears), *panic attacks* (short episodes of intense fear, rapid heartbeat, and shortness of breath), *generalized anxiety disorder* (free-floating anxiety not associated with any specific fear), and *post-traumatic stress disorder* (feelings of vulnerability and rage, plus related physical symptoms that result after experiencing trauma).

The alternative approaches listed below may help soothe and prevent anxiety, whatever its source. But people who think that they may suffer from any true anxiety disorder should see a qualified health professional for an accurate diagnosis and a discussion of more mainstream treatment options.

• **Aromatherapy:** Certain essential oils may calm you down, though the aroma that makes one person calm can agitate another person. Having an aromatherapy massage with roman chamomile or neroli oil can be particularly soothing. (See Chapter 21.)

• **Basic lifestyle changes:** Cutting back on caffeine, getting enough sleep, and exercising regularly may help prevent anxiety.

• **Biofeedback:** This practice can help train the body to relax itself at will. (See Chapter 18.)

• **Bodywork:** *Tai Chi* and other approaches can help beat stress. (See Chapter 16.)

• **Herbal remedies:** Kava, an herb extracted from the roots of a pepper plant *(Piper methysticum)*, has been used in some traditional cultures to curb anxiety for centuries and is a hot new "natural" alternative to prescription anti-anxiety drugs. Several studies suggest that kava may indeed relieve various anxiety disorders, and general anxiety as well, and, so far, side effects seem minor. (See Chapters 20 and 25.)

Valerian root *(Valeriana officinalis)* is another powerful herbal remedy for anxiety. It has a long history suggesting its powers to induce relaxation and slumber and is one of the most widely used sedatives in the world (though the latest evidence suggests that it doesn't work all that well as a sleep aid). It's also relatively safe, if used in recommended doses. (See Chapters 20 and 25.)

- **Massage and bodywork:** A back massage (even without fragrant oils) can ease anxieties, at least temporarily. So can certain forms of bodywork such as Rolfing and therapeutic touch. (See Chapter 16.)

- **Music:** This kind of therapy can help keep anxieties at bay. (See Chapter 24.)

- **Stress reduction techniques:** These techniques (including meditation, guided imagery, and hypnosis) can often help control generalized anxiety and incapacitating fears. (See Chapters 17, 18, and 19.)

Depression. More than everyday blues or sadness — which are part and parcel of normal human existence — clinical depression involves overwhelming and unrelenting sadness that interferes with daily activity, often accompanied by hopelessness, helplessness, worthlessness, apathy, and guilt. Symptoms include fatigue, sleep disorders, sexual dysfunction, dizziness, headaches, hallucinations, weight changes, and appetite changes. Untreated depression can lead to substance abuse problems and suicide attempts.

Diagnosing your own depression or deciding on your own to lay off prescribed antidepressants is a bad move — and possibly life-threatening. But if you have been diagnosed by a qualified mental health professional as having mild or moderate depression and are under professional guidance, the following alternatives may help lift your mood:

- **Basic lifestyle changes:** Getting enough sleep, exercising regularly, and eating a balanced diet shouldn't be overlooked as ways to stave off certain forms of depression.

- **Herbal remedies:** In Germany, standardized doses of St. John's wort are routinely prescribed to treat anxiety and depression, even though no one really knows how this herbal remedy works or what an optimal dose might be. And in 1996 the prestigious *British Medical Journal* published a review of 23 European studies and concluded that St. John's wort may be useful in treating mild to moderate depression, with only minimal side effects. See K. Linde, et al., "St John's wort for depression — an overview and meta-analysis of randomised clinical trials," *British Medical Journal* 313, 7052 (August 3, 1996): 253–258. (See Chapters 20 and 25.)

Ginkgo may help relieve depression in some people — at least if it's used in large, concentrated doses. But keep in mind that large doses of ginkgo can also interfere with blood clotting and should never be used with other anti-clotting medications, including aspirin. (See Chapters 20 and 25.)

The amino acid tryptophan may help relieve depression in combination with other treatments. But this substance is no longer sold in the United States because a contaminated batch caused 38 deaths and left approximately 1,500 people with a debilitating and incurable condition. (See Chapter 23.)

- **Aromatherapy:** Some people find that jasmine, rose, clary sage, or German chamomile oils used in aromatherapy can lift their mood. (See Chapter 21.)

- **Massage:** This therapy can be a relatively risk-free way to relieve depression. (See Chapter 16.)

- **Stress reduction techniques:** Deep breathing, progressive relaxation, and other methods can sometimes help lift mood. (See Chapter 17.)

Seasonal affective disorder (SAD). This term describes a form of depression that develops during the fall and winter months and disappears during the spring and summer. Although symptoms resemble those of clinical depression (see the preceding section), they recur on a seasonal basis.

SAD needs to be diagnosed by a competent mental health professional, who may suggest trying any of the following approaches (some of which aren't all that alternative anymore):

- **Acupuncture:** This and other forms of Traditional Chinese medicine may help relieve or prevent SAD. (See Chapters 9 and 15.)

- **Basic lifestyle changes:** Surrounding yourself with light or bright colors, getting outside when possible, exercising frequently, or even flying off to sunny climes (if you can) are worth thinking about, too.

- **Light therapy:** Phototherapy is often the treatment of choice for SAD, sometimes together with psychotherapy. (See Chapter 24.)

- **Massage:** This therapy can help keep any form of depression at bay. (See Chapter 16.).

- **Meditation:** This practice (including yoga) and/or guided imagery may be worth a try as well. (See Chapters 17 and 18.)

- **Polarity therapy and aromatherapy:** These approaches seem to relieve the symptoms of some people with SAD. Although none is backed by indisputable evidence, they're all probably safe to try. (See Chapters 16 and 21.)

Pain relief

Pain is something everyone knows about — and wants relief from now and then. True, pain can be a positive way for the body to signal that something is wrong — so that, ideally, something can be done to fix the problem or prevent further damage. When your finger hurts because you touch a flame, for example, pain lets you know to get your finger out of there quick. But many forms of pain are so frequent, unrelenting, or debilitating that all people want is to make them go away — and fast.

The following alternative remedies may help relieve many different forms of pain:

- **Acupuncture:** These treatments may relieve many forms of chronic pain. (See Chapter 15.)

- **Aromatherapy:** This approach may help too, or at least distract you from pain. (See Chapter 21.)

- **Biofeedback:** This practice can help you learn to reduce muscle tension and beat various forms of pain. (See Chapter 18.)

- **Craniosacral therapy:** This form of head and spinal manipulation (performed by some osteopaths, massage therapists, and chiropractors) can sometimes provide relief, especially for sciatica and for chronic neck and back pain. (See Chapters 13, 14, and 16.) And noncranial spinal manipulation can help with back pain (see the upcoming section, "Back and neck pain").

- **Exercise:** Begun with warm-up stretches, regular exercise can sometimes reduce pain by toning muscles and improving flexibility.

- **Herbal remedies:** Topical forms that may relieve pain, tenderness, and/or inflammation include those made from arnica, bromelain, cayenne, or chili peppers, as well as evening primrose oil (EPO) or gamma linolenic acid (an essential fatty acid contained in EPO). (See Chapter 20.)

- **Magnetic field therapy:** This method may help relieve some forms of intractable pain. (See Chapter 24.)

- **Massage:** This therapy, sometimes combined with deep breathing exercises, can help control many kinds of pain. (See Chapter 16.)

- **Neural therapy:** A therapist injects pain-killers *(anesthetics)* into nerve sites to restore the body's natural energy flow. Whether this approach works for the reasons it claims to, it may help relieve many kinds of chronic pain. Use it under the supervision of a trained practitioner. It can be dangerous for people with cancer, diabetes, blood-clotting disorders, kidney disease, myasthenia gravis, or individuals who are allergic to anesthetics or have certain other medical conditions.

- **Psychotherapy:** This approach is hardly alternative anymore and may help certain kinds of pain.

- **Therapeutic touch:** This approach seems to reduce the need for pain medications, at least in some studies. (See Chapter 16.)

- **Various mind-body techniques:** Relaxation, meditation, guided imagery, and hypnosis can often work quite well in relieving pain. (See Chapters 17, 18 and 19.)

Arthritis. This condition involves painful swelling and inflammation of the joints. In osteoarthritis, one of the most common forms, gradual loss of protective cartilage leaves bones to grate against each other, leading to pain and further degeneration. Susceptible joints include knees, hips, spine, thumb, hand, and big toe. In another common form of arthritis, rheumatoid arthritis (RA), membranes lining the joints become hot, swollen, and painful and ultimately may become deformed. Symptoms, which often come and go, include morning stiffness and painful wrists and knuckles. Less often, other joints — including shoulders, jaw, elbows, hips, knees, ankles, or feet — may be affected.

The following alternatives may help relieve pain or swelling from either or both of these conditions:

- **Aromatherapy:** The diluted essential oil from the thyme plant may help relieve joint pain when used as aromatherapy. (See Chapter 21.)

- **Ayurveda:** The herbal remedy curcumin (turmeric) — used in Ayurvedic medicine — may help relieve inflammation from RA if used topically. It may reduce morning stiffness and boost physical endurance if taken internally. (See Chapter 10.)

- **Herbal remedies:** Devil's claw — a remedy consisting of the roots of the *Harpagophytum procumbens* plant — may cut pain, increase range of motion, and reduce morning stiffness — but better studies need to be done to know for sure. If you do want to try it anyway, note that this herb can be quite costly.

- **Nutrition and dietary supplements:** Eating oily fish or taking fish oil supplements (EPA/DHA capsules) may reduce inflammation. Taking pantothenic acid supplements may reduce pain, disability, and stiffness, too, though understanding of effective doses, safety, and long-term effects is limited. The same is true for boron, a trace mineral, that can be toxic in high doses.

  Glucosamine or quercetin supplements may help relieve symptoms of osteoarthritis. Rich sources of glucosamine include shark, chicken, and cow cartilage; green-lipped mussels; and sea cucumbers. Because no one understands safety or long-term effects of these supplements, use them with caution. (See Chapter 23.)

Back and neck pain. Pain in these areas is extremely common and can really take the fun out of life — not to mention lead to innumerable doctor visits, lost work time (and dollars), and disability payments. Besides the general pain-relief tactics listed at the beginning of this section, the following alternatives may provide some relief:

- **Bodywork:** The Alexander technique, Pilates/Physicalmind Method, or the Feldenkrais Method may offer less painful or damaging ways to move or hold your body. (See Chapter 16.)

- **Osteopathic or chiropractic:** Manipulations may help, particularly to relieve acute low-back pain. Effectiveness for chronic pain or disk problems is less certain — but chiropractic is safer than you'd imagine and worth a try. (See Chapter 13.)

- **Yoga:** These postures may help diminish pain. (See Chapter 16.)

Headaches. Headaches can be mild or severe, occasional or continuous, and everything in between. Some are caused by serious underlying problems, others by simple tension. To be safe, sudden or severe headaches, headaches that differ from usual patterns, or headaches that worsen over days or weeks (especially in an isolated part of the head) should be evaluated promptly by an M.D. So should any headache accompanied by fever, stiff neck, speech problems, paralysis, double vision, imbalance, excruciating pain, or pain in the temple.

The following alternatives may help relieve headache pain in addition to the approaches listed earlier in this section:

- **Acupressure and shiatsu:** These techniques can target headache symptoms specifically. (See Chapter 16.)

- **Herbal remedies:** Feverfew is famous for its migraine-busting powers. (See Chapter 20.)

- **Homeopathy:** Certain headache pills may be worth a try. (See Chapter 12.)

- **Nutrition:** Some people find that avoiding certain foods — often chocolate, red wine, MSG, meats containing sodium nitrates, or cheese — prevents headaches. (See Chapter 22.)

- **Vitamins and supplements:** Taking supplements of magnesium may help prevent migraines, especially the kind associated with the menstrual cycle. (See Chapter 23.)

Muscle pain and cramps. These common pains can get you after exercise or strike without warning. Either way, the following approaches may provide relief.

- **Massage:** Sports massage and other forms of massage therapy can be extremely effective pain relievers. (See Chapter 16.)

- **Vitamins and supplements:** The amino acid derivative carnitine (often sold as L-carnitine) may help relieve pain in the legs that occurs during exercise (*intermittent claudication*). So may inositol nicotinate, a derivative of niacin (vitamin B3). (See Chapter 23.)

Some people also swear by ginkgo, calcium, or vitamin E to improve circulation and relieve leg spasms or cramps, but adequate research documenting these claims remains elusive.

Neuralgia. This term refers to nerve pain that occurs when a nerve is irritated or inflamed, and can occur for many reasons.

It includes conditions such as sciatica (back pain that radiates through a thigh and leg) and postherpetic neuralgia (which occurs after a bout of shingles). Anyone with neuralgia should call an M.D. promptly if pain is severe, involves the face, or is accompanied by a dragging foot or difficulty controlling bowel or bladder function.

The following alternative remedies may help relieve neuralgia, in addition to the general pain remedies we list at the beginning of this section:

- **Acupuncture:** These treatments can help relieve severe nerve pain. (See Chapter 15.)

- **Bodywork:** Certain forms — particularly the Alexander technique, Aston Patterning, and the Feldenkrais Method — can help train you to move, sit, and stand in less painful positions. (See Chapter 16.) So can chiropractic and osteopathy. (See Chapters 13 and 14.)

- **Magnetic field therapy:** Stationary magnets — for whatever reason — may help relieve pain. (See Chapter 24.)

- **Massage:** Deep-tissue massage may release tension in muscles that may be pressing on a nerve. (See Chapter 16.)

- **Vitamins and supplements:** Vitamin B6 or vitamin B complex may be worth a try for postherpetic neuralgia. (See Chapter 23.)

Temperomandibular jaw syndrome (TMJ). This painful condition occurs when the joints connecting the jawbone to the skull get out of alignment. Symptoms include jaw pain and sinuses, especially after moving the jaw, as well as a clicking or popping sound during chewing or yawning. Other symptoms may include frequent headaches, a mild earache, and ringing in the ears. Anyone with these symptoms should see a dentist to get an accurate diagnosis, especially because these symptoms may sometimes signal other conditions.

Many of the general pain relief approaches we list at the beginning of this section may help TMJ. Among the most effective are acupuncture, chiropractic, massage therapy, osteopathy, relaxation methods, guided imagery, and hypnotherapy. (See Chapters 13 to 18.)

Tooth and gum pain. These conditions can sometimes be relieved with certain oils used by Ayurvedic healers, acupressure, massage, or just by putting an ice pack or hot compress on the jaw. (See Chapters 10 and 16.) But if the tooth continues to throb, becomes sensitive to heat or cold, or painful, red, swollen gums or a fever develop, seeing a dentist is prudent.

Skin problems

Rashes, pimples, scales, discolorations, itches, and other skin problems can have numerous sources including contact with poison ivy or oak, allergic reactions (*eczema or contact dermatitis*), burns, scars, diaper rash, cradle cap, ringworm, infectious diseases, *vitiligo* (pale patches on the skin), or *psoriasis* (raised, pale scaly patches on the skin). Rashes on the genitals or accompanied by fever, cough, or nasal congestion should be evaluated by an M.D. — as should any slow-to-heal sore or rash (possible signs of serious underlying conditions) or any wart or mole that changes its size, shape, or color (possible signs of skin cancer).

Conventional medical treatment is the only way to go for treating skin cancer — though you can use alternative approaches to relieve the side effects, such as nausea and pain, of conventional therapies. And rashes related to infectious diseases (except perhaps chicken pox) may require conventional guidance as well, as may psoriasis. But the following treatments may be tried to relieve symptoms of many other skin problems:

- **Aromatherapy:** Lavender, clary sage, eucalyptus, niaouli, and rosemary oils may help relieve allergy-related eczema when applied to the rash, added to a bath, or even diffused through the room. (See Chapter 21.)

- **Guided imagery:** This technique may help shrink warts. (See Chapter 18.)

- **Herbal remedies:** Evening primrose oil may help relieve contact dermatitis (rashes due to allergic reactions). Applying aloe to a burn can provide prompt relief. And *Calendula* cream (often sold as a homeopathic remedy) may help relieve minor rashes. (See Chapters 12, 20, and 25.)

- **Light therapy:** Phototherapy may clear up vitiligo, psoriasis, rashes, scars, and many other skin conditions. (See Chapter 24.)

- **Stress reduction techniques:** Any method that cuts down on stress levels — including relaxation methods, guided imagery, hypnosis, meditation — may help relieve psoriasis. (See Chapters 17, 18, and 19.)

- **Traditional Chinese medicine and Ayurveda:** Healers can offer individualized treatment plans — often including dietary changes, acupuncture, and herbal remedies — to treat a variety of skin problems. (See Chapters 9 and 10.)

- **Vitamins and supplements:** Fish oil (10 to 18 grams a day for most people) may relieve red, itchy skin and psoriasis, though studies are conflicting. In any case, these supplements seem to be safe and may be worth a shot. Zinc may help people with the arthritis pain that afflicts some people with psoriasis.

  Also worth trying (even if still basically unproven) are daily supplements of cod liver oil or vitamin A for rashes, vitamin A or zinc to aid skin healing, vitamin E ointment or capsules for itching and dryness, and vitamin B complex for rashes and psoriasis.

Sleep disorders

Sleep disorders include jet lag, *sleep apnea* (brief cessations of breathing), leg cramps, *narcolepsy* (sudden sleep attacks), *bruxism* (teeth grinding), sleepwalking, and *night terrors* (terrifying visions that wake a person but are rarely remembered). Insomnia, probably the best-known sleep disorder of all, may be due to early or frequent awakenings or to trouble falling asleep. Some people are kept awake because of caffeine, medications, medical problems, emotional disorders or trauma, or a condition called "restless legs" in which creepy sensations in the calves, feet, or thighs lead them to jerk their legs uncontrollably.

Some sleep disturbances are signs of serious physical or psychological problems. That's why getting a thorough examination by a qualified M.D. is a good idea before trying to treat anything other than occasional, minor problems on your own. Sleep apnea (often characterized by loud snoring, gasping, and grunting) always requires medical attention.

The following alternatives may help you beat sleep disturbances:

- **Ayurveda:** Healers design a program of breathing exercising, massage, and meditation for your specific disorder. (See Chapter 10.)

- **Basic lifestyle changes:** Probably the best way to beat insomnia is to establish good "sleep hygiene" habits: Keep to a regular sleep-wake cycle; avoid naps; cut back on caffeine; wind down before bedtime; make the bedroom quiet, dark, and comfortable; leave the bed if you can't sleep; exercise regularly; and eat healthy regular meals.

- **Herbal remedies:** Valerian root is a widely used sedative in many countries, routinely prescribed for insomnia. Recently, though, an influential report cast doubt on valerian's powers to help people doze. Because valerian is one of the safest herbal remedies, it may be worth trying anyway. (See Chapters 20 and 25.)

  Kava is an increasingly popular herbal remedy that may help relax you — and indirectly help prevent insomnia. A cup of chamomile tea before bed may also help you nod off. (See Chapters 20 and 25.)

- **Hypnotherapy:** This method may help some people beat sleep disorders. (See Chapter 18.)

- **Stress reduction techniques:** Relaxation methods, meditation (including yoga), guided imagery, and hypnotism may help control insomnia, teeth grinding, and night terrors. (See Chapters 17, 18, and 19.)

- **Traditional Chinese medicine:** Healers may offer an individualized program — involving dietary changes, exercises, herbal remedies, and even acupuncture treatments — to relieve almost any sleep disorder. (See Chapter 9.)

- **Vitamins and supplements:** Melatonin, a natural hormone, may help you fall asleep but probably won't improve the overall length or quality of sleep. Whether melatonin can help prevent jet lag is a topic of hot debate. In any case, using melatonin means that you're manipulating a major hormone system with a little understood and poorly regulated product — one with unknown long-term effects. Use with caution! (See Chapter 23.)

We recommend avoiding the following approaches:

- **Homeopathy:** Don't use these remedies for sleep apnea, except in conjunction with mainstream therapy.

- **Sleeping pills and alcohol:** These are usually bad ideas for anything but occasional use in treating insomnia. Used excessively they can even make insomnia worse!

- **Tryptophan:** This amino acid may relieve insomnia but is no longer available in the United States because a contaminated batch several years ago led to debilities and deaths. Plus, the amount needed to induce drowsiness can make you sick to your stomach.

Smoking and other bad habits

Habits can be hard to break (that's what makes them habits!). But if you want to beat an unhealthy or just plain undesired behavior — including smoking, drinking, nail biting, or thumbsucking — various alternative approaches or combinations of approaches may help you out:

- **Acupuncture:** This treatment can play an important role in recovering from alcoholism and other substance abuse problems. (See Chapter 15.)

- **Aromatherapy:** Inhaling vapor from black pepper extract can reduce nicotine withdrawal symptoms. (See Chapter 21.)

- **Hypnotherapy:** This therapy has helped many a sufferer quit smoking, alter eating patterns, or break other undesired habits. (See Chapter 18.)

- **Nutrition:** Loading up on produce and high-fiber foods can help break bad eating habits. And cutting back on caffeine can reduce symptoms of nicotine withdrawal. (See Chapter 22).

- **Stress reduction techniques:** Relaxation methods, meditation, guided imagery, and biofeedback can help eliminate the stress on which bad habits feed. (See Chapters 17, 18, and 19.)

- **Support groups:** These resources help many people overcome smoking, alcohol and drug abuse, eating disorders, and other unwanted habits. Getting away from other smokers helps a lot, too. (See Chapter 19.)

- **Vitamins and supplements:** Taking various vitamin and mineral supplements may help smokers avoid some of the serious diseases associated with cigarettes. But evidence about any specific supplement is conflicting, and the best approach probably involves eating plenty of fruits and vegetables rich in these substances. (See Chapter 23.)

Herbal stop-smoking products claim to be "natural" alternatives to nicotine patches and gum (the more mainstream way of beating cigarette cravings). They are usually "patented" combinations of what the U.S. Food and Drug Administration considers GRAS (Generally Regarded as Safe) vitamins, minerals, and amino acids, plus herbs such as valerian root and echinacea. Even so, these products probably aren't worth your while. Why? Because the best predictor of smoking cessation is really wanting to quit — and no product, herbal or conventional, can make that happen for you.

Stomach and intestinal troubles

Tummy troubles — diarrhea, constipation, indigestion, nausea, gas (flatulence), belching, and the like — can be everyday annoyances or symptoms of serious physical or psychological disorders. If these problems continue for several months and are accompanied by abdominal pain, they may be diagnosed as *irritable bowel syndrome (spastic colon)*, probably the most common digestive disorder of all. Note that we cover some of the serious conditions that may cause digestive disturbances — including Crohn's disease and ulcerative colitis — in the section "Autoimmune disorders" under the heading of inflammatory bowel disorders.

If any digestive problem persists, becomes severe, or interferes with everyday life, a full evaluation by an M.D. is in order. See an M.D., too, if you experience bloody or black stools, dark urine, severe abdominal pain, or you find yourself losing weight, frequently passing gas, and excreting foul-smelling pale stools (a sign of a serious intestinal disorder) — or if your symptoms are accompanied by insomnia, excessive sweating, fever, coughing, or wheezing. A burning sensation in the upper middle abdomen, sometimes accompanied by other digestive problems, can signal an ulcer (a hole in the stomach lining or other part of the digestive tract) and needs to be evaluated and treated by an M.D.

Below are various alternative approaches that can relieve many digestive woes:

- **Acupressure or shiatsu:** These therapies may alleviate gas pains fast, as well as improve digestion in general and relieve constipation and indigestion. (See Chapter 16.)

- **Acupuncture:** Treatments can help keep nausea at bay and relieve pain associated with irritable bowel syndrome. (See Chapter 15.)

- **Aromatherapy:** Just inhaling certain essential oils can relieve indigestion. Peppermint or rosemary oils work for many people, but you may have to do some experimenting. (See Chapter 21.)

- **Ayurveda:** Healers may tailor a treatment plan — including dietary changes, exercise and meditation techniques, and even sound or music therapy — to remedy various digestive problems. (See Chapters 10 and 24.)

- **Chiropractic:** These treatments — though probably not just spinal adjustments alone — may provide some relief. (See Chapter 13.)

- **Herbal remedies:** Drinking chamomile, ginger, or peppermint tea may calm an upset stomach, relieve gas pains, and reduce nausea. Chili peppers seem to relieve digestive troubles in some people and cause them in others. (See Chapter 20.) Getting a little licorice root down your throat can help heal ulcers. Be sure to use the kind with the glycyrrhizic acid removed, because this is the ingredient that seems to cause serious side effects often associated with licorice (including high blood pressure). And don't expect too much help from eating licorice candy, much of which contains very little of the real thing. (See Chapter 20.)

- **Homeopathy:** Digestive aids may be worth a try for specific symptoms. (See Chapter 12.)

- **Massage:** Gentle massage can often relieve indigestion. (See Chapter 16.)

- **Nutrition and supplements:** Diet can make a huge difference in many stomach and intestinal problems. If you just avoid overeating, you can often prevent indigestion, gas, and bloating. Eating more fiber can help either diarrhea or constipation. Drinking warm lemon juice or eating prunes may relieve constipation, and limiting the diet to dry toast, bananas, applesauce, and rice can help diarrhea. Many people with irritable bowel syndrome find that cutting back on dietary fats provides relief. Avoiding beans, alcohol, spicy foods, or fermented foods may help minimize gas pains or indigestion. And, of course, if the trouble is due to a food allergy, avoiding the problem food is an obvious solution. (See Chapter 22.) Psyllium, or other "natural laxatives," can help the stool absorb water and so prevent or relieve constipation and so may powdered flaxseed. Enzyme supplements may help certain people who get sick after eating dairy products or beans. (See Chapter 4.)

- **Stress reduction techniques:** Get stress under control, and many tummy troubles let up. Relaxation methods, guided imagery, and meditation can all help. (See Chapters 17 and 18.)

- **Yoga:** The postures may provide relief from gas and bloating. (See Chapter 16.) And getting regular exercise of any sort can stave off many digestive troubles.

Weight loss

Eating less and exercising continue to be the safest, most effective ways of getting and keeping off excess pounds. But many people who need (or want) quicker, easier answers turn to potent medications to rev up the metabolism and burn fat quickly — sometimes with serious, even lethal, side effects. So it's no wonder that certain alternative providers are promoting "natural" versions of these prescription remedies (some of which are now banned) and billing them as side-effect free.

D-42 Best-Bet Alternatives for Specific Conditions _____

Here's the real story on some of the most popular alternative weight-loss products on the market:

- **Amino acids such as phenylalanine and L-carnitine:** Bottled as weight-loss products, these supplements supposedly help control food cravings while lifting mood. Although theoretically possible, no one yet has shown that these products help people lose weight — or studied their long-term safety records. (See Chapter 23.)

- **Chromium (chromium picolinate) supplements:** These products are probably wastes of money. Oddly, many promise to speed up your metabolism and to make it work more efficiently — a contradiction in terms, because an efficient metabolism works more slowly so that the body can subsist on fewer calories. So far no credible study proves that chromium supplements can spur weight loss — plus some studies suggest that they may lead to anemia, mental impairment, or kidney problems. (See Chapter 23.)

- **Herbal weight-loss products:** Generally, avoid these products, not only because no evidence proves that they work, but because using them can be dangerous. Usually these products combine St. John's wort (an antidepressive herb) with ephedra (a natural stimulant and appetite suppressant), also known as ma huang. Ephedra has a track record of causing nervousness, insomnia, headaches, high blood pressure, irregular heart beat, heart attack, stroke, psychosis, and even death. Right now, the U.S. Food and Drug Administration is considering banning it or at least requiring a warning label. (See Chapter 20.)

You'll put your time and money to better use with the following alternative weight control aids, coupled with old-fashioned exercise and dietary restrictions:

- **Acupuncture:** The treatments may help control food addictions and cravings. (See Chapter 15.)

- **Aromatherapy:** Sometimes sniffing vanilla, orange, peppermint, or cinnamon can help take the place of eating it. (Ever notice how many bath and body products tout delectable fragrances, offering vicarious pleasure to folks who deny themselves foods? People who would never touch whipped cream douse their hair with frothy mousse; people who would never touch dessert rub vanilla-scented oils into their skin!) Other aromas may just plain relax or energize you, providing sensual pleasure as you "deprive" yourself of cakes and candies. Of course, if the aromas get your juices flowing and send you to the bakery, better stay away! (See Chapter 21.)

- **Basic lifestyle changes:** Regular exercise and a healthy diet are the best ways to go, whether you regard these tactics as mainstream, alternative, or just plain disappointing. There's just no getting around it: The combination of eating a variety of foods (emphasizing vegetables, fruits, and whole grains) and moderating fat, sugar, and alcohol consumption is not only a way to lose weight but — for most people — a healthy way to live. (See Chapter 22.)

- **Homeopathy:** The weight-loss remedies may not work any better than herbal products, but they're almost certainly safer to try. And if using them helps you eat more healthily (for whatever reason), they may be worth the investment. (See Chapter 12.)

- **Hypnotherapy:** This practice can help you beat food cravings, at least temporarily. (See Chapter 18.)

- **Meditation:** This practice can help take your mind off food and help you discover other pleasures. So may other mind-body methods such as relaxation techniques, guided imagery, and yoga (which, in some cases, can also be a good way to get more exercise). (See Chapters 17 and 18.)

Women's health

Women's health is a huge area that includes conditions unique to women or that affect women differently than men. In this section, we describe some of the health issues — related to women's reproductive organs — that are often amenable to alternative therapies.

Breast cancer. Breast cancer is an often lethal form of cancer that has reached epidemic proportions in many developed nations, including the United States. Although no one fully understands the reasons for its extraordinary growth, many researchers cite lifestyle changes, including better nutrition (which may account for earlier first menstrual periods that, in turn, increase lifetime exposure to estrogen), delayed childbearing, and possibly increased exposure to cancer-causing chemicals or foods. Some of the increase may also be due to better detection methods.

Many women discover that they have breast cancer only after having a mammogram — a screening test that all women should have on a regular basis after the age of 40 or so, and earlier if they have a family history of breast cancer. Other women discover a lump in a breast on their own, sometimes as a result of a monthly breast self-evaluation (a good idea for all women). The vast majority of breast lumps are noncancerous — but any lump should be evaluated by a physician because the

earlier breast cancer is discovered, the greater the chances of cure.

No one with breast cancer should rely on alternative therapies alone to treat the condition. But the following approaches may be used together with conventional therapy or may play a role in breast cancer prevention:

- **Acupuncture:** Treatments can reduce nausea from chemotherapy and radiation. (See Chapter 15.)

- **Exercise:** Regular, moderate exercise may help lower the odds of developing breast cancer.

- **Hypnotherapy:** This therapy is often relieves pain that may follow mainstream therapies. (See Chapter 18.)

- **Mind-body approaches:** Guided imagery, meditation, and yoga probably won't make cancer disappear but can make coping with fear, grief, and anger easier. These approaches may also help reduce pain, nausea, vomiting, insomnia, and other side effects of mainstream treatment. (See Chapters 17 and 18.)

- **Nutrition:** Eating more soy-based foods may help prevent breast cancer. Miso, soybeans, tempeh, tofu, and some soy milks contain compounds called isoflavones that act as natural estrogens (*phytoestrogens*). Although the estrogen in hormone replacement therapy (see the section, "Hormone replacement therapy") may increase the risks of breast cancer, phytoestrogens seem to reduce the risk — and probably lower the risk of heart disease and osteoporosis to boot. Interestingly, Japanese women who eat large quantities of soy-based foods have much lower rates of heart disease, hip fractures, and breast cancer than American women.

D-44 Best-Bet Alternatives for Specific Conditions _____

A lowfat, low-calorie diet may reduce the chance of developing breast cancer — but evidence remains elusive. The same is true for taking supplements of antioxidant vitamins such as beta-carotene and vitamins C and E. For now, the best bet (for healthy living in general as well as breast cancer prevention) remains eating a balanced diet rich in fruits, vegetables, and whole grains. (See Chapter 22.)

Restricting alcohol consumption to two or fewer drinks per week may lower risks of developing breast cancer, particularly in younger women.

- **Support groups:** Participation in groups of other breast cancer patients may not only improve the quality of life for breast cancer patients but, in some cases, may even increase life expectancy. (See Chapter 19.)

Cervical dysplasia. This condition occurs when cells in the cervix (the opening to the uterus at the top of the vagina) grow abnormally. Although these abnormally growing *(dysplastic)* cells often revert to normal on their own, they may sometimes become cancerous (cervical cancer) if not treated. Fortunately, regular PAP smears detect most cases early, which makes cervical cancer one of the most preventable cancers.

Often women with cervical dysplasia experience no symptoms at all, and they find out about this condition only when the results of a Pap smear show an abnormality. (Symptoms of cervical cancer may include abnormal vaginal bleeding and pelvic pain.) If Pap smear results do come back abnormal, a woman should discuss mainstream treatment options with her clinician. These options may include more tests to examine the cervix, removal of the abnormal cells, or just plain watchful waiting.

Some alternative approaches may help as well but are no substitutes for regular Pap smears or conventional medicine:

- **Basic lifestyle changes:** Limiting sexual partners and using a diaphragm or condom together with spermicidal creams or jellies may help prevent cervical dysplasia, which is often associated with the sexually-transmitted human papilloma virus (HPV). Avoiding cigarettes can reduce the chances of cervical dysplasia, as well as help prevent dysplasia from developing into cancer.

- **Nutrition, vitamins, and supplements:** Supplementing certain vitamins — especially vitamins A and C, and folic acid — may prevent dysplasia and perhaps prompt dysplastic cells to revert to normal. A diet rich in fruits and vegetables may work just as well — and is a good idea anyway. (See Chapters 22 and 23.)

- **Stress reduction techniques:** Relaxation and meditation can relieve stress that often arises while waiting for test results or enduring pelvic examinations and procedures. (See Chapters 17 and 18.)

Endometriosis and pelvic pain. Women may develop pain in the lower abdominal region (pelvic pain) for many reasons, including pelvic inflammatory disease (PID, an infection of the reproductive organs), cancer, uterine fibroids (abnormal growths), ectopic pregnancy (which occurs when the embryo grows outside the uterus), a twisted or ruptured ovarian cyst, impending miscarriage, bladder infection, menstrual cramps, *adhesions* (scar tissue), and *endometriosis* (a condition in which tissue normally lining the uterus grows in other places). Many of these conditions require conventional medical care, so pelvic pain needs to be evaluated by an M.D.

Although not cures for serious causes of pelvic pain (including endometriosis, PID, uterine fibroids, or cancers), many alternatives may relieve pain:

- **Acupuncture:** The treatments may significantly reduce pain. (See Chapter 15.)

- **Basic lifestyle changes:** Limiting sexual partners and practicing "safer sex" (by using condoms, diaphragms, spermicidal jellies and creams, and the like) can reduce the chances of contracting a sexually transmitted disease and related pelvic pain.

- **Chiropractic:** Manipulations may help as well, though more studies need to be done to know for sure. (See Chapter 13.)

- **Herbal remedies:** Various herbs purport to treat endometriosis, but right now the evidence for their safety and efficacy remains too scant to recommend any specifically. The same is true for nutritional supplements such as vitamins, minerals, and essential fatty acids (such as gamma linolenic acid and evening primrose oil). Stay tuned.

- **Nutrition:** Eating cranberries or drinking cranberry juice can help prevent urinary tract infections. (See Chapter 20.)

- **Stress reduction techniques:** Relaxation methods, meditation, and guided imagery can zap stress that can contribute to pelvic pain. (See Chapters 17 and 18.)

Hormone-replacement therapy (HRT). Sometimes called *estrogen replacement therapy,* HRT during and after menopause (the cessation of menstrual periods) is a topic of hot debate in women's health care. Accumulating evidence suggests that supplements of the hormone estrogen (often in combination with the hormone progesterone) can help relieve menopausal symptoms (such as hot flashes and vaginal dryness) and may also help prevent heart disease, osteoporosis, and possibly even Alzheimer's disease and other conditions. On the other hand, taking these hormones may slightly increase the risks of breast cancer and, if estrogen is not combined with progesterone, uterine (endometrial) cancer. Plus, some women object to hormone supplementation for philosophical reasons.

As a result, various alternatives to synthetic hormones are widely promoted to help relieve menopausal symptoms and/or prevent osteoporosis and heart disease in women:

- **Basic lifestyle changes:** Avoiding cigarette smoking — and cutting back on alcohol and caffeine consumption — may lower the risk of osteoporosis (the loss of bone mass that may increase the risk of serious fractures). So may avoiding rapid weight loss and excessive thinness. Regular weight-bearing exercise (such as brisk walking, hiking, jogging, dancing, jumping rope, stair climbing, weight training, or tennis) can help build bone mass and so reduce the risk of osteoporosis.

- **Herbal remedies:** Black cohosh or dong quai helps some women with menopausal symptoms. (See Chapter 20.)

A new "natural progesterone" pill made out of the Mexican wild yam has just been approved in the United States as a treatment for irregular menstrual periods — and it's being evaluated as an alternative to the synthetic progesterone *(progestins).* This pill may help prevent uterine lining from building up abnormally (a risk factor for uterine cancer) and, unlike progestins, won't decrease levels

D-46 Best-Bet Alternatives for Specific Conditions

of HDL cholesterol (the so-called good cholesterol). But it may produce the same side effects as synthetic progesterones (including vaginal bleeding, weight gain, mood swings, and headaches.)

Nonprescription creams made from "natural" progesterone may relieve for vaginal dryness and don't cause the same side effects as either natural or synthetic progesterone pills. Although these creams can't be relied on to prevent uterine cancer, a new prescription gel made from natural progesterone seems to be absorbed better through the skin and may someday become a viable alternative to progesterone pills (natural or synthetic), though it's quite costly.

Avoiding most other over-the-counter "HRT alternatives" (unless under the supervision of a qualified practitioner) is probably smart: Most of these have never been tested for efficacy and may contain mysterious and potentially dangerous substances.

- **Nutrition:** Soy-based foods such as tempeh, tofu, soy powder, and soy milk may help reduce hot flashes (though usually not as well as HRT). So may supplements of the natural estrogens (phytoestrogens) contained in many of these foods. They also may help prevent heart disease and stroke by preventing plaque from accumulating in arteries (atherosclerosis), perhaps just as well as conventional HRT, though neither approach works too well in reducing plaque that has already accumulated. (See Chapter 22.)

- **Stress reduction techniques:** Relaxation exercises, guided imagery, meditation, prayer, or any tactic that elicits the relaxation response or reduces stress may help relieve hot flashes. (See Chapters 17, 18, and 19.)

- **Support groups:** Social support can not only provide ideas about coping with menopausal symptoms and age-associated changes but may actually help reduce physical symptoms. (See Chapter 19.)

- **Vitamins and supplements:** Calcium and perhaps vitamin D may help prevent and even relieve osteoporosis. Adding lowfat milk powder to soups and sauces isn't a bad idea either. Premenopausal women need at least 1,000 milligrams of calcium per day; adolescent, pregnant, and breastfeeding women need 1,200 milligrams and postmenopausal women not taking HRT need 1,500 (those taking HRT need 1,000). Calcium carbonate is usually the cheapest and best absorbed form of calcium, and should be taken with food. Many women, especially those who are older, sick, or poorly nourished also need to take vitamin D supplements (400 to 800 IU per day) because calcium cannot be absorbed without enough vitamin D. (See Chapter 23.)

We recommend avoiding DHEA (dehydroepiandrosterone) pills as a way to treat menopausal symptoms, reverse aging, and the like. Not only is there little evidence of benefits, but DHEA may decrease evidence of HDL cholesterol, which in turn may increase a woman's risk of heart attack and lead to serious side effects including masculinization and liver damage. (See Chapter 23.)

Infertility and pregnancy loss. The inability to become pregnant or deliver a healthy newborn (due to repeated pregnancy loss) isn't always a women's health problem; in fact, for 40 percent of couples, the problem lies with the man, and in 20 percent of couples, factors in both the man and woman account for the problem. But many women do have conditions that make it difficult, if not impossible, for them to bear children, including endometriosis, pelvic inflammatory disease, sexually transmitted disease, hormone imbalances, growths in the uterus (polyps or fibroids), advanced age, and many unknown factors.

Some of these problems cannot be corrected by any approach known to humankind. Others are amenable to high-tech, expensive, and often emotionally wrenching feats of modern medicine. But in a surprising number of cases, lower-key alternatives may help:

- **Acupuncture:** The treatments may be worth a try, if only because some women credit acupuncture with helping them get pregnant.

- **Basic lifestyle changes:** Avoiding cigarettes may help improve the chances of conception. Avoiding illegal drugs may help regulate secretion of hormones important for ovulation (the release of an egg from the ovary) and the build-up of lining in the uterus.

  Eating a balanced diet and maintaining a normal weight can help regulate hormone production. (See Chapter 22.)

  Limiting sexual partners, using condoms and spermicides, and practicing "safer sex" may reduce the odds of contracting sexually transmitted diseases that often underlie infertility.

  If you want children, plan to bear them in your 20s and 30s if possible. Fertility decreases with age.

- **Stress reduction techniques:** Meditation, yoga, mindfulness, guided imagery, relaxation exercises, and any other stress-busters may help some infertile women become pregnant. The same techniques can help women cope with grief, anger, guilt, and other emotions often associated with pregnancy loss or infertility. (See Chapters 17 and 18.)

- **Support groups:** Involving other women who are infertile or who have experienced pregnancy loss may be invaluable in terms of both emotional and spiritual uplift and concrete ideas about new treatments and/or accepting infertility. (See Chapter 19.)

Pregnancy, childbirth, and breastfeeding. Conceiving, gestating, and delivering a healthy normal baby can pose innumerable health concerns for women, and many of these concerns can be helped with alternative approaches. Any pregnant woman should contact a physician promptly, though, if she experiences heavy vaginal bleeding, persistent vomiting, severe abdominal pain, ruptured "bag of waters," or — during the last three months of pregnancy — swollen hands or face, continuous headaches, or blurred vision. After childbirth, the following symptoms also warrant a call to the doctor: persistent pain around the genitals, foul-smelling vaginal discharge, high fever, a hot or painful breast, nausea, vomiting, painful urination, chest pain, or cough.

The following alternatives may provide relief for some common pregnancy-related problems:

- **Acupuncture:** Treatments can relieve nausea and vomiting of morning sickness. They may also stimulate the uterus to contract in women past their due dates. (See Chapter 15.)

- **Aromatherapy:** Using jasmine oil may help stimulate milk production in breastfeeding women. (See Chapter 21.)

D-48 Best-Bet Alternatives for Specific Conditions _____

- **Guided imagery:** This has become a common, essentially mainstream, approach to help women tolerate the pain of labor and delivery. Various relaxation techniques and meditation approaches can help, too. (See Chapters 17 and 18.)

- **Herbal remedies:** Ginkgo, hawthorn, or horse chestnut may help relieve varicose veins or hemorrhoids that often occur during pregnancy. Pregnant women should avoid taking any herbal remedy internally, though, except under the supervision of a qualified clinician. (See Chapter 20.)

  Raspberry leaf tea is a tried-and-true tonic for many pregnancy woes according to many herbalists. But try to avoid taking any "remedy" — except good nutrition and a basic multivitamin — during the first trimester of pregnancy, when the fetus is forming basic organ systems.

  Bromelain, an herbal remedy derived from the pineapple plant, may help relieve pain and swelling after an *episiotomy* (a surgical incision made next to the vagina to prevent tearing during delivery). (See Chapter 20.)

- **Massage:** This therapy may help relieve varicose veins. (See Chapter 16.)

- **Stress reduction techniques:** Any mind-body approach that reduces negative stress — including relaxation exercises, meditation, yoga, or guided imagery — can encourage the production of breast milk. (See Chapters 17 and 18.)

- **Vitamins and supplements:** Taking fish oil supplements may help prevent premature birth. Eating oily fish such as salmon, mackerel, sardines, or bluefish several times a week may help, too, but pregnant women are probably better off with supplements because fish may contain levels of mercury and other contaminants that put a growing fetus at risk. (See Chapter 23.)

Premenstrual syndrome. This common condition is characterized by any of several symptoms that recur 5 to 15 days before menstruation begins and usually let up after the first day or two of bleeding. Common symptoms include mood swings, headaches, bloating, breast swelling and pain, weight gain, insomnia, hot flashes, nausea, constipation, diarrhea, food cravings, irritability, anxiety, anger, depression, nervousness, pelvic pain, back pain, muscle pain, joint swelling, and acne.

Many alternative approaches may ease the symptoms of PMS:

- **Aromatherapy:** Lavender, Roman chamomile, neroli, or clary sage oils often help relieve mood swings, anxiety, irritability, and other negative emotions. (See Chapter 21.)

- **Basic lifestyle changes:** Regular exercise and healthy sleeping and eating habits can sometimes keep symptoms at bay. Regular aerobic exercise can lessen the symptoms of PMS and menstrual problems in general, by slightly decreasing hormone levels (but don't do it to the point that you stop menstruating — as often happens with women who lose too much body fat).

- **Herbal remedies:** Supplements of evening primrose oil, or the essential fatty acids it contains (linolenic and gamma linolenic) may relieve breast and other premenstrual pain. (See Chapter 20.)

- **Nutrition:** Avoiding certain foods — especially chocolate — may help reduce food cravings in some women. Other women find relief from eating more protein and complex carbohydrates; cutting back on caffeine, alcohol, and/or sugar; and/or eating smaller, more frequent meals. Eating an extremely lowfat diet (with under 15 percent of daily calories from fat) may help relieve premenstrual breast pain. (See Chapter 22.)

- **Stress reduction techniques:** Relaxation, meditation, and yoga may help control moodiness, depression, anger, irritability, and anxiety. (See Chapters 17 and 18.)

- **Traditional Chinese medicine:** Healers may recommend certain herbal remedies to ease numerous PMS symptoms. (See Chapter 9.)

- **Support groups:** A group, especially one led by a psychotherapist, may provide coping strategies and help reduce the severity of symptoms. (See Chapter 19.)

- **Vitamins and supplements:** Taking supplements of calcium (1,000 milligrams a day), magnesium (200 milligrams a day during the second half of the menstrual cycle), vitamin B6 (50 to 200 milligrams a day), and vitamin E (150 to 400 IU a day) seems to help relieve depression or breast pain in some women. Taking magnesium may also help prevent premenstrual migraine headaches. (See Chapter 23.)

Vaginal irritation and infections. Pain, swelling, redness, and itching of the vagina or vulva are extremely common. They can be caused by poor hygiene, physical trauma, retained foreign objects (tampons, diaphragms, and so on), hormone changes (due to birth control pills, HRT, pregnancy, or menopause), diabetes, douching, sexually transmitted diseases (STDs), infections, or even psychological factors. When vaginal irritation is accompanied by abnormal vaginal discharge, it may be called *vaginitis,* a term that includes common

vaginal infections such as yeast infections, trichomonas, bacterial vaginosis, and cytologic vaginosis.

Any vaginal or vulvar irritation that persists for more than a few days or that is accompanied by severe pain, abnormal bleeding, rash, or fever should be evaluated by a qualified clinician to rule out the possibility of STDs, toxic shock syndrome, and other conditions that require conventional therapy.

The following alternative approaches may help provide relief for vaginal itching, soreness, and/or abnormal discharge:

- **Herbal remedies:** Certain topical botanical remedies — including tea tree oil, echinacea, garlic, goldenseal, and calendula — may relieve irritation, though not necessarily any more safely or effectively than any other nonprescription cream. Cranberries may help prevent urinary tract infections that sometimes irritate the vulva. (See Chapters 20 and 25.)

- **Homeopathy:** These remedies may be worth a try for minor vaginal irritation. (See Chapter 12.)

- **Hygiene:** Practicing the standard rules is the best line of defense. Included are keeping the vulva clean, dry, and cool; wiping from front to back after a bowel movement; getting enough rest; eating a balanced diet; using a vaginal lubricant if necessary; and avoiding douching, which can predispose women to vaginal infections. Limiting sexual partners, using spermicides and condoms, and following guidelines for "safer sex" in general can help prevent sexually transmitted diseases, although some women develop vaginal irritation from spermicides. Sitz baths with or without epsom salts can provide welcome relief from pain and itching.

D-50 Best-Bet Alternatives for Specific Conditions _____

- **Psychotherapy:** This type of treatment may help relieve some forms of vaginal pain, although it's hardly considered an alternative approach these days.

- **Stress reduction techniques:** Minimizing negative stress can help prevent vaginal irritation or reduce pain from them. These techniques include relaxation exercises, meditation, yoga, hypnotherapy, and guided imagery. (See Chapters 17 and 18.)

No credible evidence backs the common claim that coffee, alcohol, sugar, refined carbohydrates, or any other food predisposes women to vaginal infections or that cutting back on these substances helps cure them. Nor is there any reason to think that eating yogurt has any merit in treating vaginal irritation, though go ahead and eat it if it pleases your palate.

Part VIII
The Part of Tens

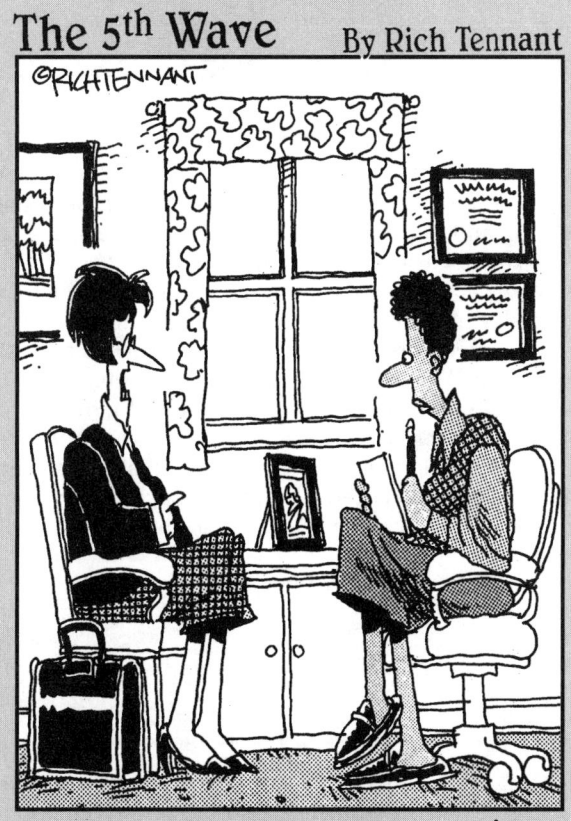

The 5th Wave   By Rich Tennant

"I think my body's energy centers
ARE well balanced. I keep my pager
on my belt, my cell phone in my right
pocket, and my palmtop computer in
my inside left breast pocket."

In this part . . .

We get an extra chance here to fill you in on some fun and important facts we didn't have space to cover in detail earlier in the book. We spell out just which alternatives are almost always safe to try, and which ones are risky. We also fill you in on some "hot" herbs and dietary supplements that are taking the world's pharmacies by storm. Want to know more about echinacea, garlic, ginkgo, dong quai, kava, saw palmetto, or valerian? How about androstenedione and creatine, the stuff the athletes are swallowing like candy? Or substances that have whole books written about them such as 5-HTP, St. John's wort, and ginseng? You're in the right place.

Chapter 25

Ten Herbs Everyone's Talking About

. . . .

In This Chapter

▶ Finding out about herbs that you have to know to be "in the know"

▶ Separating the reality from the hype

▶ Using these herbs safely — and deciding when not to use them

. . . .

*T*his chapter introduces you to ten of the top "superstar" herbs that are taking the health world (and drugstore shelves) by storm. Some of these herbs may help relieve everyday ailments with fewer side effects than conventional therapies — and, often, at a much lower cost. Others rest their claims more on tradition — or the efforts of slick marketers — than on scientific evidence. But one thing is certain: You have to know a little something about every one of these herbs if you're going to make it through the next cocktail party without drowning in a sea of misinformation and hype. This chapter gives you the scoop in no time.

Aloe

Traditional folklore has it that a little gel taken from the aloe *(Aloe vera, Aloe barbadensis*, or *Aloe vulgaris)* plant can help soothe burns and speed wound healing — and the folklore apparently has it right, at least when it comes to burns. Whether aloe speeds wound healing is more uncertain, particularly in healthy, young people, whose bodies are pretty darn good at healing themselves. However, aloe may indeed be useful in speeding up healing in elderly people, who typically have problems with slow wound healing due to bed sores, diabetes, or circulation problems. Even better, aloe doesn't have any known serious side effects or dangerous interactions with other medications — though swallowing dried juice from the aloe plant can get your bowels moving a little faster than you may like.

Aloe's ability to trigger healing may turn out to be even more useful. Already the U.S. Department of Agriculture has sanctioned aloe as a cancer treatment for dogs and cats (although it is not yet safe for injection into human beings). But so far aloe's promise in treating anything but wounds and burns remains largely unexplored territory.

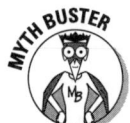

One caveat: Using commercial aloe products may not bring you the same relief as squirting a little gel out of your home-grown aloe plant. That's because aloe may lose some of its healing powers during storage, or the commercial products may contain minuscule quantities of aloe.

Dong Quai

With baby boomers hitting menopause, it's no wonder that dong quai (*Angelica polymorpha* or *Angelica sinensis*) is getting a ton of press. This remedy (also known as dang gui or tang kuie) has been used in China for generations to treat menopausal symptoms such as hot flashes and night sweats, plus relieve menstrual distress and irregularity. But, oddly, most Western women don't have good luck with it, perhaps because dong quai needs to be used alongside other traditional Chinese herbs and other techniques. Expecting it to act like a magic bullet — vanquishing symptoms at the pop of a pill — may be unrealistic.

Whether it helps, dong quai needs to be used with considerable caution — and, ideally, under the guidance of a practitioner skilled in traditional Chinese medicine. In some people, doing quai may lead to skin rashes or light sensitivity. And it's just plain dangerous for pregnant woman — so if there's any chance that your menstrual "irregularity" is actually due to pregnancy, take a pregnancy test before trying dong quai.

Echinacea

Don't be surprised if someone suggests trying echinacea the next time you find yourself under the weather. One of the hottest herbs around, this remedy is derived from the purple coneflower, a member of the lowly daisy family native to the central United States. Increasing evidence suggests that this little plant may stimulate the immune system and help you keep cold and flu symptoms at bay if you take it after the first sneeze or cough. It may even help prevent recurrent infections (including urinary and ear infections). And applying echinacea as a topical cream may relieve insect bites, eczema, cold sores, burns, psoriasis, and hard-to-heal wounds.

If you're not using the right form, part, or species of this herb, don't count on results. The best studies documenting echinacea's power were done in Germany and used an injectable form of the herb — a form not available in the United States (where most people take echinacea by mouth). Those results don't mean that other forms don't work — but there are no guarantees until better data come in.

For now, try sticking to standardized extracts packaged by reputable manufacturers. Only buy from vendors who can assure you that their products are unadulterated. Alcohol/water extract tinctures are usually your best bets (just look for these words on the package). And make sure that the product you purchase contains the part of the echinacea plant that has been shown to work (the recently dried whole plant of the *Echinacea angustifolia* or *Echinacea purpurea,* or roots of the *Echinacea pallida*).

Don't take echinacea for longer than eight weeks at a time, or it may lose its effects. Of course, if you're one of those people who keeps good records, you could try taking it for up to eight weeks during peak cold season, lay low for about a month, and then start dosing yourself again if necessary.

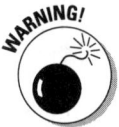

Echinacea is a relatively safe herb, but it may cause allergic reactions, especially in people allergic to plants in the daisy family. And it should never be used (without consent of an M.D.) by pregnant women or by anyone with tuberculosis, autoimmune disorders, or other serious diseases that stress the immune system (including HIV infection, cancer, and diabetes). If you have a problem with recurrent infections, getting a physical examination before you start treating yourself with echinacea is a smart move.

Garlic

Everyone knows that garlic is good at keeping vampires (and friends) away — but garlic may also be good at keeping disease (especially heart disease) away as well. In fact, the same chemical that gives garlic its distinctive odor and flavor (allicin) seems key to this herb's health benefits.

Allicin can lower levels of cholesterol and triglycerides in the bloodstream (at least in adults) — and so perhaps the lower risk of heart disease. This little herb appears to be able to do lots of other neat tricks, too — including thinning the blood, and maybe preventing and reversing the build-up of plaque on artery walls *(atherosclerosis)* that can lead to heart attacks. It may also help destroy disease-causing microbes, lower blood pressure, and even reduce the risks of certain types of cancer. (By the way, onions and leeks contain chemicals similar to allicin, so they may have similar abilities.)

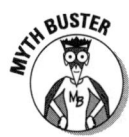

But before you start wolfing down the pesto sauce, keep in mind that no one so far has proved that eating garlic is going to lower your chances of heart disease, cancer, or any other condition. No one knows if cutting or crushing garlic reduces its potency. Plus, if you want results, you'll have to eat the garlic raw (or take garlic pills), because cooking destroys allicin. In fact, you have to eat about 5 to 20 cloves every day to reduce atherosclerosis and 1 clove a day to lower cholesterol levels. And even though garlic is about as safe as any herb can be, large doses can cause serious bleeding problems if used with aspirin or other blood-thinning drugs.

Still, if you're battling high cholesterol and/or high triglycerides, you may want to talk to your clinician about garlic. If chomping on vast quantities of raw garlic or taking garlic powder tablets disturbs your stomach or your friends, try odorless enteric-coated tablets of freeze-dried garlic. These tablets allow you to get the garlic beyond your stomach before any of the allicin escapes.

Ginkgo

If your health problems are related to sluggish blood circulation, an extract from the leaves of the ornamental ginkgo *(Ginkgo biloba)* tree may help. The ginkgo tree has been the source of many Chinese medicines for thousands of years. And, today, people are getting really excited because concentrated extracts from ginkgo leaves have been shown to improve blood flow through the arteries and veins — and so may help treat many conditions associated with reduced circulation, especially in older people, including short-term memory loss, thinking disorders, dizziness, ringing in the ears, and head-aches. Ginkgo may also help relieve *intermittent claudication,* a condition in which the legs become painful during walking or other exercise.

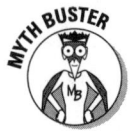

But perhaps you've heard that ginkgo can cure Alzheimer's disease, turn you into an Einstein, or at least improve memory, alertness, concentration, and energy in just about anyone. Here the evidence is less convincing. Yes, ginkgo may improve thinking or relieve mental disorders related to blocked arteries (which block blood flow to the brain) — but it probably won't help if your problems have other roots (or if you just want to be smarter or more alert).

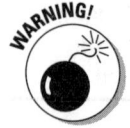

Ginkgo is also very good at keeping blood from clotting. Although this property may help prevent some kinds of heart attacks, it may also cause dangerous internal bleeding in people already taking anticlotting (blood-thinning) medications, including aspirin. In recommended doses, ginkgo rarely causes serious side effects, and even in very large doses, most effects can easily be reversed simply by stopping the herb or reducing doses.

Ginseng

Ginseng — also known as Asian, Chinese, or Korean ginseng — is an herbal remedy that comes from the roots of the *Panax ginseng* plant. It is often confused with American ginseng (sometimes also called just plain ginseng —

which explains the confusion), which comes from the roots of the *Panax quinquefolius,* a North American species of *Panax.* Adding to the confusion is a third ginseng, Siberian ginseng *(Eleutherococcus senticosus),* which some advocates say works better and more safely than Asian ginseng.

In traditional Chinese medicine, ginseng (of the Asian variety) is a kind of cure-all — a prized "tonic" with powers to boost energy and vitality, promote resistance to disease, and restore male sexual potency. In fact, the name *Panax* comes from the word *panacea,* which means cure-all. More recently, Westerners have turned to this drug as an immune-system stimulant, physical and mental energy booster, and as a specific antidote for diabetes, menopausal symptoms, ulcers, depression, and many other stress- or age-related conditions.

A vast sea of literature describes and applauds these effects — but, amazingly, very little decent scientific evidence backs them up. Most of the studies so far have been poorly designed, so that no one could determine whether results were due to ginseng, some other stimulant it was mixed with, or the power of suggestion. Better data may come in soon — but many of ginseng's supposed effects (such as increasing resistance to disease or stress) are indirect and so nearly impossible to prove using the standards of Western science (see Chapter 3).

On the plus side, ginseng in recommended doses is probably safe for most healthy people — though anyone with asthma, emphysema, fibrocystic breast disease, blood clotting disorders, hormonal abnormalities, or heart beat irregularities should consult a physician, as should pregnant or breastfeeding women. And if you're tired all the time, don't be foolish — go see a doctor. The problem could be something simple and treatable such as anemia or low thyroid hormone.

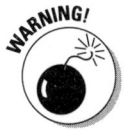

Even though ginseng is supposedly a treatment for diabetes, no one with this disease should use it without medical guidance because it may lead to low blood sugar. People with high blood pressure should generally avoid Asian ginseng *(Panax ginseng)* in particular because it may raise blood pressure. Some people using ginseng have reported side effects such as insomnia, irritability, diarrhea, and skin rashes, though no one's really sure which species — or the amount — of ginseng they were using.

If you do decide to try ginseng, you should ideally buy whole ginseng root to make sure that you're getting all the active ingredients — but the cost can be prohibitive. If you're using ginseng as a preventive tonic (kind of like a daily multivitamin), paying over $20 an ounce may not sit too well. Your other option is to go with a commercial product, but confirm that you're getting actual ginsenosides (one of the main active ingredients in ginseng root). Many products with "ginseng" on the label contain little or none of the real thing — and often the amount varies from brand to brand, or even batch to batch.

Traditional healers say that anyone taking Asian ginseng on a regular basis should take a 1 to 2-week break every 2 to 3 weeks. People taking Siberian ginseng can go 5 to 7 weeks before taking a 1-to-2 week break.

Kava

Kava isn't quite as much of a household word as some of the other herbs in this chapter — but it's getting to be one, and quick. This herbal remedy, derived from the root and stem of a South Pacific plant called *Piper methysticum,* is being sold as an anxiety-reliever, or — in the United States, where it cannot legally make any health claims for itself — as a way to relax, achieve bliss, or beat the "yuppie blues." Kava also has the power to get people high, but you probably won't hear much about that from the folks trying to push it as a "natural" alternative to conventional tranquilizers and sedatives.

Clearly, kava does something to the body — probably due to its natural muscle relaxants *(kavalactones).* But just what kava does and how it does it remains largely unexplored. So do basic issues such as safe and effective dosage and long-term safety, plus questions about how kava interacts with other drugs. For now, all we have to go on are a few German studies suggesting that this herb may help relieve anxiety. What we don't know is whether kava relieves anxiety better — or more safely — than any other remedy.

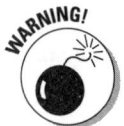

Take too much kava, and you may end up reeling. (Remember, some people use it as a recreational drug or an aphrodisiac.) And use it too long, and your skin may start to peel or dry out.

Saw Palmetto

Until the 1950s, conventional M.D.s in the United States used a plant that grows in the southern United States and the West Indies called the saw palmetto or dwarf palm *(Serenoa repens)* to treat bladder infections and enlargement of the prostate. Even today, saw palmetto is widely prescribed in Europe to treat men with benign prostatic hypertrophy (BPH), a noncancerous enlargement of the prostate gland. And throughout the Western world, saw palmetto is a top-selling alternative treatment for a whole host of conditions, including BPH, impotence, asthma, and even undesirably small breasts.

Recent studies show that chemicals in the ripe berries of the saw palmetto do have some demonstrable effects in a test tube — including mimicking the female hormone estrogen and counteracting male sex hormones. And some small, short-term European studies have suggested that saw palmetto may help relieve the symptoms of mild and moderate BPH just about as well as conventional drugs — and without the cost and nasty side effects. But other equally credible studies show that saw palmetto works no better than a placebo. And so far, no credible data backs claims that it can treat asthma or bronchitis, boost sex drive and endurance, increase sperm production, or enlarge women's breasts.

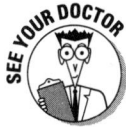

For now, the most prudent way to use saw palmetto is to talk to your doctor about it if you have BPH. Although no one knows for sure whether it will help, this herb seems to be safe for virtually anyone (in fact, it was a popular food among southeastern Native Americans), and side effects seem to be minimal. Long-term effects remain unknown.

Make sure that any product you purchase contains extracts from the fresh or partially dried ripe fruits (often labeled as *fatty acids* or *lipophilic extracts*) — the part of the saw palmetto that works. And don't bother sipping saw palmetto teas, which will have little effect because the active chemicals dissolve poorly in water.

St. John's Wort

St. John's wort *(Hypericum perforatum)* is a yellow-flowered perennial plant that may help treat mild or moderate depression — with minimal side effects. We hate to be killjoys, but — despite the fairly convincing evidence that this stuff may do some good — right now we can't in good faith recommend using this herb except under the supervision of an M.D. who is treating the depression.

This advice is particularly true in countries (including the United States), where extracts sold in herbal remedies are not tested for safety or efficacy, or standardized. But even in countries with better quality controls (such as Germany), and where St. John's wort is already routinely prescribed to treat anxiety and depression, this herb is not a remedy you want to be using on your own. That's partly because no one fully understands how it works, how it affects people long-term, or what doses work optimally. Also, depression is simply not the kind of problem that anyone should be diagnosing or treating alone. Untreated depression can not only lead to disabling symptoms but, in severe cases, suicide.

Don't get us wrong: St. John's wort is a powerful, promising herb, and it almost certainly has important benefits to offer to the many people suffering from depression. But until better data come in (including those from the first U.S. clinical trial, currently underway, for use of this herb in treating moderate depression), we suggest that you use St. John's wort only as part of a professionally-guided treatment plan. Try to purchase products that contain 0.3 percent hypericin extract (hypericin is thought to be the active chemical in St. John's wort), the amount used in most of the studies showing that this stuff actually works.

Safety first — treating herbs with respect

Whatever the label says — an herbal remedy that works is a drug. Period. And because many herbal products have not gone through rigorous testing for safety and efficacy or quality control procedures for purity and consistency, the burden is on the consumer. That's why — however promising — you have to think of every one of these remedies as a "drug," and treat it with considerable respect. (For more details on using herbal remedies safely and effectively, see Chapter 20.)

St. John's wort also seems to have antiviral, antibacterial, and anticancer properties when activated by light. These properties suggest that this herb — or, more likely, the chemical hypericin it contains — may someday be useful in treating AIDS, brain tumors, hepatitis, cancers, and other serious diseases. But we're still years off from having any definitive data on these uses.

Valerian

Valerian *(Valeriana officinalis)* is an old stand-by sedative, used for thousands of years in many countries to treat anxiety, hysteria, and insomnia. Even today it's a common ingredient in many European over-the-counter drugs. Recent studies confirm the calming properties of this herb, made from the roots and rhizomes of the valerian plant — also known as the garden heliotrope. And if used in recommended doses (usually under 450 milligrams a day for under 2 weeks), it rarely causes any serious side effects. So it's no wonder that valerian is one of the world's most popular herbs.

Throwing a wet blanket on all this good news is a recent statement issued by the United States Pharmacopeia (a nonprofit group of scientists aiming to set and disseminate quality standards for health care products) stating that no credible evidence proves that valerian root is an effective sleep-aid. Other experts (including German health authorities) beg to differ — as do many people who argue, quite logically, that if valerian has the ability to tranquilize, it probably helps at least some people get to sleep. In any case, if basic sleep hygiene isn't working for you (see Part VII), valerian may be worth a try — and is certainly safer than sleeping pills or even melatonin, a widely promoted but still little-understood hormone that may help promote sleep (see Chapter 23).

Most people prefer to use valerian in capsule form because teas, tinctures, and bath oils made with this stuff can reek. Using valerian together with alcohol or other central nervous system depressants may be dangerous (although no one has ever reported any problem). And overdoses of valerian may lead to irregular heart rhythms, headaches, nausea, blurred vision, or excitability.

Chapter 26

Ten More Supplements Worth Knowing

*W*e cover the big-time supplements in Chapter 23 — vitamins, minerals, and other natural substances that may well do you some good, plus a lot of hyped-up stuff that most people don't need. If you want to know more about DHEA, coenzyme Q-10, zinc, antioxidant vitamins, melatonin, and more, check out that chapter.

But it seems like every time we turn around, another intriguing supplement hits the stores (and sometimes the headlines). That's why we're including this chapter, which lists what we like to think of as the second-string supplements. They may not be quite popular enough to make the top-ten list, but their status could change any day now. Chances are that some of these supplements will become household words in the near future. This chapter gives you the bottom line on these supplements so you'll know what you're up against when you stand facing a row of products that no one ever mentioned in school.

One more thing: Before you get excited about *any* supplement, take some time to think about your expectations. Do you plan to take this supplement for the rest of your life — or long-term? Is this a reasonable plan? If you plan to stop taking the supplement at some point, what happens then? Thinking about these issues will reduce your chances of disappointment down the line.

5-HTP

A few years back, the amino acid tryptophan (L-tryptophan) was sold as a treatment for insomnia, depression, obsessive/compulsive behavior, stress, and premenstrual syndrome (PMS). The body converts tryptophan to serotonin, a neurotransmitter that carries signals from one cell to the next and helps control mood, behavior, appetite, and sleep patterns. But tryptophan was banned permanently in the United States when a contaminated batch poisoned hundreds of people.

Today, tryptophan is making a stunning comeback as 5-HTP (5-hydroxytryptophan), another form of tryptophan that is also converted into serotonin by the body. According to a rash of new books and articles, 5-HTP is supposed to be a natural form of "serotonin" — a rather bizarre idea because serotonin itself *is* natural. But no matter. This supplement, already popular in Europe, is taking the United States by storm as a potential cure for depression, anxiety, overeating, PMS, fibromyalgia, anxiety, insomnia, Parkinson's disease, and migraine headaches — anything linked to low levels of serotonin. Supposedly, 5-HTP works faster than St. John's wort, right now the leading "natural" antidepressant on the alternative market. And (though more studies need to be done) 5-HTP may even have antioxidant properties — and so perhaps help prevent age-related deterioration.

Advocates say that because the 5-HTP used in today's supplements is extracted from a natural source, the seed of the African griffonia plant, it may not be as vulnerable to contamination as were those notorious vials of L-tryptophan. But just as this book went to press, Mayo Clinic researchers published a study in *Nature Medicine* showing that they had found worrisome levels of the same contaminants in 5-HTP that caused the L-tryptophan problems years ago. Whether these findings were a fluke or a widespread problem remains to be seen. See B. L. Williamson, et al., *Nature Medicine* 4,9 (September 1998): 983.

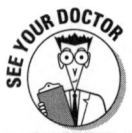

If you're suffering from depression or any other potentially serious medical disorder, get an accurate diagnosis from an M.D. before trying to treat yourself with 5-HTP or any other substance.

Androstenedione

Androstenedione hit the headlines recently when home run leader Mark McGwire admitted to using it. Banned by the International Olympic Committee, the NFL, and the NCAA, this supplement is still permitted in baseball — and is supposed to boost energy and (if combined with exercise) build muscle strength.

A natural hormone converted by the body to testosterone (the masculinizing hormone), androstenedione does — in high enough doses — help build muscles. But whether it's effective in the doses generally prescribed is an open question. And safety is an even bigger question. That's why many — but not all — health food stores currently ban this supplement.

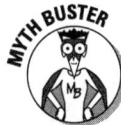

Make no mistake. Androstenedione is a steroid hormone. The U.S. FDA may call it a "dietary supplement," and hucksters may deny that it's a "drug" or a "hormone" till they're blue in the face — but they're just plain wrong.

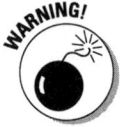

Some critics say that androstenedione in recommended amounts (about 100 milligrams a day) doesn't do much, except maybe make you more aggressive for an hour or so. But other critics say that athletes are tempted to assume that more is better, and that the higher doses they take could lead to big troubles down the line. No one can say what these troubles are yet, but past experience has shown that people who took other forms of testosterone developed tumors, cholesterol problems, and heart disease years later.

Whatever you decide, fueling yourself with androstenedione is going to cost you between $25 and $40 for a bottle of 60 (100 milligram) capsules. We think that's a fairly hefty price to pay for a big unknown.

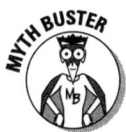

Frankly, expensive supplements or "natural" hormones do not make someone a significantly better athlete. Mark McGwire is not an awesome power-hitter because he takes an androgen precursor from a health food store. And we doubt that Roger Maris was taking something fancy back in 1961.

Blue-Green Algae

No question about it: Blue-green algae *(spirulina)* is packed with loads of vitamins, minerals, and other goodies. This so-called "super seaweed" or "superfood" particularly shines in providing beta-carotene (an antioxidant), vitamin B-12, gamma linolenic acid, and protein and amino acids, all stuff known to do the body good. Plus, it may contain other protective *phytochemicals,* natural substances that help prevent disease. That's why supplement manufacturers are pushing blue-green algae powders, tablets, and fruit drinks as a way to strengthen your immune system, prevent cancer, lower cholesterol, treat arthritis, cut viral infections, and clean out your intestines.

Even so, if you're well-nourished and have access to other (cheaper) sources of protein, blue-green algae should probably be low on your priority list — at least until better results from clinical trials come in. Right now no one (except the blue-green algae gurus) knows just what (if anything) the phytochemicals in blue-green algae do, and researchers are equally unsettled about the risks and benefits of beta-carotene supplements. Worse, the form of B-12 found in blue-green algae happens to be the kind that human beings can't metabolize. And, finally, although blue-green algae's other drawing card, gamma linolenic acid, may indeed help prevent heart disease and relieve arthritis, this essential fatty acid only occurs in one species of blue-green algae — not necessarily the one (out of the many thousands of other species) that happens to be in the supplement you buy.

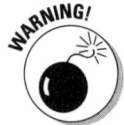

Given that a month's worth of blue-green algae can put you out over 50 bucks and that many commercial preparations have been contaminated with toxins, this supplement just doesn't have much in its favor — unless you're severely malnourished.

Creatine

Creatine *(creatine monohydrate)* is a substance normally made by the liver that helps muscles release and regenerate energy. So it stands to reason that loading up on this stuff could help improve your performance on the soccer field or tennis court.

And, yes, in theory, loading your muscles with extra creatine may indeed improve your performance in any kind of short-duration, high-intensity exercise — such as sprinting or weight-lifting. Many athletes swear by it, too, but no one knows whether creatine or just the "belief in creatine" explains the effects. Note, though, that — even in theory — this kind of *creatine-loading* can't help you with any kind of high-endurance exercise — such as running the Boston Marathon. And, in any case, no one knows for sure whether creatine can help anyone or how much you need to take to see results.

No one knows about long-term effects of creatine either (including possible kidney damage)— which makes this supplement potentially risky. Some users have reported muscle cramps and possible dehydration.

Grape Seed Extract

People in France not only enjoy cream sauces in bounty but generally exercise less and smoke more than people in most other countries. And yet they have a relatively lower death rate from heart disease. The explanation for this "French Paradox" could lie in the wine without which no true French meal would be complete — red wine in particular. That's because red wine contains certain biologically active chemicals *(bioflavonoids* or *flavonoids)* that, in a test tube, scavenge chemicals (free radicals) that mess up your cholesterol balance and damage your genes, cells, and tissues.

The seeds and skins of the grapes used to make red wine are loaded with these bioflavonoids. So it's no surprise that grape seed extract is a rising star, both as a pill and as a supplement to various foods and drinks. It's promoted as a way to stave off heart disease and keep the aging process at bay.

Of course, noting that grape seed extract has certain chemical properties is a far cry from concluding that it's going to keep your body from falling apart. Maybe it will — but we're waiting for better research before drawing any final conclusions.

In the meantime, eating foods laced with grape seed oil probably won't hurt you, nor will taking pills if you want to give it a try. Just make sure that you avoid products in which the manufacturer extracted the grape seed using cancer-causing (and environmentally damaging) chemicals; stick to the stuff extracted with water or alcohol.

Homocysteine Formulas

The homocysteine "formulas" you may have seen advertised are picking up on the hot new hypothesis that too much homocysteine, which is an amino acid naturally occurring in the body, may increase your risk of heart disease. Note that we said "hypothesis," which is not at all the same as a generally accepted theory.

Even if you do buy into the homocysteine-heart disease connection, there are cheaper ways to get your homocysteine levels in check. The fancy homocysteine formulas are actually nothing but a complex of B vitamins that control levels of homocysteine in your body. Buying B vitamins alone, or taking a multivitamin, is a much more frugal way to achieve the same effects.

Lecithin and Inositol

Lots of people want to sell you lecithin, an important chemical required for numerous bodily functions. It's found in many different foods, including baked goods, margarine, chocolate, and many other high-fat, high-cholesterol foods. Forms of lecithin made from defatted soybean oil are also available in supplemental powders, pills, and capsules — all prominent items in most health food stores.

What can supplemental lecithin do for you? Not much, if you go by credible research studies. Supplement manufacturers claim that lecithin can boost your memory and lower your cholesterol, plus make you more disease-resistant and energetic. Some alternative healers insist lecithin supplements can help relieve symptoms of multiple sclerosis and chronic fatigue syndrome. But so far most of the talk is theoretical.

Some nutritionally-oriented practitioners recommend high doses of inositol (one of the constituents of lecithin) for chronic fatigue syndrome, depression, attention-deficit hyperactivity disorder (ADHD), and other conditions. This approach may help, but large and long-term studies are once again lacking.

On the plus side, lecithin is one of the safest supplements around. So if you want to see how it works for your mother's Alzheimer's symptoms or how well it lowers your cholesterol levels, it could be worth trying. Just don't expect miracles.

Lycopene

Everyone knows that fresh produce is good for you — and lycopene may be one of the reasons why. A chemical compound found in tomatoes, watermelon, red grapefruit pulp, and other red-colored produce, lycopene may help prevent prostate, breast, skin, and cervical cancers.

The best way to get your lycopene — and other potentially cancer-fighting compounds that may go along with it — is to eat your fruits and veggies (at least five servings a day). Two to three servings a week in lycopene-rich tomatoes (including tomato sauce) may help cut your risk of prostate cancer in particular. But if your diet is less than ideal, taking a supplement containing lycopene probably can't hurt (most of these are labeled as "prostate formulas" or "men's health formulas" even though lycopene may help prevent women's health problems, too). Meanwhile, expect to hear more about lycopene in the near future.

Pycnogenol

Pycnogenol is a mixture of bioflavonoids (natural health-promoting chemicals) derived from the pine tree and other evergreens. Right now it is being heavily promoted as a treatment for heart disease, cancer, AIDS, arthritis, and other serious conditions because it has antioxidant properties: the power to scavenge the free radicals that damage cells and tissues. Advocates have also dubbed pycnogenol to be a veritable fountain of youth that can smooth skin, shrink varicose veins, maintain collagen, ease pain, calm allergies, improve eyesight, boost memory, relieve ulcers, increase joint flexibility, and more.

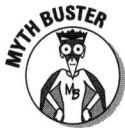

This stuff sounds pretty great — but wait! Unfortunately, most of the claims are based on wishful thinking more than solid evidence. Promoters often look at a list of conditions linked to free radical damage and then just assume that pycnogenol (which does seem to blast free radicals *in a test tube*) must, therefore, help them. Few, if any, convincing trials have been done involving actual human beings who have been helped with this stuff — and comparing them to similar people who haven't used it.

In short, it's way too early in the game to make pycnogenol your miracle drug — but keep your eye out for future research.

Selenium

Selenium is an essential mineral that the human body requires in tiny amounts (see Chapter 23). It also happens to be an antioxidant — which is why some people are excited about it. Antioxidants protect cells and tissues from damage, the kind of damage that can lead to arthritis, cancers, and heart disease. As it turns out, people with certain cancers and heart disease do seem to have abnormally low levels of selenium, and in some countries with high levels of selenium in the soil, cancer rates are strikingly low.

Such discoveries make selenium sound like something worth investigating. But it's a huge leap from these findings to the conclusion that selenium supplements (such as selenium picolinate or selenium citrate) will actually *prevent* cancer or heart disease. After all, it's possible that selenium levels fall in people only *after* they get sick — or that low selenium levels reflect the presence (or absence) or some other crucial and as-yet-unknown factor. Similarly, some other factor in the countries with high-selenium soil may explain their lower cancer rates.

Real answers are still years away. But, for now, adding a little selenium to your life probably isn't going to hurt you. Even so, it's probably best to get it from food sources such as whole grains, eggs, garlic, mushrooms, lean meats, and seafood.

If you do take supplements (other than multivitamins), make sure that you're under a doctor's supervision because selenium can be highly toxic in high doses (over 200 micrograms a day). Early signs of overdose are a metallic or garlicky taste in your mouth, fragile or discolored nails, dizziness, or nausea.

Chapter 27
Ten "Low-Risk" Alternatives

In This Chapter

▶ Cheap, easy, and safe treatments

▶ Treatments that mix well with conventional therapies

▶ When — if ever — to avoid these alternatives

Contrary to popular belief, the word "alternative" is not synonymous with safe, gentle, or low-risk. As we describe in many sections throughout this book, plenty of alternative approaches can be just as risky, even riskier, than conventional medicine.

But many alternative approaches are cheap, easy, and safe. Most of these approaches are mind-body techniques and can be tried by virtually anyone — often anywhere and anytime. Others are tried-and-true home remedies or hands-on approaches that many nonmedical folks have used for centuries, even before good data started rolling in showing their effectiveness.

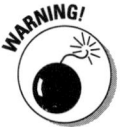

This chapter describes ten "low-risk" alternatives that have great odds of making you feel better and low odds of harming you. But none of these alternatives should be considered a cure, or even a stand-alone treatment. You're best off thinking of them mainly as adjuncts to conventional care. And remember that *any* alternative therapy is "high risk" if it keeps you from getting conventional medical care for a serious condition. Plus, expecting any unproven alternative to cure you puts you at risk for disappointment, not to mention feelings of regret and failure. Thanks to David Eisenberg, M.D., for many of the ideas in this chapter — see David Eisenberg, M.D., "Advising Patients Who Seek Alternative Medical Therapies," *Annals of Internal Medicine* 127 (July 1, 1997): 61–69.

Homeopathy

Homeopathy is a system of healing that uses extremely diluted portions of natural substances to cure symptoms of disease. Whether they actually cure diseases is a matter of hot debate. But chances are virtually nil that these highly diluted solutions will hurt you. In fact, homeopathic remedies contain so little of the so-called active substance that, from the point of view of mainstream science, they are nothing but water or alcohol.

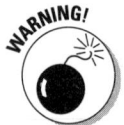

Homeopaths do report that patients often seem to get worse initially, before expected improvements set in. But don't worry about that. This phenomenon is usually mild, self-limited, and anticipated by the practitioner. (See Chapter 12 for more information on homeopathic remedies.)

Massage Therapy

Getting a little hands-on — whether in the form of hugging, Swedish massage, or more exotic massage practices — can do the body, mind, and spirit a world of good. And, in most cases, a little touching is virtually risk-free, especially when performed by a reputable and well-trained therapist. Even during pregnancy, massage can be quite safe, assuming that it is performed by a therapist well-versed in the art of pregnancy massage.

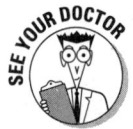

People with certain serious medical conditions (including infections, cancer, blood clots, peptic ulcers, enlarged livers or spleens, and high blood pressure) should consult an M.D. before engaging in massage therapy (see Chapter 16).

Prayer

Surely praying to get better, or praying that someone else gets better, isn't going to hurt any. Plus, it's about as inexpensive and simple an approach as anyone could ask for. And, hey, it may even help (although the data right now about prayer's effect on health is still largely anecdotal).

Just about the only caveat anyone ever gives about prayer is that it shouldn't ever be used as a substitute for conventional medical care. One of us just read in the paper this morning about parents who sat around praying while they watched their toddler slowly choke to death on a banana. This kind of prayer is clearly not the "low-risk" form (see Chapter 19).

Spiritual Healing

Going to regular religious services or just taking a "spiritual" approach to life may help prevent and maybe even treat some diseases. And, even if it doesn't, having a hopeful, peaceful, contented attitude — which is how "spirituality" is usually defined — is a pretty desirable way to go through life (see Chapter 19).

Many forms of traditional medicine from around the world also rely largely on spiritual healing, which may, in part, explain why so many people are turning to Native American medicine, Latin American medicine, Tibetan medicine, and the like for new ideas about health care. Many of these traditions include herbal remedies, massage therapies, and exotic rituals, but they all rest on a spiritual foundation.

Relaxation Techniques

We suppose that a burglar could sneak into your kitchen one day while you're off relaxing, or one of your kids could decide to decorate the living room wall in purple crayon. But, basically, you can't beat relaxation techniques for cheap, safe, and simple ways to feel better. Taking ten minutes a day to breathe deeply, vanquish everyday worries, and just focus on yourself — how could anyone see any problem with that?

Even better, discovering how to relax and get some of the negative stress out of your life can have measurable effects on the amount of physical suffering you do. Relaxation may not cure a serious disease or work as a stand-alone treatment, but it can soothe the symptoms of many different stress-related conditions — and, considering that many, if not most, conditions afflicting modern humanity have at least some stress component, this is no mean feat. Plus, getting the stress out of your life may well help keep your resistance up, reducing your chances of getting sick in the first place (see Chapter 17).

Meditation and Yoga

Meditation is a lot like relaxation when it comes to risk. Because meditation is actually a form of relaxation technique, this statement should hardly come as a surprise. Virtually all meditation techniques (including yoga) involve freeing your mind from intrusive and troubling thoughts by breathing slowly and deeply and focusing on a calming image, phrase, or sound. And, as a reward, you may find yourself less anxious and more comfortable, and perhaps even relieved of nagging pain, coughs, and other serious physical ailments.

The only reason that meditation is slightly more risky than at-home relaxation techniques is that you may have to pay to take a class in it, especially if you want to explore some of the more formal methods (such as Zen or transcendental meditation). Or you may have to shell out a few bucks for books or tapes on meditation techniques. And you run the risk of wasting your time and/or money on a lousy instructor. But, all things considered, this risk is worth taking when you weigh it against all the ways that meditating can make you feel better and can even make coping with serious ailments easier.

Yoga is a slightly riskier form of meditation, simply because it involves physical exercises. Even so, the risks are negligible, especially if you're working with a well-trained teacher and skipping the less common, more aggressive forms of yoga (see Chapter 17).

Biofeedback

Okay, biofeedback is not a "cheap" method. It can cost you a bundle, in fact, because if it's going to work, you'll probably have to go back to a trained therapist for numerous sessions at close to $150 a pop. In each of these sessions, you'll be hooked up (electronically) to a machine that measures a basic body function over which you normally have no voluntary control — breathing rate, pulse, temperature, or blood pressure, for example. But by observing visual or auditory feedback from the machine as these automatic functions change in your body, you gradually learn to control them at will. As a result, you can eventually discover how to command pain, stress, or blood pressure with your thoughts, and, as a result, relieve symptoms of a wide variety of disorders.

Cost aside, biofeedback is one of the safest approaches to health. And it's so well accepted among mainstream doctors for certain applications that we hesitate to call it alternative (see Chapter 18).

Guided Imagery

All you need to do guided imagery is an active imagination and a little peace and quiet. The idea is to think about your body combating cancer cells or microorganisms, working or moving less painfully, or wiping away all stress and anxiety. And, with enough practice, just imagining these events may make you feel better and may even improve your physical well-being or skills — even if it won't cure cancer or obliterate serious conditions. The latter feats may be possible but so far have never been documented with any kind of credible scientific evidence.

Guided imagery can make conventional treatments and surgical procedures easier to tolerate. Plus, it can be a great way to relax, as well as a useful adjunct to treatment for chronic pain, menstrual problems, high blood pressure, cold and flu symptoms, allergies, and many other disorders (see Chapter 18).

Hypnosis

Hypnosis is "low-risk?" Isn't hypnosis the method of mad scientists who put innocent people into trances and then, using the power of suggestion, transform them into uncontrollable axe-murderers? Well, no, of course not. Such scenarios may have been popular on the vaudeville stage, but in reality hypnosis is a well-accepted and perfectly innocuous form of therapy that has helped many people break bad habits, control pain, relieve allergies and asthma, and rid their lives of excess stress and anxiety. For many years now, hypnotism has even been accepted as a valid treatment by the mainstream medical community.

Yes, getting hypnotized can cost you a bit of money if you're working with a professional hypnotherapist (which is usually a good idea, especially if you're using hypnotherapy to treat serious problems). But for safety, you'd be hard pressed to find any kind of therapy — conventional or alternative — that gives you so much bang for the buck. People suffering from psychiatric disorders should never try hypnosis without first consulting a psychiatrist familiar with the effects of hypnosis on their particular disorder (see Chapter 18).

Hydrotherapy

If you use water in any way to promote your health, you're using hydrotherapy. Whether you steam your face or soak your feet, ice a sprain, luxuriate in a whirlpool, apply hot or cold compresses to a sore spot, or irrigate your insides with douches or enemas, you're using hydrotherapy. Even taking a bath, swimming in a pool, or drinking an herbal tea counts.

So, what's so alternative about hydrotherapy? Sometimes nothing. Conventional medicine advocates water power all the time as a form of relaxation and as a way to relieve painful and swollen body parts. But many naturopaths (see Chapter 11) and other alternative practitioners say that water can do a lot more for you, ranging from "cleaning out" your intestines to curing cancer, arthritis, chronic fatigue syndrome, and other serious ailments. Expecting water to work these kinds of miracles is *not* low-risk. But the vast majority of hydrotherapy approaches are.

You can, and probably already do, use many kinds of hydrotherapy as part of your daily life. Hey, even if you just wash your face, you're using water to good effect (and may even be able to stave off acne and other skin conditions).

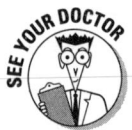 Always check with your doctor before using any kind of heat or cold therapy (including sitting too long in warm baths) if you're pregnant, paralyzed, or suffering from frostbite, or if you have circulatory disorders, diabetes, atherosclerosis, or a condition that makes it difficult for you to sense temperature with your hands and feet.

Home Remedies

Home remedies (sometimes called folk remedies) are simply treatments used by ordinary people (or lay healers) rather than professional healers. Many of these treatments emphasize herbs and other natural products, as well as the importance of family, religion, and emotions in healing. People rely on home remedies when they can't (or won't) use a doctor or if they feel that their problem is something they can handle themselves.

Folk or home remedies aren't necessarily inconsistent with what conventional medicine tells you to do — but they got there first. Conventional medicine took them on because they worked. Some remedies, we admit, are downright kooky — such as the Russian folk remedy we discovered on the Internet that advises people with bad sore throats to breathe on a frog until they pass their problem to him. (The one about drinking a glass of spiced-up vodka to soothe an upset tummy, however, sounds rather intriguing.)

The kind of home remedies that many of us are used to often involve easy, cheap, and sensible things that we all do almost instinctively. When Grandma says to eat slowly (so you won't belch), she's practicing a form of home medicine. And if you take a hot bath to relieve an ache, drink soda to ease a queasy stomach, or run your burned hand under cold water, you're doing it, too!

Appendix

Information Resources

• •

*T*his appendix lists organizations that can help provide more information about many of the alternative approaches we describe in this book — and, quite often, help you find qualified practitioners in your area. Although most of the organizations are located in English-speaking countries — and mainly in the United States — we include international organizations whenever possible. (Obviously, listing a source for every country on the planet would fill every page of this book.) But often a single telephone call to these groups can lead you to a good information source in your part of the world.

One word of warning: Health organizations are notorious for changing addresses and telephone numbers (and sometimes even names) at the drop of a hat. We've made every effort to make this list accurate at the time this book was published, but we can't predict the future. If you have trouble reaching any of these groups, a telephone call to the local directory assistance will often help you locate them. And anyone comfortable with the World Wide Web can track down these groups (and other useful sources of information) in seconds flat. (If you're not comfortable with the Web, get a copy of *The Internet For Dummies,* 5th Edition, by John R. Levine, Carol Baroudi, and Margaret Levine Young, published by IDG Books Worldwide, Inc.)

Acupressure

Acupressure Institute, 1533 Shattuck Ave., Berkeley, CA 94709, 800-442-2232 or 510-845-1059.

Acupuncture

American Academy of Medical Acupuncture, 5820 Wilshire Blvd., Suite 500, Los Angeles, CA 90036, 213-937-5514.

American Association of Oriental Medicine (formerly American Association of Acupuncture and Oriental Medicine), 433 Front St., Catasauqua, PA 18032, 610-266-1433.

National Certification Commission for Acupuncture and Oriental Medicine, 11 Canal Center Plaza, Suite 300, Alexandria, VA 22314, 703-548-9004.

The British Medical Acupuncture Society, Newton House, Newton Ln., Whitley, Warrington, Cheshire, U.K. WA4 4JA, 1925-730727.

European Federation of Modern Acupuncture, 59 Telford Crescent, Leigh, Lancashire, U.K. WN 5LY, 1942-678092.

Australian Acupuncture and Chinese Medicine Association Ltd., P.O. Box 5142, West End, Brisbane, Australia 4101, 800-025-334 (within Australia) or 617-3846-5866 (outside Australia).

Alternative and Complementary Medicine (General)

Office of Alternative Medicine (OAM) Information Clearinghouse, National Institutes of Health (NIH), 6120 Executive Blvd., EPS Suite 450, Rockville, MD 20892, 301-402-2466.

Richard and Hinda Rosenthal Center for Alternative/Complementary Medicine, College of Physicians and Surgeons at Columbia University, 630 W. 168th St., New York, NY 10032, 212-543-9550.

The British Register of Complementary Practitioners, P.O. Box 194, London, U.K. SE16 1QZ.

The Institute for Complementary Medicine, Unit 15, Tavern Quay, Commercial Centre, Rope St., London, U.K. SE16 1TX, 171-237-5165.

Australian Traditional Medicine Society, P.O. Box 1027, Meadowbank, NSW, Australia 2114, 9809-6800.

Applied Kinesiology

International Board of Applied Kinesiology, 6405 Metcalf Ave., Suite 503, Shawnee Mission, KS 66202, 913-384-5336.

Aromatherapy

National Association for Holistic Aromatherapy, P.O. Box 17622, Boulder, CO 80308-0622, 800-566-6735.

Pacific Institute of Aromatherapy, P.O. Box 6723, San Rafael, CA 94903, 415-479-9121.

Association of Medical Aromatherapists, 11 Park Circus, Glasgow, U.K. G84 8NF, 141-332-4924.

International Society of Professional Aromatherapists, 82 Ashby Road, Hinkley, Leicester, U.K. LE10 1AG, 1455-637987.

Ayurveda

American Association of Ayurvedic Sciences, 2115 112th Ave., NE, Bellevue, WA 98004, 425-453-8022.

Ayurvedic Institute, 11311 Menaul NE, Suite A, Albuquerque, NM 87112, 505-291-9698.

Biofeedback

Association for Applied Psychophysiology and Biofeedback, 10200 W. 44th Ave., Suite 304, Wheat Ridge, CO 80033-2840, 800-477-8892 or 303-422-8436.

Bodywork (Asian)

American Oriental Bodywork Therapy Association, Laurel Oak Corporate Center, Suite 408, 1010 Haddonfield-Berlin Rd., Voorhees, NJ 08043, 609-782-1616.

Bodywork (General)

Associated Bodywork and Massage Professionals, 28677 Buffalo Park Rd., Evergreen, CO 80439, 800-458-2267.

National Certification Board for Therapeutic Massage and Bodywork, 8201 Greensboro Dr., Suite 300, McLean, VA 22102, 800-296-0664.

Chelation Therapy

American Board of Chelation Therapy, 1407-B N. Wells, Chicago, IL 60610, 800-356-2228.

Chinese Medicine

American Association of Oriental Medicine, 433 Front St., Catasauqua, PA 18032, 610-266-1433.

National Certification Commission for Acupuncture and Oriental Medicine (NCCAOM), 11 Canal Center Plaza, Suite 300, Alexandria, VA 22314, 703-548-9004.

Chiropractic

American Chiropractic Association, 1701 Clarendon Blvd., Arlington, VA 22209, 703-276-8800.

International Chiropractors Association, 1110 N. Glebe Rd., Suite 1000, Arlington, VA 22201, 703-528-5000.

The British Association for Applied Chiropractic, The Old Post Office, Cherry St., Stratton Audley, Nr. Bicester, Oxon, U.K. 0X6 9BA, 1869-27111.

British Chiropractic Association, 29 Whitley St., Reading, Berks, U.K. RG2 0EG, 1734-757557.

Energy Medicine (General)

International Society for the Study of Subtle Energies and Energy Medicine (ISSSEEM), 356 Goldco Cir., Golden, CO 80401, 303-425-4625.

Environmental Medicine

Environmental Health Center, 8345 Walnut Hill Ln., Suite 205, Dallas, TX 75231, 214-368-4132.

Guided Imagery

The Academy for Guided Imagery, P.O. Box 2070, Mill Valley, CA 94942, 650-493-4430.

Herbal Remedies

See also Naturopathy and Chinese Medicine

American Botanical Council, P.O. Box 144345, Austin, TX 78714, 512-331-8868.

The American Herbalists Guild, P.O. Box 70, Roosevelt, Utah, 84066, 435-722-8434.

Herb Research Foundation, 1007 Pearl St., Suite 200, Boulder, CO 80302, 800-748-2617 or 303-449-2265.

International Register of Herbalists and Aromatherapists, 32 King Edward Rd., Swansea, U.K. SA1 4LL, 1792-655886.

National Institute of Medical Herbalists, 56 Longbrook St., Exeter, U.K. EX4 6AH, 1392-426022.

Holistic Medicine (General)

American Holistic Health Association, P.O. Box 17400, Anaheim, CA 92817-7400, 714-779-6152.

American Holistic Medical Association, 6728 Old McBean Village Dr., McLean, VA 22101, 919-787-5146.

Australasian College of Natural Therapies, 57 Foveaux St., Surry Hills, NSW, Australia 2010, 02-9211-7744.

Homeopathy

British Institute of Homeopathy and College of Homeopathy, 520 Washington Blvd., Suite 423, Marina Del Ray, CA 90292, 310-306-5408.

The National Center for Homeopathy, 801 North Fairfax St., Suite 306, Alexandria, VA 22314, 703-548-7790.

The British Institute of Homeopathy, 1495 St. Joseph Blvd., Gloucester, Ontario, Canada K1C 7K9, 613-830-4759.

The International Register of Homoeopathic Practitioners, 32 King Edward Rd., Swansea, U.K. SA1 4LL, 1792-655886.

The United Kingdom Homeopathic Medical Association, 6 Livingstone Rd., Gravesend, Kent, U.K. DA12 5DZ, 1474-560336.

Humor Therapy

American Association for Therapeutic Humor, 222 S. Meramec, Suite 303, St. Louis, MO 63105, 314-863-6232.

Hypnosis and Hypnotherapy

The American Society of Clinical Hypnosis, 2200 E. Devon Ave., Suite 291, Des Plaines, IL 60018, 847-297-3317.

International Medical and Dental Hypnotherapy Association, 4110 Edgeland, Suite 800, Royal Oak, MI 48073, 800-257-5467 (outside Michigan) or 313-549-5594.

The National Guild of Hypnotists, P.O. Box 308, Merrimack, NH 03059, 603-429-9938.

London College of Clinical Hypnotherapists, 229a Sussex Gardens, Lancaster Gate, London, U.K. W2 2RL, 171 402 9037.

National Central Register of Advanced Hypnotherapists, 28 Finsbury Rd., London, U.K. N4 2JX, 171-359-6991.

Light Therapy

Society for Light Treatment and Biological Rhythms, 10200 W. 44th Ave., Suite 304, Wheat Ridge, CO 80033-2840, 303-424-3697.

Magnetic Field Therapy

Bio-Electro-Magnetics Institute, 2490 W. Moana Ln., Reno, NV 89509, 702-827-9099.

Massage Therapy

American Massage Therapy Association, 820 Davis St., Suite 100, Evanston, IL 60201-4444, 847-864-0123.

National Certification Board for Therapeutic Massage and Bodywork, 8201 Greensboro Dr., Suite 300, McLean, VA 22102, 800-296-0664 or 703-610-9015.

Touch Research Institute, University of Miami School of Medicine, Department of Pediatrics, P.O. Box 016820, Miami, FL 33101, 305-243-6781.

The Massage Training Institute, 24 Highbury Grove, London, U.K. N5 2EA, 171-266-5313.

Association of Massage Therapists, P.O. Box 1248, Bondi Junction, Australia NSW 2022, (02) 4959-4706. U.S./Canadian International Public Relations 352-795-2081.

Association of Remedial Masseurs, 120 Blaxland Rd., Ryde, Australia 2112, 9807-4769.

Meditation

Center for Spiritual Awareness, P.O. Box 7, Lake Rabun Rd., Lakemont, GA 30552-0007, 706-782-4723.

Maharishi International University, 1000 N. 4th St., Fairfield, IA 52557, 555-472-7000.

Himalayan Institute of Canada, 371 Berkeley St., Toronto, Ontario, Canada M5A 2X8, 416-960-5062.

Himalayan Institute of Great Britain, 70 Claremont Rd., West Ealing, London, U.K. WI3 ODG, 181-991-8090.

Mind-Body Medicine (General)

The Center for Mind-Body Studies, 5225 Connecticut Ave. NW, Suite 414, Washington, DC 20015, 202-966-7338.

The Mind-Body Medical Center, Deaconess Hospital, Deaconess Rd., Boston, MA 02215, 617-632-9525.

Music Therapy

National Association for Music Therapy, 8455 Colesville Rd., Suite 1000, Silver Spring, MD 20910, 301-589-3300.

Canadian Association for Music Therapy (Association de Musicothérapie du Canada), Wilfrid Laurier University, Waterloo, Ontario, Canada N2L 3C5, 519-884-1970 ext. 6828.

British Society for Music Therapy, 25 Rosslyn Ave., East Barnet, Herts, U.K. EN4 8DH, 181-368-8879.

Naturopathy

American Association of Naturopathic Physicians, 601 Valley St., Suite 105, Seattle, WA 98109, 206-298-0126.

American Naturopathic Medical Association, P.O. Box 96273, Las Vegas, NV 89193, 702-897-7053.

Homeopathic Academy of Naturopathic Physicians, P.O. Box 69565, Portland, OR 97201, 503-795-0579.

Canadian Naturopathic Association, P.O. Box 4520, Station C, Calgary, Alberta, Canada T2T 5N3, 403-244-4487.

General Council and Register of Naturopaths, Goswell House, 2 Goswell Road, Street, Somerset, U.K. BA16 0JG, 1458-840072.

The Incorporated Society of Registered Naturopaths, 293 Gilmerton Rd., Kingston Coach House, Edinburgh, U.K. EH16 5UT, 31-664-3435.

Nutrition

American Dietetic Association, 216 W. Jackson Blvd., Suite 800, Chicago, IL 60606, 800-366-1655.

Nutrition Education Association, P.O. Box 20301, Houston, TX 77225, 713-665-2946.

U.S. Department of Agriculture Center for Nutrition Policy and Promotion, 1120 20th St. NW, Suite 200, North Lobby, Washington, DC 20036, 202-418-2312.

Society for the Promotion of Nutritional Therapy (SPNT), P.O. Box 47, Heathfield, East Sussex, U.K. TN21 8ZX, 1435-867007.

Orthomolecular Medicine

Linus Pauling Institute of Science and Medicine, 440 Page Mill Rd., Palo Alto, CA 94306, 650-327-4064.

Osteopathy

American Academy of Osteopathy, 3500 DePauw Blvd., Suite 1080, Indianapolis, IN 46268, 317-879-1881.

American Osteopathic Association, 142 East Ontario St., Chicago, IL 60611, 800-367-4895 or 312-202-8000.

British Osteopathic Association, Langham House East, Mill Street, Bedfordshire, U.K. LU1 2NA, 1582-488455.

Natural Therapeutic Osteopathic Society and Register, 14 Marford Rd., Wheathampstead, Herts, U.K. AL4 8AS, 1582-833950.

Osteopathic Information Service, OIS at the General Osteopathic Council, Room 432, Premier House Room 432, 10 Greycoat Pl., London Victoria, U.K. SW1P 13B, 171-799-2442.

Oxygen and Ozone Therapy

Ocean Hyperbaric Center, Ocean Medical Center, 4001 Ocean Dr., Suite 105, Lauderdale-by-the-Sea, FL 33308, 954-777-4000.

International Association for Oxygen Therapy, P.O. Box 1360, Priest River, IA 83856, 208-448-2504.

Qi Gong

Qigong Institute/East-West Academy of Healing Arts, 450 Sutter St., Suite 2104, San Francisco, CA 94108, 415-788-2227.

Reflexology

American Academy of Reflexology, 606 E. Magnolia Blvd., Suite B, Burbank, CA 91501, 818-841-7741.

The Philip Salmon Reflexology Information Centre, Research House, P.O. Box 131, Fraser Rd., Greenford, Middlesex, U.K. UB6 7DX, 181-810-5644.

Relaxation Techniques

The Mind-Body Medical Institute, 110 Francis St., Suite 1A, Boston, MA 02215, 617-632-9525.

Shiatsu

See also Bodywork (Asian)

The European Shiatsu Network, Highbanks, Lockeridge, Marlborough, Wiltshire, U.K. SN8 4TQ, 1672-861362.

The Shiatsu Society, 31 Pullman Ln., Godalming, Surrey, U.K. GU7 1XY, 1483-860771.

Sound Healing

Sound and Listening Learning Center, 2701 E. Camelback, Suite 205, Phoenix, AZ 85016, 602-381-0086.

Sound Healers Association, P.O. Box 2240, Boulder, CO 80306, 303-443-8181.

Spiritual Healing

National Federation of Spiritual Healers, Old Manor Farm Studio, Church St., Sunbury-on-Thames, Middlesex, U.K. TW16 6RG, 1932-783164.

Therapeutic Touch

National League for Nursing, 350 Hudson St., New York, NY 10014-4584, 800-669-1656 or 212-989-9393.

Nurse Healers Professional Associates, Inc., 1211 Locust St., Philadelphia, PA 19107, 215-545-8079.

Yoga

American Yoga Association, 513 S. Orange Ave., Sarasota, FL 34236, 941-953-5859.

International Association of Yoga Therapists, 20 Sunnyside Ave. Ste. A243, Mill Valley, CA 94941, 415-332-2478.

British Wheel of Yoga, 1 Hamilton Place, Boston Rd., Sleaford, Lincolnshire, U.K. NG34 7ES, 1529-306859.

Index

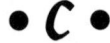

● **C** ●

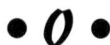

• *O* •

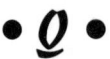
• Q •

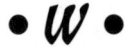

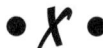

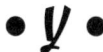

Notes

Notes

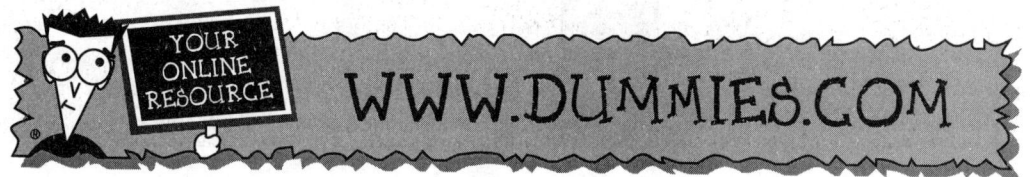

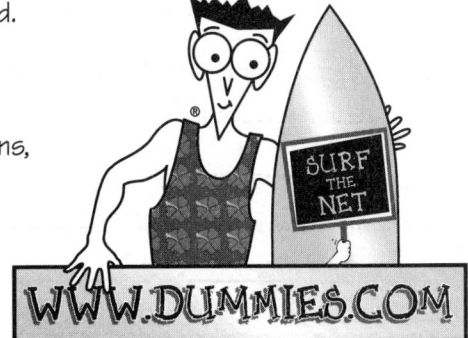
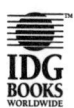

IDG BOOKS WORLDWIDE
BOOK REGISTRATION

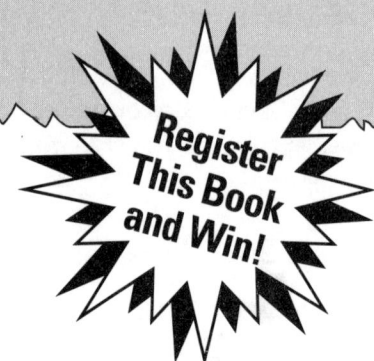

We want to hear from you!

Visit **http://my2cents.dummies.com** to register this book and tell us how you liked it!

- ✔ Get entered in our monthly prize giveaway.

- ✔ Give us feedback about this book — tell us what you like best, what you like least, or maybe what you'd like to ask the author and us to change!

- ✔ Let us know any other ...*For Dummies*® topics that interest you.

Your feedback helps us determine what books to publish, tells us what coverage to add as we revise our books, and lets us know whether we're meeting your needs as a ...*For Dummies* reader. You're our most valuable resource, and what you have to say is important to us!

Not on the Web yet? It's easy to get started with *Dummies 101*®: *The Internet For Windows*® *98* or *The Internet For Dummies*®, 5th Edition, at local retailers everywhere.

Or let us know what you think by sending us a letter at the following address:

...*For Dummies* Book Registration
Dummies Press
7260 Shadeland Station, Suite 100
Indianapolis, IN 46256-3945
Fax 317-596-5498

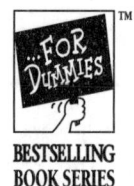

**BESTSELLING
BOOK SERIES
FROM IDG**